Post-Transplant Lymphoproliferative Disorders

Vikas R. Dharnidharka
Michael Green • Steven A. Webber
Ralf Ulrich Trappe
Editors

Post-Transplant Lymphoproliferative Disorders

Second Edition

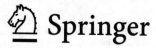 Springer

Editors
Vikas R. Dharnidharka
Washington University School of Medicine
and St. Louis Children's Hospital
Saint Louis, MO
USA

Michael Green
UPMC Children's Hospital of Pittsburgh
University of Pittsburgh Medical Center
Pittsburgh, PA
USA

Steven A. Webber
Vanderbilt University Medical Center
Nashville, TN
USA

Ralf Ulrich Trappe
Ev. Diakonie-Krankenhaus Bremen
German PTLD Study Group
Bremen
Germany

ISBN 978-3-030-65405-4   ISBN 978-3-030-65403-0   (eBook)
https://doi.org/10.1007/978-3-030-65403-0

This Springer imprint is published by the registered company Springer Nature Switzerland AG
The registered company address is: Gewerbestrasse 11, 6330 Cham, Switzerland

We dedicate this book to the clinicians and scientists who came before us, who cared for transplant patients, and began the work of understanding the problem of PTLD; to the transplant recipients and their families that we care for who motivate these efforts; and to the colleagues we work with to provide care to our patients.

Finally, we want to give a special thank you to our families and friends who put up with us and supported our efforts in preparing this book, and in all things:

Pushpa, Ramnath, Dimple, Shrey, and Ria;

Jenny, Dave, Erin, Molly, and Allison and my granddaughter Lyla;

Hannah and Katie;

Hanno, Heiner, Nina, and Petra.

PTLD Book Second Edition Preface

When we wrote the first edition of this book on post-transplant lymphoproliferative disorders more than a decade ago, we recognized that the topic was of interest to a limited audience. As such, we did not know whether the inaugural edition would ever have a successor. To our pleasant surprise, the chapter downloads averaged about a 1000/year over the next 9 years, a heartening result. Combined with the significant influx of new knowledge in the field over the intervening time, we were very happy that Springer agreed to publish a second edition.

For this second edition, the three original editors welcome Dr. Ralf Trappe as an editor. Dr. Trappe was the lead investigator on some of the most important PTLD trials conducted in the last 10 years, including the PTLD-1 trial and its offshoots. In this second edition, we have added a completely new part on PTLDs after hematopoietic stem cell transplantation. Many new authors covering a wider range of countries across the world have contributed their expertise.

PTLD transcends multiple disciplines and demands a team approach to improve knowledge and treatment. The highly experienced internationally recognized authors have updated every part, plus added many new chapters, including on genetic abnormalities in virus and host seen in PTLDs. The newest PTLD classifications and current treatment paradigms that reflect recently conducted international trials are fully incorporated. As technologies have advanced, we provide the state-of-the-art new diagnostic and prognostic information.

Post-Transplant Lymphoproliferative Disorders is designed to be a comprehensive reference guide that will be of great value to oncologists and all transplant professionals (surgeons, nephrologists, cardiologists, hepatologists/gastroenterologists, pulmonologists, infectious disease specialists, pathologists) as well as interns and residents in training in these specialties. This book will provide these professionals with comprehensive and up-to-date information that will guide their management of transplant patients before and after transplant, with and without PTLD.

St. Louis, MO, USA   Vikas R. Dharnidharka
Pittsburgh, PA, USA   Michael Green
Nashville, TN, USA   Steven A. Webber
Bremen, Germany   Ralf Ulrich Trappe

Contents

Contributors

Upton D. Allen Department of Paediatrics, Division of Infectious Diseases, The Hospital for Sick Children, University of Toronto, Toronto, ON, Canada

Catherine M. Bollard Center for Cancer and Immunology Research, Children's National Health System, Washington, DC, USA

Department of Pediatrics, George Washington University School of Medicine, Washington, DC, USA

Department of Microbiology, Immunology and Tropical Medicine, George Washington University School of Medicine, Washington, DC, USA

Catherine Burton Division of Infectious Diseases, Department of Pediatrics, University of Alberta, Edmonton, AB, Canada

Sophie Caillard Nephrology-Transplantation Department, Hôpitaux Universitaires de Strasbourg, Strasbourg, France

Sylvain Choquet Department of Clinical Hematology, APHP-Sorbonne University, Pitié-Salpêtrière Hospital, Paris, France

Patrizia Comoli Pediatric Hematology/Oncology and Cell Factory, IRCCS Fondazione Policlinico San Matteo, Pavia, Italy

Vikas R. Dharnidharka Division of Pediatric Nephrology, Hypertension and Pheresis, Washington University School of Medicine, St. Louis, MO, USA

Daan Dierickx Department of Hematology, University Hospitals Leuven, Leuven, Belgium

Anne I. Dipchand Labatt Family Heart Centre, Hospital for Sick Children, Department of Paediatrics, University of Toronto, Toronto, ON, Canada

Carlos O. Esquivel Department of Surgery, Division of Abdominal Transplantation, Stanford School of Medicine, Stanford, CA, USA

Maher K. Gandhi Blood Cancer Research Group, Mater Research, University of Queensland, Translational Research Institute, Brisbane, QLD, Australia

Department of Haematology, Princess Alexandra Hospital, Brisbane, QLD, Australia

Allan R. Glanville The Lung Transplant Unit, St. Vincent's Hospital, Sydney, NSW, Australia

Michael Green Departments of Pediatrics, University of Pittsburgh School of Medicine, UPMC Children's Hospital of Pittsburgh, Pittsburgh, PA, USA

Departments of Surgery, University of Pittsburgh School of Medicine, UPMC Children's Hospital of Pittsburgh, Pittsburgh, PA, USA

Division of Infectious Diseases, UPMC Children's Hospital of Pittsburgh, Pittsburgh, PA, USA

Thomas G. Gross Department of Pediatrics, University of Colorado School of Medicine, Center for Cancer and Blood Diseases, Children's Hospital Colorado, Aurora, CO, USA

Britta Höcker Department of Pediatrics I, University Children's Hospital of Heidelberg, Heidelberg, Germany

Mitchell E. Hughes Abramson Cancer Center, University of Pennsylvania, Philadelphia, PA, USA

Ajai Khanna Division of Transplant Surgery, UPMC Children's Hospital of Pittsburgh, Pittsburgh, PA, USA

Department of Surgery, University of Pittsburgh School of Medicine, Pittsburgh, PA, USA

Charlotte Lees Blood Cancer Research Group, Mater Research, University of Queensland, Translational Research Institute, Brisbane, QLD, Australia

Princess Alexandra Hospital Southside Clinical Unit, Faculty of Medicine, University of Queensland, Translational Research Institute, Brisbane, QLD, Australia

Britta Maecker-Kolhoff Hannover Medical School, Pediatric Hematology and Oncology, Hannover, Germany

Olivia M. Martinez Department of Surgery/Division of Transplantation and Stanford Immunology, Stanford University School of Medicine, Stanford, CA, USA

George V. Mazariegos Division of Transplant Surgery, UPMC Children's Hospital of Pittsburgh, Pittsburgh, PA, USA

Department of Surgery, University of Pittsburgh School of Medicine, Pittsburgh, PA, USA

Michael McDonald Department of Medicine, Advanced Heart Failure and Transplant Program, Peter Muck Cardiac Centre/UHN Transplant, Division of Cardiology, Toronto, ON, Canada

Lauren P. McLaughlin Center for Cancer and Immunology Research, Children's National Health System, Washington, DC, USA

Department of Pediatrics, George Washington University School of Medicine, Washington, DC, USA

Diana M. Metes University of Pittsburgh School of Medicine, Thomas E. Starzl Transplantation Institute, Pittsburgh, PA, USA

Jutta K. Preiksaitis Division of Infectious Diseases, Department of Medicine, University of Alberta, Edmonton, AB, Canada

Cliona M. Rooney Center for Cell and Gene Therapy, Baylor College of Medicine, Houston Methodist Hospital and Texas Children's Hospital, Houston, TX, USA

Dan L. Duncan Comprehensive Cancer Center, Children's National Health System, Washington, DC, USA

Department of Pediatrics, Baylor College of Medicine, Houston, TX, USA

Department of Immunology, Baylor College of Medicine, Houston, TX, USA

Department of Virology, Baylor College of Medicine, Houston, TX, USA

Rayne H. Rouce Center for Cell and Gene Therapy, Baylor College of Medicine, Houston Methodist Hospital and Texas Children's Hospital, Houston, TX, USA

Dan L. Duncan Comprehensive Cancer Center, Children's National Health System, Washington, DC, USA

Françoise Smets Pediatrics, Cliniques universitaires Saint-Luc – UCLouvain, Brussels, Belgium

Jan Styczynski Department of Pediatric Hematology and Oncology, Collegium Medicum, Nicolaus, Copernicus University Torun, Jurasz University Hospital, Bydgoszcz, Poland

Steven H. Swerdlow University of Pittsburgh School of Medicine, Division of Hematopathology, UPMC-Presbyterian, Pittsburgh, PA, USA

Ralf Ulrich Trappe Department of Hematology and Oncology, Christian-Albrechts-University Kiel, Kiel, Germany

Division of Hematology and Oncology, Department of Medicine, DIAKO Ev. Diakonie-Krankenhaus Bremen, Bremen, Germany

Donald E. Tsai Abramson Cancer Center, University of Pennsylvania, Philadelphia, PA, USA

Gary Visner Department of Pediatrics, Boston Children's Hospital, Harvard Medical School, Boston, MA, USA

Steven A. Webber Department of Pediatrics, Vanderbilt University School of Medicine, Monroe Carell Jr. Children's Hospital at Vanderbilt, Nashville, TN, USA

Introduction and History

Vikas R. Dharnidharka, Michael Green, Steven A. Webber, and Ralf Ulrich Trappe

Introduction

Posttransplant lymphoproliferative disorders (PTLDs) remain a major and feared complication of solid organ and hematopoietic stem cell transplantation. PTLDs are at once both the "bad" and the "fascinating" in organ and stem cell transplantation: "bad" since they represent an unwanted complication of transplantation, with significant morbidities and mortality, and "fascinating" since this heterogenous group

V. R. Dharnidharka (✉)
Division of Pediatric Nephrology, Hypertension and Pheresis, Washington University School of Medicine, St. Louis, MO, USA
e-mail: vikasd@wustl.edu

M. Green
Departments of Pediatrics, University of Pittsburgh School of Medicine, UPMC Children's Hospital of Pittsburgh, Pittsburgh, PA, USA

Departments of Surgery, University of Pittsburgh School of Medicine, UPMC Children's Hospital of Pittsburgh, Pittsburgh, PA, USA

Division of Infectious Diseases, UPMC Children's Hospital of Pittsburgh, Pittsburgh, PA, USA
e-mail: Michael.green@chp.edu

S. A. Webber
Department of Pediatrics, Vanderbilt University School of Medicine, Monroe Carell Jr. Children's Hospital at Vanderbilt, Nashville, TN, USA
e-mail: steve.a.webber@vumc.org

R. U. Trappe
Department of Hematology and Oncology, Christian-Albrechts-University Kiel, Kiel, Germany

Division of Hematology and Oncology, Department of Medicine, DIAKO Ev. Diakonie-Krankenhaus Bremen, Bremen, Germany
e-mail: rtrappe@gwdg.de

© Springer Nature Switzerland AG 2021
V. R. Dharnidharka et al. (eds.), *Post-Transplant Lymphoproliferative Disorders*,
https://doi.org/10.1007/978-3-030-65403-0_1

of diseases, in many cases, results from lost immune control of a long-lived virus that has infected the body's cells, leading to uncontrolled proliferation of the infected cell. However, an increasing number of cases do not harbor this virus, leading to many new questions about alternative pathogenic mechanisms behind the development of cancer in populations that are immune suppressed. Thus, PTLD straddles not only the disciplines of organ and stem cell transplantation but also the related areas of immunology, infectious diseases, and oncology. The related areas of immune response, infection, and malignancy are basic processes involved in a large percentage of all diseases in the general population. The study of PTLD, therefore, has led to advances that have ramifications beyond just transplantation, enhancing our understanding of how the body's immune system deals with any long-lived microbe, especially when placed in non-physiological situations such as allogeneic organ and stem cell transplantation.

When the organ transplant field began in the 1950s and 1960s, the focus was on how to prevent acute rejection of the allograft by the recipient's immune system. The concepts that (1) a virus could be long-lived in a latent form in an organ being transplanted and (2) this virus would have far-reaching consequences because of use of therapeutic immune suppression were well beyond people's imagination at the time. Occasional cases of PTLDs were seen in the late 1960s and early 1970s, beginning with the first reports by Dr. Thomas Starzl in 1968 in a written discussion of Murray's transplant results [1], referring to the malignancies as "reticulum cell sarcomas." The B-cell lymphoid origin and the link to the Epstein-Barr virus became apparent later.

As more cases were reported, this disease presented many more complexities than originally thought. Back then, PTLDs were considered as a rare nuisance, a necessary but very infrequent evil of the good all of us were trying to do [2]. Many investigators seized on the opportunity provided by this experiment of nature (and man). "Lightening" of immunosuppression, as shown by Starzl in his seminal Lancet series [3], seemed enough in some cases to cause tumor regression and eliminate the hopelessness of the word lymphoma. What our transplant community did not anticipate then was that as newer and more potent immunosuppressive agents were developed and introduced, the PTLD frequency would increase, responses would be suboptimal, and more strategies would be needed. PTLD thus developed into a major complication of transplantation, such that its study has become a discipline unto itself. The amount of knowledge and information accumulated over these last five decades did not fit within the confines of medical journal review articles, hence the need that we felt for this book.

Historical Perspective

The linkage of PTLD to EBV was initially made serendipitously but then confirmed through several types of investigations. Less than a decade after the introduction of immunosuppression, an increased risk of cancer in renal allograft recipients and five cases of malignant lymphoma were reported [4, 5]. In the 1970s it was reported that the incidence of malignant lymphomas arising in patients with genetically determined immunodeficiency diseases (e.g., congenital immunodeficiency, ataxia telangiectasia, X-linked lymphoproliferative (XLP) syndrome) and in immunosuppressed renal allograft recipients was increased [6–10]. There were many hypotheses about the causes including impaired immune surveillance, chronic antigenic stimulation, reactivation of latent oncogenic herpesviruses, and direct oncogenic effects of immunosuppressive drugs, but none were proven [11]. By 1980, malignant lymphomas had been described in kidney, liver, heart, bone marrow, and thymic epithelial transplant recipients, as reviewed by Hanto et al. in 1985 [12].

The Epstein-Barr Virus

In 1964 the Epstein-Barr virus (EBV) was identified by electron microscopy in cultured cells from African Burkitt's lymphoma (BL) biopsies [13]. Over the next two decades, EBV was shown to transform B lymphocytes inducing a polyclonal proliferation in vitro [14] and in vivo [15] and to cause infectious mononucleosis (IM) in humans [16] and a fatal lymphoproliferative disorder in cotton-top marmosets [17] and was linked to BL [18], nasopharyngeal carcinoma (NPC), and the lymphoproliferative disorders (LPD) occurring in patients with XLP [8, 9].

The Serendipitous Intersection of Immunosuppression and EBV

In May 1976, a patient at the University of Minnesota underwent a living donor kidney transplant 1 month after his college roommate developed IM. The recipient died 4 weeks later of a rapidly progressive and invasive polyclonal LPD associated with an elevated heterophil antibody titer, a rise in the anti-VCA (viral capsid antigen) IgM and IgG titers, and a polyclonal increase in serum immunoglobulins. This was thought to represent a case of severe fatal IM transmitted from the roommate, but also had features suggestive of an aggressive lymphocytic malignancy and was reported at a pathology meeting because of the unusual morphologic features and polyclonality [19]. Subsequent cases in other renal transplant recipients were soon observed. The clinical and pathologic presentation and subsequent clinical course in these patients were varied, providing early evidence of the range of histology, progression, and outcome of these lesions. The unusual clinical presentations, pathologic findings, and hint of a role for EBV led to a great interest in studying these and additional patients over the next 2 years [20–24].

Initial Studies of "Posttransplant Lymphoma"

The initial analyses of the patient with possible IM and two new patients with oropharyngeal lesions raised many questions. The former patient had an invasive and fatal lymphoproliferative disorder that behaved, and had many characteristics of, an aggressive lymphoma, but was polyclonal, not monoclonal. Was it an EBV infection (i.e., fatal IM) accelerated by immunosuppression (a form of iatrogenic XLP) or an unusual manifestation of an aggressive lymphoma? Two subsequent patients had on initial biopsy an invasive polymorphic B-cell hyperplasia that in one patient evolved into a polymorphic B-cell lymphoma with characteristics of a monoclonal malignancy (see below). Again the question was whether these were infectious in origin or an unusual presentation of a malignant lymphoma?

Cell marker studies done by immunofluorescence for surface (sIg) and cytoplasmic immunoglobulin (cIg) and immunoperoxidase staining for kappa (κ) and lambda (λ) light chains demonstrated on the initial biopsies of these two patients that they were both polyclonal proliferations. Clonal cytogenetic abnormalities in one patient, however, suggested the development of a malignant cell clone not yet identifiable morphologically or by cell marker studies. Tissue from both patients demonstrated EBV-specific sequences. With a reduction of immunosuppression, lesions in both of these patients resolved. However, the second patient developed generalized lymph node disease which on biopsy had changed morphologically and now manifests features more characteristic of a malignant lymphoma and, as in the first patient, now contained a subpopulation of cells with cytogenetic abnormalities. This patient subsequently developed widespread disease and died.

Where Are We Now?

Since the publication of the first edition of this book in 2009, much new knowledge has been gained. The editors were pleasantly surprised to note that the first edition had accumulated more than 11,000 chapter downloads, consistently spread out over a 10-year period. We therefore saw potential for an updated version of the book, to incorporate all the new knowledge available. This second edition has many new features. We have created a separate new section on PTLD after hematopoietic stem cell transplantation (HSCT) and welcome a fourth editor Dr. Trappe to spearhead this section. Many chapters are written by specialists from across the world with complimentary expertise in either organ transplantation or oncology or adult and pediatric medicine.

Drs. Swerdlow and Webber present the definitions and pathological classification currently in use, which incorporates genetic and molecular information that is continually being updated under the auspices of the World Health Organization. Dr. Martinez discusses the current state of knowledge with respect to EBV biology and the pathogenesis of PTLD, an ever-changing field. Drs. Gandhi and Lees review the newer knowledge on genetic mutations and gene expression analyses in PTLDs. Dr. Metes presents the knowledge about immune responses to EBV in immunocompromised hosts. Drs. Preiksaitis and Burton provide an exhaustive overview of Epstein-Barr virus PCR technology and the caveats involved in the assay and its interpretation.

In the solid organ transplant section, Dr. Dharnidharka details the epidemiological aspects, including the changing incidence over time and the relationship to immunosuppression. Drs. Allen and Dierickx present the myriad clinical features possible, which forces transplant clinicians to keep PTLD in the differential diagnoses in so many situations. Drs. Trappe and Webber discuss the therapeutic options currently available and the evidence on which their usage is based. Drs. Green and Choquet then summarize the very important topic of EBV disease and PTLD prevention. Drs. Tsai and Hughes explore the prognostic factors reported so far.

In the new section on HSCT, Drs. Dharnidharka and Gross review the risk and prognostic factors for PTLD after HSCT. Drs. Dierickx and Maecker-Kolhoff present a short chapter on clinical presentations of PTLD after HSCT. Drs. Comoli and Styczynski then discuss the management options for PTLD after HSCT, which are somewhat different than after SOT. The last chapter in this section covers the preemptive and prevention approaches, where EBV-specific cytotoxic T cells have made a major impact, particularly in the setting of PTLD after stem cell transplant.

Several organ subspecialists then summarize the epidemiology, presentation, and treatment of PTLD in recipients of heart (Dr. Anne Dipchand), lung (Dr. Drs. Glanville and Visner), liver (Drs. Smets and Esquivel), intestine (Drs. Mazariegos and Khanna), and kidney (Drs. Caillard and Hocker). Finally, we end by summarizing much that is still unknown and the directions required for future research to solve this perplexing and many-faceted disease.

This book should be of value to transplant professionals in all disciplines including transplant surgery, oncology, hematopoietic stem cell transplant, nephrology, immunology, infectious disease, hepatology, cardiology, pulmonology, and pathology. We wish to thank all the authors that have contributed their expert knowledge and hard work to this text and also wish to offer our thanks to Springer for recognizing the need for a second edition.

Acknowledgments Sections of the history of PTLD were taken from a different chapter written by Douglas Hanto in the first edition of the book.

References

1. Murray JE, Wilson RE, Tilney NL, Merrill JP, Cooper WC, Birtch AG, et al. Five years' experience in renal transplantation with immunosuppressive drugs: survival, function, complications, and the role of lymphocyte depletion by thoracic duct fistula. Ann Surg. 1968;168(3):416–35. Discussion by Starzl TE, p. 33–34
2. Nalesnik MA, Makowka L, Starzl TE. The diagnosis and treatment of posttransplant lymphoproliferative disorders. Curr Probl Surg. 1988;25(6):367–472.
3. Starzl TE, Nalesnik MA, Porter KA, Ho M, Iwatsuki S, Griffith BP, et al. Reversibility of lymphomas and lymphoproliferative lesions developing under cyclosporin-steroid therapy. Lancet. 1984;1(8377):583–7.
4. McKhann CF. Primary malignancy in patients undergoing immunosuppression for renal transplantation. Transplantation. 1969;8:209–12.
5. Penn I, Hammond W, Brettschneider L, Starzl TE. Malignant lymphomas in transplantation patients. Transplant Proc. 1969;1(1):106–12.
6. Penn I. Malignancies associated with immunosuppressive or cytotoxic therapy. Surgery. 1978;83(5):492–502.

7. Spector BD, Perry GS 3rd, Kersey JH. Genetically determined immunodeficiency diseases (GDID) and malignancy: report from the immunodeficiency--cancer registry. Clin Immunol Immunopathol. 1978;11(1):12–29.
8. Purtilo DT. Pathogenesis and phenotypes of an X-linked recessive lymphoproliferative syndrome. Lancet. 1976;2(7991):882–5.
9. Purtilo DT, DeFlorio D Jr, Hutt LM, Bhawan J, Yang JP, Otto R, et al. Variable phenotypic expression of an X-linked recessive lymphoproliferative syndrome. N Engl J Med. 1977;297(20):1077–80.
10. Gatti RA, Good RA. Occurrence of malignancy in immunodeficiency diseases. A literature review. Cancer. 1971;28(1):89–98.
11. Matas AJ, Simmons RL, Najarian JS. Chronic antigenic stimulation, herpesvirus infection, and cancer in transplant recipients. Lancet. 1975;1(7919):1277–9.
12. Hanto DW, Frizzera G, Gajl-Peczalska KJ, Simmons RL. Epstein-Barr virus, immunodeficiency, and B cell lymphoproliferation. Transplantation. 1985;39(5):461–72.
13. Epstein MA, Achong B. The Epstein-Barr Virus. New York: Springer Verlag; 1979.
14. Rosen A, Gergely P, Jondal M, Klein G, Britton S. Polyclonal Ig production after Epstein-Barr virus infection of human lymphocytes in vitro. Nature. 1977;267(5606):52–4.
15. Robinson JE, Brown N, Andiman W, Halliday K, Francke U, Robert MF, et al. Diffuse polyclonal B-cell lymphoma during primary infection with Epstein-Barr virus. N Engl J Med. 1980;302(23):1293–7.
16. Henle G, Henle W. The virus as the etiologic agent of infectious mononucleosis. In: Epstein M, Achong B, editors. The Epstein-Barr Virus. New York: Springer Verlag; 1979. p. 297–320.
17. Frank A, Andiman WA, Miller G. Epstein-Barr virus and nonhuman primates: natural and experimental infection. Adv Cancer Res. 1976;23:171–201.
18. Klein G. Lymphoma development in mice and humans: diversity of initiation is followed by convergent cytogenetic evolution. Proc Natl Acad Sci U S A. 1979;76(5):2442–6.
19. Hertel B, Rosai J, Dehner P, Simmons R. Lymphoproliferative disorders in organ transplant recipients. Lab Investig. 1977;36:340.
20. Hanto DW, Frizzera G, Purtilo DT, Sakamoto K, Sullivan JL, Saemundsen AK, et al. Clinical spectrum of lymphoproliferative disorders in renal transplant recipients and evidence for the role of Epstein-Barr virus. Cancer Res. 1981;41(11 Pt 1):4253–61.
21. Hanto DW, Frizzera G, Gajl-Peczalska J, Purtilo DT, Klein G, Simmons RL, et al. The Epstein-Barr virus (EBV) in the pathogenesis of posttransplant lymphoma. Transplant Proc. 1981;13(1 Pt 2):756–60.
22. Frizzera G, Hanto DW, Gajl-Peczalska KJ, Rosai J, McKenna RW, Sibley RK, et al. Polymorphic diffuse B-cell hyperplasias and lymphomas in renal transplant recipients. Cancer Res. 1981;41(11 Pt 1):4262–79.
23. Hanto DW, Sakamoto K, Purtilo DT, Simmons RL, Najarian JS. The Epstein-Barr virus in the pathogenesis of posttransplant lymphoproliferative disorders. Clinical, pathologic, and virologic correlation. Surgery. 1981;90(2):204–13.
24. Hanto DW, Gajl-Peczalska KJ, Frizzera G, Arthur DC, Balfour HH Jr, McClain K, et al. Epstein-Barr virus (EBV) induced polyclonal and monoclonal B-cell lymphoproliferative diseases occurring after renal transplantation. Clinical, pathologic, and virologic findings and implications for therapy. Ann Surg. 1983;198(3):356–69.

Part I
Biology and Pathology

Definitions and Pathology of PTLD

2

Steven H. Swerdlow and Steven A. Webber

Introduction

Definition

Post-transplant lymphoproliferative disorders (PTLDs) are defined by the World Health Organization as "lymphoid or plasmacytic proliferations that develop as a consequence of immunosuppression in a recipient of a solid organ or stem cell allograft" [1]. An association with Epstein-Barr virus (EBV) is frequent but not required. It is important to exclude other causes of lymphoid/plasmacytic proliferations that can occur in immunocompromised hosts, such as chronic inflammatory responses to infection or rejection in the allograft.

General Pathologic Features and Classification

The post-transplant lymphoproliferative disorders (PTLD) demonstrate a spectrum of pathologic appearances that vary in terms of their degree of resemblance to other reactive and neoplastic lymphoid and plasmacytic proliferations, in terms of their cytologic composition and cell(s) of origin, and in terms of whether or not they are associated with EBV. Specifically, it should be noted that EBV positivity is not required for the diagnosis of a PTLD, that about 20–40% of cases are EBV negative

S. H. Swerdlow (✉)
University of Pittsburgh School of Medicine, Division of Hematopathology,
UPMC Presbyterian, Pittsburgh, PA, USA
e-mail: swerdlowsh@upmc.edu

S. A. Webber
Department of Pediatrics, Vanderbilt University School of Medicine,
Monroe Carell Jr. Children's Hospital at Vanderbilt, Nashville, TN, USA
e-mail: steve.a.webber@vumc.org

© Springer Nature Switzerland AG 2021
V. R. Dharnidharka et al. (eds.), *Post-Transplant Lymphoproliferative Disorders*,
https://doi.org/10.1007/978-3-030-65403-0_2

9

which is higher than seen in the past, and that the EBV negative cases include more monomorphic PTLD and more PTLD of T-cell origin [2–4]. Rare cases have been associated with HHV-8 [5]. Most, but not all, PTLDs in solid organ transplant patients are of host origin, whereas they are of donor origin in bone marrow/stem cell transplant patients. It is important to exclude other specific (or non-specific) lymphoid or plasmacytic proliferations prior to diagnosing PTLD, since transplant patients are also at risk for other infectious or inflammatory processes. In addition, infiltrates associated with rejection in the allograft should not be confused with PTLD.

In order to deal with this wide spectrum of PTLD, a consensus classification has evolved from those originally suggested by Frizzera et al., Nalesnik et al., Knowles et al., a Society for Hematopathology slide workshop, and others [6–13]. The current classification of the PTLD is part of the 2016 WHO classification of hematopoietic and lymphoid tumors (Table 2.1) [1, 14].

In brief, the non-destructive PTLDs show findings that could be seen in reactive proliferations in immunocompetent hosts: the *polymorphic PTLDs* are the most unique-appearing and demonstrate heterogeneous populations of lymphocytes and plasma cells with architectural destruction of the underlying tissues and are not easily categorized as one of the standard lymphomas that occur in immunocompetent hosts; the *monomorphic* PTLDs generally resemble one of the transformed B-cell

Table 2.1 WHO classification of PTLD [1, 14]

Non-destructive PTLDs
Plasmacytic hyperplasia
Infectious mononucleosis
Florid follicular hyperplasia
Polymorphic PTLD[a]
Monomorphic PTLDs[b]
B-cell neoplasms
Diffuse large B-cell lymphoma, NOS
Burkitt lymphoma
Plasma cell myeloma
Plasmacytoma
Other[c]
T-cell neoplasms
Peripheral T-cell lymphoma, NOS
Hepatosplenic T-cell lymphoma
Other
Classic Hodgkin lymphoma PTLD

[a]EBV-positive mucocutaneous ulcer which might resemble a polymorphic PTLD should be separately designated
[b]Classify according to lymphoma they resemble
[c]Indolent small B-cell lymphomas arising in transplant recipients are not included among the PTLDs, with the exception of EBV-positive extranodal marginal zone lymphoma of mucosa-associated lymphoid tissue (MALT lymphoma)

lymphomas, a plasma cell neoplasm, or T/NK-cell lymphoma; and *classic Hodgkin lymphoma* PTLDs fulfill the same criteria as those for classic Hodgkin lymphoma in immunocompetent hosts. *EBV-positive mucocutaneous ulcer* is another polymorphic proliferation that can be seen in the post-transplant setting and should be separately designated [15, 16]. It was introduced as a new provisional entity into the 2016 WHO classification [14, 17]. With the exception of EBV+ extranodal marginal zone lymphomas of mucosa-associated lymphoid tissue (MALT lymphoma), the small B-cell lymphomas are not considered PTLD even if occurring in transplant patients. This is both for historical reasons and because the standardized incidence ratios are either not increased or only moderately elevated in solid organ transplant recipients [1, 18–20].

While one should try to categorize the PTLD as precisely as possible, and note if they are EBV positive or negative, there is a spectrum of changes ranging from the non-destructive lesions to polymorphic to B-cell monomorphic lesions making precise classification sometimes impossible and reproducibility questionable. Furthermore, individual patients may have different types of PTLD, sometimes clonally unrelated or even with a different cell of origin, either simultaneously at the same or different sites or subsequently. In some cases, recurrences may show evidence of progression from a less destructive or more polymorphic PTLD to one that is more lymphoma-like, including B-cell or T-cell monomorphic PTLD or even Hodgkin lymphoma [4, 21].

Differential Diagnosis

Before diagnosing a PTLD, it is important to exclude the possibility of some other type of lymphoid or plasmacytic proliferation that simply happens to be occurring in a patient post-transplantation or, if the biopsy is from the allograft, exclude the possibility of rejection. Features that would favor the diagnosis of a PTLD over rejection (and over many, but not all, other types of inflammatory infiltrates) include the presence of expansile nodules or a mass lesion, numerous transformed cells, lymphoid atypia, a very B-cell-rich infiltrate, extensive serpiginous necrosis in the infiltrate, a high proportion of plasma cells and finding numerous EBV+ cells. Not all of these features, however, will be present in a PTLD, and one must also be aware of cases with both rejection and a PTLD. Diagnosis, thus, of the PTLD requires a multiparameter approach that also must take into account the clinical setting. Non-destructive lesions without a high proportion of transformed cells at extranodal sites other than the tonsils or spleen, even if EBV+, are generally not diagnosed as a PTLD, but rather as an inflammatory process, such as EBV hepatitis or EBV enteritis. Nevertheless, these extranodal infiltrates may precede PTLD, be associated with PTLD at other sites, and get treated like a PTLD with reduction in immunosuppression, frequently with resolution [22–24].

It should be noted that finding a small proportion of EBV-positive cells in a lymphoid proliferation is not pathognomonic of a PTLD. Likewise, although the subject is too extensive to review here, there are transplant patients with chronically elevated peripheral blood EBV loads who never develop a PTLD, although in some settings it may put them at higher risk for one [25, 26]. Following peripheral blood EBV loads has been useful in trying to recognize the earliest signs of a PTLD so they can be treated more successfully; however, the findings are not absolute, and the best way to monitor EBV loads remains to be determined [25, 27, 28]. This topic is covered in more detail in Chaps. 6, 11, and 17.

Multiparameter Approach to the Diagnosis of PTLD

The diagnosis and classification of PTLD require handling nodal or extranodal biopsies of potential cases using a standard protocol that provides for histologic sections and fresh material for flow cytometric immunophenotypic studies (if possible) (Table 2.2). In some instances, sending fresh tissue for classical cytogenetic studies may also be of interest, and if possible, snap freezing a small portion of tissue may be worthwhile for certain molecular studies [29, 30].

Adequate evaluation requires morphologic review, at least limited immunophenotypic studies, and an Epstein-Barr virus-encoded RNA (EBER) in situ hybridization stain to assess EBV status (immunostain for EBV-LMP1 is satisfactory if positive). Depending on these results and those of classical cytogenetic studies (if performed), genotypic studies (usually looking for a demonstrably clonal B-cell or T-cell population), and/or cytogenetic fluorescence in situ hybridization (FISH) studies (looking for one of the lymphoma-associated translocations or numerical abnormalities) may be required to arrive at a precise diagnosis. Gene expression profiling studies have provided interesting new information about PTLD but are not of diagnostic or prognostic utility at the current time [31, 32]. Mutational studies are also of interest, but again are not a part of current clinical practice.

Non-destructive PTLDs

The non-destructive PTLDs are defined as lymphoid/plasmacytic proliferations in the post-transplant setting that do not efface the underlying architecture, usually do produce mass lesions, and do not have another explanation, such as a specific non-EBV-associated infectious disorder. These lesions were previously known as "early

Table 2.2 Recommendations for tissue-based diagnosis of PTLD

1. Excisional biopsy preferred over fine needle aspiration or needle core, when feasible.
2. Histopathologic and immunophenotypic evaluation, similar to "lymphoma workup" in an immunocompetent host.
3. EBER in situ hybridization stain for EBV essential.
4. Molecular/cytogenetic testing often helpful and essential in a subset of cases.
5. Diagnosis requires categorization of PTLD based on the 2016 WHO classification and statement of whether the PTLD is EBV+. Cases of M-PTLD must be evaluated and classified based on the type of lymphoma they most closely resemble.

PTLD"; however, the name was changed because there was confusion with PTLD of varied types that occurred "early" after transplantation. In fact, these non-destructive lesions may occur many months to years after transplantation [33]. There are three types of non-destructive PTLDs that are currently recognized. It is advisable to use these diagnoses cautiously given the non-specificity of the histologic/immunophenotypic findings, at least in the absence of extensive EBV. Some, however, have specifically argued that transplant patients can have enlarged tonsils with marked follicular hyperplasia and EBV+ cells who do not have a PTLD and never develop one [34]. In contrast to many PTLDs that occur in extranodal sites, the classic non-destructive cases are found most commonly in lymph nodes and tonsils. In the absence of underlying tissue destruction in a biopsy of an extranodal site, particularly if there is a paucity of EBV+ cells (defined in one study of children after small bowel transplantation as not more than 15 EBV+ cells/"field") [24], the diagnosis of a PTLD should only be made with great caution. As noted above, even if there is EBV positivity, non-destructive infiltrates, such as in the liver or bowel, are conventionally designated as EBV hepatitis or EBV enteritis, respectively.

Plasmacytic Hyperplasia (PCH)

Histopathology
Lymph nodes demonstrate intact sinuses with a proliferation of predominantly small lymphocytes and plasma cells with few transformed cells[1] (Fig. 2.1a, b). Caution is advised as, especially if EBV cannot be documented, the changes are totally non-specific.

Ancillary Studies
PCH either is usually non-clonal or at best only has a very small clonal population sometimes only documentable with EBV terminal repeat Southern blot analysis (Fig. 2.1c, d). Cytogenetic or oncogene abnormalities are not expected.

Infectious Mononucleosis (IM) PTLD

Histopathology
Although underlying architectural features are retained, there is a polymorphous lymphoplasmacytic proliferation often in lymph nodes or tonsils/adenoids with more numerous transformed cells/immunoblasts than seen in PCH (Fig. 2.2a, b). Distinction from infectious mononucleosis in the normal host is impossible.

---

[1] Transformed lymphoid cells are relatively large, usually with a round to oval nucleus with one or more nucleoli and basophilic cytoplasm as seen on a Wright-Giemsa-type stain. They resemble lymphocytes that have been exposed to a mitogen.

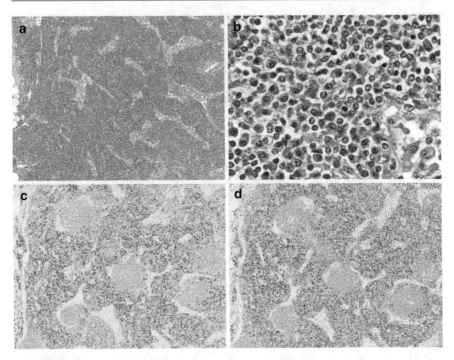

Fig. 2.1 Plasmacytic hyperplasia, lymph node. (**a**) Note there is architectural preservation with many open sinuses. (**b**) There are many plasma cells and some small lymphocytes but few transformed cells. Note the open sinus at the lower right. The (**c**) kappa and (**d**) lambda immunohistochemical stains demonstrate polytypic plasma cells. The scattered follicles are negative. (Unless otherwise noted all figures are hematoxylin and eosin stained sections)

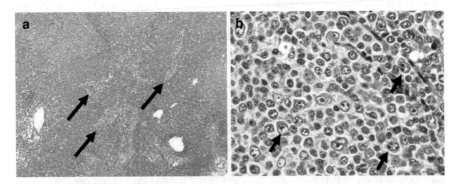

Fig. 2.2 Infectious mononucleosis PTLD, lymph node. (**a**) There is a more florid mostly diffuse proliferation in this lymph node that still demonstrates intact paler sinuses (arrows). (**b**) The proliferation is polymorphic and includes more transformed cells/immunoblasts (arrows) than in plasmacytic hyperplasia. The plasma cells were polytypic

Ancillary Studies

IM PTLD are typically EBV positive and do not demonstrate phenotypic aberrancies. Some cases have small clonal or oligoclonal lymphoid populations, and occasional cases are reported with simple clonal cytogenetic abnormalities [21, 30].

Florid Follicular Hyperplasia

Histopathology

These cases are indistinguishable from non-specific florid follicular hyperplasias in the normal host but should be mass-forming lesions. They are reported not to have significant expansion of interfollicular areas and few interfollicular immunoblasts/transformed cells. Distinction from totally non-specific FH may be impossible especially in the absence of significant numbers of EBV+ cells or other abnormalities, and there will be a gray zone between these cases and IM PTLD.

Ancillary Studies

Immunophenotypic studies are non-diagnostic, and most cases fail to demonstrate a clonal lymphoid population by any method. Occasional cases are reported to demonstrate simple clonal cytogenetic abnormalities [30].

Polymorphic PTLD

Polymorphic (P) PTLDs traditionally are destructive polymorphic lymphoplasmacytic proliferations that do not fulfill the criteria for a typical lymphoma as seen in immunocompetent hosts. These PTLDs are common in children after solid organ transplantation but form a minority of the PTLDs observed in adults. They are also more commonly seen in the first few years after transplantation (especially when associated with primary EBV infection in children) but may still be observed in late-onset cases years after transplantation. When originally defined, ancillary studies were very limited so P-PTLDs were defined in terms of their polymorphism (lymphoid cells of varied size and shape and at different maturational stages) in contrast to the more uniform transformed cell proliferations that defined the monomorphic (M) PTLD. With the increasing use of more ancillary studies, many classic P-PTLDs may have at least some features that do suggest a traditional lymphoma, such as easily identified clonal plasma cells in addition to B-cell clones identified by molecular studies. In addition, some M-PTLDs share features commonly associated with P-PTLD such as pleomorphism or more numerous smaller lymphocytes (see below) so that there is now more of a gray zone between these two categories of PTLD, and it is clear that there is a lack of uniformity in the way P-PTLD is used. There is also a gray zone between some P-PTLD and IM-PTLD, particularly in tonsils. Cases of EBV+ mucocutaneous ulcer should be separately designated.

Histopathology

There is destruction of the underlying lymph node or other parenchymal tissue architecture by a diffuse polymorphic proliferation of lymphocytes of varying size, shape, and degree of transformation plus plasma cells (Fig. 2.3a, b). The transformed cells/immunoblasts may be "atypical" and resemble classic Reed-Sternberg cells (Fig. 2.3c). The infiltrates may be angiocentric and angiodestructive and, in the lung, may resemble lymphomatoid granulomatosis. Geographic (serpiginous) areas of necrosis are seen in about one third of cases. The separately designated EBV+ mucocutaneous ulcers are ulcerated polymorphic proliferations in the skin, oral mucosa, or intestine, often with many large transformed cells and Reed-Sternberg-like cells with admixed lymphocytes, histiocytes, plasma cells and eosinophils, and a rim of smaller lymphocytes at their periphery [17]. Angioinvasion and necrosis may also be present. Some more closely resemble a diffuse large B-cell lymphoma.

Ancillary Studies

Typically, immunophenotypic studies demonstrate an admix of variably sized B cells and heterogeneous T cells (Fig. 2.3d, e). Major light chain restricted B-cell populations are not expected; however, light chain restricted plasma cell populations are found in some cases that most people would still include in this category, and genotypic studies will demonstrate variably sized B-cell clones in virtually all cases. *BCL6* mutations that in part are physiologic are reported in some polymorphic PTLD; however, while abnormalities in tumor suppressor genes and oncogenes have been reported, they are much less common than in M-PTLD [8, 32, 35, 36]. Some cases have cytogenetic abnormalities [29, 30]. Many, but not all, cases are EBV+ (Fig. 2.3f).

EBV+ mucocutaneous ulcer typically has prominent large CD20+, IRF4/MUM1+, and CD30+ B cells that may be CD15+, as well as admixed EBV− T cells that are most dense at the periphery of the lesion [15]. Monoclonal immunoglobulin rearrangements are seen in less than half of the cases, and there are often oligoclonal or restricted T-cell populations. They typically lack EBV DNA in the peripheral blood [16].

Monomorphic PTLD

The monomorphic PTLD are a heterogeneous group of lymphoid/plasmacytic proliferations that fulfill the criteria for one of the lymphomas or plasma cell neoplasms that are recognized in the immunocompetent host. While EBV+ MALT lymphomas are now accepted as a form of M-PTLD, other small B-cell lymphomas are not [1, 20]. While classically defined as being composed predominantly of numerous transformed lymphoid cells at one maturational stage (hence monomorphic), they may show pleomorphism, have plasmacytic differentiation, be composed of sheets of

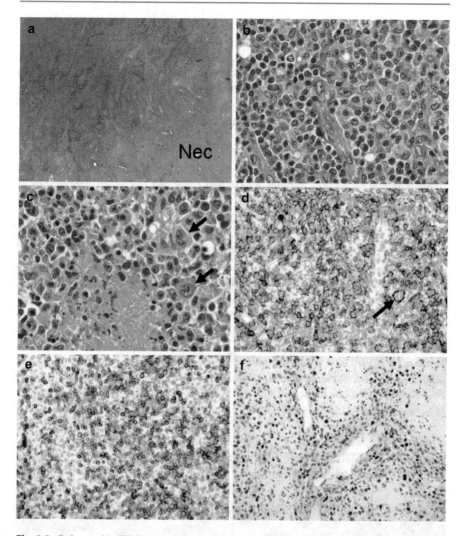

Fig. 2.3 Polymorphic PTLD, lymph node. (**a**) There is diffuse architectural effacement and extensive areas of eosinophilic geographic necrosis (Nec). (**b**) The lymphoid cells vary in size and shape and degree of transformation. There are also admixed histiocytes and eosinophils. (**c**) Atypical immunoblasts are seen especially around the necrotic areas (arrows). (**d**) There are many CD20+ B cells including the atypical/Reed-Sternberg-like cells (arrows). (**e**) There are also many admixed CD3+ T cells. (**f**) Many of the cells are EBV+ as seen in this EBER in situ hybridization stain

light chain restricted plasma cells, or, in the case of monomorphic T-cell PTLDs, be composed of quite heterogeneous T-cell populations as long as they would fulfill the criteria for a lymphoid neoplasm. They are all expected to be monoclonal, and it is among the monomorphic T-cell PTLDs that the greatest frequency of EBV negative cases will be found (about 70%). M-PTLD is the predominant pathology observed in adult transplant recipients.

Monomorphic B-Cell PTLD

The majority of the monomorphic PTLD resemble one of the types of diffuse large B-cell lymphoma, not otherwise specified, with smaller numbers resembling Burkitt lymphoma, plasma cell myeloma, or another type of plasma cell neoplasm. Cases of the new provisional entity, Burkitt-like lymphoma with 11q aberration, may be over-represented among transplant patients, but are not common [1, 37].

Histopathology

The most common monomorphic B-cell M-PTLDs are of the diffuse large B-cell lymphoma (DLBCL), not otherwise specified type, and are usually composed of sheets of large transformed cells growing with an infiltrative and/or destructive pattern and sometimes showing angiocentricity (Fig. 2.4a, b). There may be pleomorphism, and plasmacytic differentiation may be present in some cases. These cases do not have uniform morphologic features, and some B-cell M-PTLD may fulfill the criteria for one of the other large B-cell lymphomas, such as intravascular large B-cell lymphoma or plasmablastic lymphoma (Fig. 2.5) [38, 39]. Less frequently, they are of Burkitt type and composed of sheets of intermediate-sized transformed cells with amphophilic cytoplasm and a starry sky appearance due to the scattered tingible body macrophages that contain phagocytized apoptotic debris (Fig. 2.6). Some may resemble a Burkitt lymphoma but lack *MYC* translocations and have 11q aberrations [37]. Other cases are composed of a sheet of plasma cells as seen in plasma cell myeloma or a non-myelomatous plasmacytoma (Fig. 2.7a, b). These two situations must be distinguished just as they would be in an immunocompetent host, with an expected different approach to therapy [40–42].

Ancillary Studies

Most cases are CD20 positive. Except in cases that lack immunoglobulin expression, immunophenotypic studies should show light chain class restriction and a

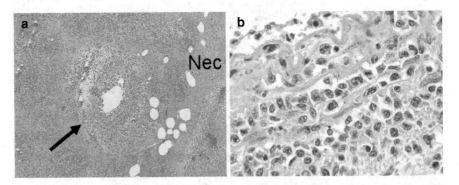

Fig. 2.4 Monomorphic B-cell PTLD, diffuse large B-cell lymphoma, not otherwise specified type, small intestine. (**a**) Note the angioinvasion (arrow) and foci of eosinophilic necrosis (Nec). (**b**) There are numerous transformed cells that marked as B cells in the vessel wall. Even here the cells are not completely monotonous

Fig. 2.5 Monomorphic B-cell PTLD, plasmablastic lymphoma type, sinus contents. Note the anaplastic-appearing plasmacytic cells that were CD20−, CD138+, kappa+, and EBV+

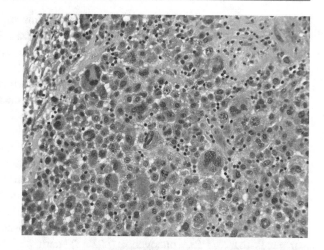

Fig. 2.6 Monomorphic B-cell PTLD, Burkitt lymphoma type, duodenum. There is a diffuse proliferation of transformed lymphoid cells and a starry sky appearance from the scattered tingible body macrophages (arrows). The cells had a typical Burkitt lymphoma phenotype (CD10+, BCL6+, BCL2−, Ki-67 numerous positive cells) and a *MYC* translocation

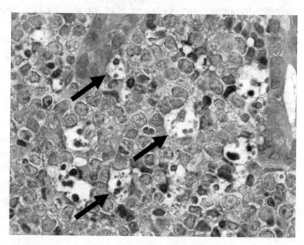

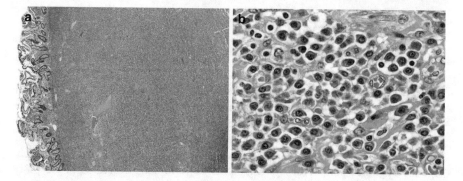

Fig. 2.7 Monomorphic B-cell PTLD, plasmacytoma type, small intestine. (**a**) Note the large mass lesion. (**b**) In most areas the mass was composed of a sheet of monotypic plasma cells. Cases like this must be distinguished from visceral involvement by plasma cell myeloma

more detailed phenotype like that seen in the neoplasms they resemble. The DLBCL may have either a germinal center type or non-germinal center phenotype with the former phenotype more common among the EBV-negative cases [43]. The prognostic importance of this distinction in the post-transplant setting is not well-established, but it still might have therapeutic implications. Burkitt lymphomas usually have a CD20+, CD10+, BCL6+, and BCL2− phenotype. The plasma cell neoplasms usually lack B-cell-associated markers and are CD138+ with cytoplasmic light chain class restriction. EBV is present in a majority of cases but a significant minority is negative.

Genotypic studies can be used to confirm the monoclonality of these PTLDs; however, they are usually unnecessary for diagnostic purposes. Caution is advised as clonal T-cell receptor rearrangements may also be present in the absence of a coexistent T-cell PTLD [44]. Among the common types of PTLD, the B-cell M-PTLDs are the ones most likely to demonstrate abnormalities of tumor suppressor genes (e.g., *TP53*), oncogenes (*N-RAS*), perhaps *BCL6* mutations, aberrant somatic hypermutation (e.g., of *MYC* or *RHO/TTF*), and translocations such as of *MYC* (a feature of Burkitt lymphomas) [8, 32, 35]. Cytogenetic abnormalities, including some (not universally agreed upon) recurrent abnormalities, are more common than in the other types of B-cell-rich PTLD [29, 30]. In addition to finding some recurrent abnormalities associated with conventional lymphomas, such as involving *MYC*, trisomies 9 and 11 have been found by some with trisomy 11 also associated with other EBV-associated neoplasms [29, 45]. EBV+ PTLDs have been reported to have fewer genetic/mutational abnormalities than EBV− cases which may show more features like the DLBCL in immunocompetent hosts which they resemble [46, 47]. Nevertheless, at least limited differences are reported between even EBV- PTLD and DLBCL arising in immunocompetent hosts, with more differences found in comparison with the EBV+ PTLD [36]. Although not consistently found, at least two gene expression profiling studies have shown differences between EBV+ and EBV− PTLD, consistent with mutational differences [31, 36, 46, 48].

Monomorphic T/NK-Cell PTLD

Monomorphic T/NK-cell PTLDs account for only about 7–15% of PTLD in Western countries and appear to be more common in Japan [4]. They are defined as post-transplant lymphoid proliferations that fulfill the criteria for one of the T/NK-cell neoplasms recognized in the WHO classification and hence are often not composed of monomorphic large transformed cells [1]. The T/NK-cell PTLDs most commonly resemble peripheral T-cell lymphoma, not otherwise specified, with cases of hepatosplenic T-cell lymphoma another one of the more common types seen. Many of the recognized peripheral T-cell lymphomas have been described in the post-transplant setting including, among others, T-cell lymphoblastic leukemia/lymphoma, T-cell large granular lymphocyte leukemia, adult T-cell leukemia/lymphoma, mycosis fungoides, Sézary syndrome, and cutaneous and other anaplastic large cell lymphomas (ALK+ and ALK−) [4]. Occasional lymphomas of natural killer cells, including extranodal NK/T cell lymphoma, nasal type, are also reported. Only about one third of T-cell PTLD are EBV positive.

Histopathology

The histopathology of the T/NK-cell PTLD is very variable but should be the same as for the varied T-cell lymphomas seen in immunocompetent hosts. These cases may be confused with polymorphic PTLD or other reactive proliferations because many T/NK-cell lymphomas can appear heterogeneous and include many admixed reactive elements. Some features to look for, in addition to a destructive growth pattern, include prominent cytologically atypical lymphoid cells or, in some cases, very numerous transformed lymphoid cells (like in other monomorphic PTLD) (Fig. 2.8a). A discussion of the histopathology of T-cell lymphomas is beyond the scope of this chapter [1].

Ancillary Studies

Ancillary studies are critical in the diagnosis of the T-cell PTLD. Immunophenotypic studies are useful to exclude findings that would suggest one of the other types of PTLD (e.g., abnormal B cells); to document that the cells of concern mark as T cells (pan-T-cell and T-cell subset marker expression) or natural killer (NK) cells (surface CD3−, CD5−, CD56+); and, in some cases, to demonstrate a population with an aberrant T-cell phenotype (e.g., "loss" of one or more pan-T-cell markers) or expansion of a T-cell subset that is either usually not present in large numbers or is present on cells that clearly appear neoplastic based on their cytologic features and growth pattern (Fig. 2.8b). For example, finding that an intrasinusoidal neoplastic T-cell infiltrate in the liver lacks T-cell receptor beta chain expression and is positive with TIA-1 but not granzyme B helps make the diagnosis of a hepatosplenic T-cell

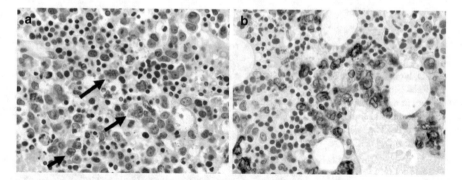

Fig. 2.8 Monomorphic T-cell PTLD, peripheral T-cell lymphoma, not otherwise specified type (cytotoxic), bone marrow. (**a**) There is a patchy interstitial infiltrate composed of very large cells with irregular nuclear contours (arrows) in the marrow biopsy. (**b**) The very abnormal cells are more easily seen in this CD3 immunohistochemical stain that identifies T cells (and natural killer cells). A clonal T-cell receptor beta chain rearrangement was documented by Southern blot analysis. EBV was not detected

lymphoma type T-PTLD. Molecular studies (PCR analyses looking for clonal T-cell receptor gene rearrangements) are also very important to help identify the presence of a clonal T-cell population remembering that clonal populations can be seen in the setting of infectious mononucleosis [49] and in some B-cell PTLD [44] and that natural killer cell neoplasms will be negative. Both chromosomal abnormalities and oncogene and epigenetic modifier gene mutations are commonly found and reported to be similar to those in T-cell lymphomas arising in immunocompetent hosts [50].

Classic Hodgkin Lymphoma PTLD

Classic Hodgkin lymphoma PTLD is strictly defined and must fulfill the criteria for classic Hodgkin lymphoma in an immunocompetent host. Caution is advised as cells resembling Reed-Sternberg cells are seen in many different types of PTLD, most of which are not of Hodgkin type. So-called "Hodgkin-like" PTLDs are no longer included with the classic Hodgkin PTLD and are to be categorized in whatever other PTLD category they best fit in [51].

Histopathology

Post-transplant classic Hodgkin lymphoma most typically shows at least partial architectural effacement by a proliferation of variable numbers of small lymphocytes, plasma cells, eosinophils, and histiocytes, together with diagnostic Reed-Sternberg cells and Reed-Sternberg variants (Fig. 2.9). Most cases in the transplant setting fulfill the criteria for the mixed cellularity type. Whether post-transplant Hodgkin lymphoma has any unique features is difficult to assess given the difficulty sometimes in distinguishing it from other PTLD with Hodgkin-like features.

Fig. 2.9 Mixed cellularity classic Hodgkin lymphoma PTLD, lymph node. There are Reed-Sternberg cells (arrow) in a sea of small lymphocytes and some plasma cells. The Reed-Sternberg cells were CD20−, CD15+, and CD30+

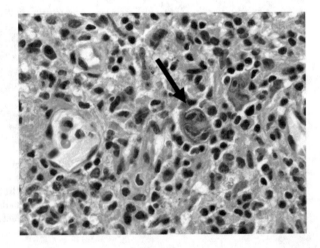

Ancillary Studies

Immunohistochemical studies are critical, particularly given the resemblance of many other types of PTLD to classic Hodgkin lymphoma. In the most definite cases, the Reed-Sternberg cells are CD15+, CD30+, CD20−, and CD45− with the majority of the surrounding small lymphocytes of T-cell type. It is expected that, as in immunocompetent hosts, the Reed-Sternberg cells are also either OCT2 (POU2F2) or BOB.1 (POU2AF1) negative – a feature that may be helpful in the presence of some CD20 staining or an absence of CD15 expression. The neoplastic cells should also be weakly positive for PAX5 in most cases and positive for IRF4/MUM1. Almost all cases have been EBV+. Genotypic studies may demonstrate clonal B cells in some cases.

Take-Home Pearls

- The PTLDs include many different types of lymphoid and plasmacytic proliferations that are associated with the Epstein-Barr virus in about 60–80% of cases. Some cases may be driven by other forms of chronic antigenic stimulation.
- Classification of the PTLD is important and is best accomplished by working up potential cases as one would a potential lymphoma. Categorization requires knowledge about the WHO criteria both for the PTLD and for lymphomas in general.
- In spite of one's best efforts, some cases may be difficult to categorize because there are gray zones between the different types of PTLD, particularly those of non-destructive, polymorphic, and monomorphic B-cell types.
- There is no sharp border between a PTLD and an overt lymphoma in the post-transplant setting.
- It is always important to exclude the possibility of some other type of lympho-plasmacytic proliferation including rejection prior to making the diagnosis of a PTLD. In rare cases there may be both rejection and a PTLD.

References

1. Swerdlow SH, Campo E, Harris NL, Jaffe ES, Pileri SA, Stein H, et al., editors. WHO classification of tumours of haematopoietic and lymphoid tissues. Revised 4th ed. IARC: Lyon; 2017.
2. Leblond V, Davi F, Charlotte F, Dorent R, Bitker MO, Sutton L, et al. Posttransplant lymphoproliferative disorders not associated with Epstein-Barr virus: a distinct entity? J Clin Oncol. 1998;16(6):2052–9.
3. Nelson BP, Nalesnik MA, Bahler DW, Locker J, Fung JJ, Swerdlow SH. Epstein-Barr virus-negative post-transplant lymphoproliferative disorders – a distinct entity? Am J Surg Pathol. 2000;24(3):375–85.
4. Swerdlow SH. T-cell and NK-cell posttransplantation lymphoproliferative disorders. Am J Clin Pathol. 2007;127(6):887–95.

5. Kapelushnik J, Ariad S, Benharroch D, Landau D, Moser A, Delsol G, et al. Post renal transplantation human herpesvirus 8-associated lymphoproliferative disorder and Kaposi's sarcoma. Br J Haematol. 2001;113(2):425–8.

6. Frizzera G, Hanto DW, Gajl-Peczalska KJ, Rosai J, McKenna RW, Sibley RK, et al. Polymorphic diffuse B-cell hyperplasias and lymphomas in renal transplant recipients. Cancer Res. 1981;41(11 Pt 1):4262–79.

7. Harris NL, Ferry JA, Swerdlow SH. Posttransplant lymphoproliferative disorders: summary of society for hematopathology workshop. Semin Diagn Pathol. 1997;14(1):8–14.

8. Knowles DM, Cesarman E, Chadburn A, Frizzera G, Chen J, Rose EA, et al. Correlative morphologic and molecular genetic analysis demonstrates three distinct categories of posttransplantation lymphoproliferative disorders. Blood. 1995;85(2):552–65.

9. Locker J, Nalesnik M. Molecular genetic analysis of lymphoid tumors arising after organ transplantation. Am J Pathol. 1989;135(6):977–87.

10. Ho M, Jaffe R, Miller G, Breinig MK, Dummer JS, Makowka L, et al. The frequency of Epstein-Barr virus infection and associated lymphoproliferative syndrome after transplantation and its manifestations in children. Transplantation. 1988;45(4):719–27.

11. Shapiro RS, McClain K, Frizzera G, Gajl-Peczalska KJ, Kersey JH, Blazar BR, et al. Epstein-Barr virus associated B cell lymphoproliferative disorders following bone marrow transplantation. Blood. 1988;71(5):1234–43.

12. Swerdlow SH. Posttransplant lymphoproliferative disorders: a working classification. Curr Diagn Pathol. 1997;4:29–36.

13. Swerdlow SH. Classification of the posttransplant lymphoproliferative disorders: from the past to the present. Semin Diagn Pathol. 1997;14(1):2–7.

14. Swerdlow SH, Campo E, Pileri SA, Harris NL, Stein H, Siebert R, et al. The 2016 revision of the World Health Organization classification of lymphoid neoplasms. Blood. 2016;127(20):2375–90.

15. Dojcinov SD, Venkataraman G, Raffeld M, Pittaluga S, Jaffe ES. EBV positive mucocutaneous ulcer--a study of 26 cases associated with various sources of immunosuppression. Am J Surg Pathol. 2010;34(3):405–17.

16. Hart M, Thakral B, Yohe S, Balfour HH Jr, Singh C, Spears M, et al. EBV-positive mucocutaneous ulcer in organ transplant recipients: a localized indolent posttransplant lymphoproliferative disorder. Am J Surg Pathol. 2014;38(11):1522–9.

17. Gaulard P, Swerdlow SH, Harris NL, Sundstrom C, Jaffe ES. EBV-positive mucocutaneous ulcer. In: Swerdlow SH, Campo E, Harris NL, Jaffe ES, Pileri SA, Stein H, et al., editors. WHO classification of tumours of haematopoietic and lymphoid tissues. Revised 4th ed. Lyon: IARC; 2017. p. 307–8.

18. Clarke CA, Morton LM, Lynch C, Pfeiffer RM, Hall EC, Gibson TM, et al. Risk of lymphoma subtypes after solid organ transplantation in the United States. Br J Cancer. 2013;109(1):280–8.

19. Knight JS, Tsodikov A, Cibrik DM, Ross CW, Kaminski MS, Blayney DW. Lymphoma after solid organ transplantation: risk, response to therapy, and survival at a transplantation center. J Clin Oncol. 2009;27(20):3354–62.

20. Gibson SE, Swerdlow SH, Craig FE, Surti U, Cook JR, Nalesnik MA, et al. EBV-positive extranodal marginal zone lymphoma of mucosa-associated lymphoid tissue in the posttransplant setting: a distinct type of posttransplant lymphoproliferative disorder? Am J Surg Pathol. 2011;35(6):807–15.

21. Wu TT, Swerdlow SH, Locker J, Bahler D, Randhawa P, Yunis EJ, et al. Recurrent Epstein-Barr virus-associated lesions in organ transplant recipients. Hum Pathol. 1996;27(2):157–64.

22. Randhawa PS, Jaffe R, Demetris AJ, Nalesnik M, Starzl TE, Chen YY, et al. Expression of Epstein-Barr virus-encoded small RNA (by the EBER-1 gene) in liver specimens from transplant recipients with post-transplantation lymphoproliferative disease. N Engl J Med. 1992;327(24):1710–4.

23. Randhawa PS, Markin RS, Starzl TE, Demetris AJ. Epstein-Barr virus-associated syndromes in immunosuppressed liver transplant recipients. Clinical profile and recognition on routine allograft biopsy. Am J Surg Pathol. 1990;14(6):538–47.

24. Finn L, Reyes J, Bueno J, Yunis E. Epstein-Barr virus infections in children after transplantation of the small intestine. Am J Surg Pathol. 1998;22(3):299–309.
25. Bingler MA, Feingold B, Miller SA, Quivers E, Michaels MG, Green M, et al. Chronic high Epstein-Barr viral load state and risk for late-onset posttransplant lymphoproliferative disease/lymphoma in children. Am J Transplant. 2008;8(2):442–5.
26. Green M, Soltys K, Rowe DT, Webber SA, Mazareigos G. Chronic high Epstein-Barr viral load carriage in pediatric liver transplant recipients. Pediatr Transplant. 2009;13(3):319–23.
27. Green M, Reyes J, Webber S, Rowe D. The role of antiviral and immunoglobulin therapy in the prevention of Epstein-Barr virus infection and post-transplant lymphoproliferative disease following solid organ transplantation. Transpl Infect Dis. 2001;3(2):97–103.
28. Tsai DE, Douglas L, Andreadis C, Vogl DT, Arnoldi S, Kotloff R, et al. EBV PCR in the diagnosis and monitoring of posttransplant lymphoproliferative disorder: results of a two-arm prospective trial. Am J Transplant. 2008;8(5):1016–24.
29. Djokic M, Le Beau MM, Swinnen LJ, Smith SM, Rubin CM, Anastasi J, et al. Post-transplant lymphoproliferative disorder subtypes correlate with different recurring chromosomal abnormalities. Genes Chromosomes Cancer. 2006;45(3):313–8.
30. Vakiani E, Nandula SV, Subramaniyam S, Keller CE, Alobeid B, Murty VV, et al. Cytogenetic analysis of B-cell posttransplant lymphoproliferations validates the World Health Organization classification and suggests inclusion of florid follicular hyperplasia as a precursor lesion. Hum Pathol. 2007;38(2):315–25.
31. Craig FE, Johnson LR, Harvey SA, Nalesnik MA, Luo JH, Bhattacharya SD, et al. Gene expression profiling of Epstein-Barr virus-positive and -negative monomorphic B-cell post-transplant lymphoproliferative disorders. Diagn Mol Pathol. 2007;16(3):158–68.
32. Vakiani E, Basso K, Klein U, Mansukhani MM, Narayan G, Smith PM, et al. Genetic and phenotypic analysis of B-cell post-transplant lymphoproliferative disorders provides insights into disease biology. Hematol Oncol. 2008;26(4):199–211.
33. Nelson BP, Wolniak KL, Evens A, Chenn A, Maddalozzo J, Proytcheva M. Early posttransplant lymphoproliferative disease: clinicopathologic features and correlation with mTOR signaling pathway activation. Am J Clin Pathol. 2012;138(4):568–78.
34. Meru N, Davison S, Whitehead L, Jung A, Mutimer D, Rooney N, et al. Epstein-Barr virus infection in paediatric liver transplant recipients: detection of the virus in post-transplant tonsillectomy specimens. Mol Pathol. 2001;54(4):264–9.
35. Cesarman E, Chadburn A, Liu YF, Migliazza A, Dalla-Favera R, Knowles DM. BCL-6 gene mutations in posttransplantation lymphoproliferative disorders predict response to therapy and clinical outcome. Blood. 1998;92(7):2294–302.
36. Menter T, Juskevicius D, Alikian M, Steiger J, Dirnhofer S, Tzankov A, et al. Mutational landscape of B-cell post-transplant lymphoproliferative disorders. Br J Haematol. 2017;178(1):48–56.
37. Ferreiro JF, Morscio J, Dierickx D, Marcelis L, Verhoef G, Vandenberghe P, et al. Post-transplant molecularly defined Burkitt lymphomas are frequently MYC-negative and characterized by the 11q-gain/loss pattern. Haematologica. 2015;100(7):e275–9.
38. Borenstein J, Pezzella F, Gatter KC. Plasmablastic lymphomas may occur as post-transplant lymphoproliferative disorders. Histopathology. 2007;51(6):774–7.
39. Morscio J, Dierickx D, Nijs J, Verhoef G, Bittoun E, Vanoeteren X, et al. Clinicopathologic comparison of plasmablastic lymphoma in HIV-positive, immunocompetent, and posttransplant patients: single-center series of 25 cases and meta-analysis of 277 reported cases. Am J Surg Pathol. 2014;38(7):875–86.
40. Perry AM, Aoun P, Coulter DW, Sanger WG, Grant WJ, Coccia PF. Early onset, EBV(−) PTLD in pediatric liver-small bowel transplantation recipients: a spectrum of plasma cell neoplasms with favorable prognosis. Blood. 2013;121(8):1377–83.
41. Karuturi M, Shah N, Frank D, Fasan O, Reshef R, Ahya VN, et al. Plasmacytic post-transplant lymphoproliferative disorder: a case series of nine patients. Transpl Int. 2013;26(6):616–22.

42. Richendollar BG, Hsi ED, Cook JR. Extramedullary plasmacytoma-like posttransplantation lymphoproliferative disorders: clinical and pathologic features. Am J Clin Pathol. 2009;132(4):581–8.
43. Johnson LR, Nalesnik MA, Swerdlow SH. Impact of Epstein-Barr virus in monomorphic B-cell posttransplant lymphoproliferative disorders: a histogenetic study. Am J Surg Pathol. 2006;30(12):1604–12.
44. Ibrahim HA, Menasce LP, Pomplun S, Burke M, Bower M, Naresh KN. Presence of monoclonal T-cell populations in B-cell post-transplant lymphoproliferative disorders. Mod Pathol. 2011;24(2):232–40.
45. Chan WY, Chan AB, Liu AY, Chow JH, Ng EK, Chung SS. Chromosome 11 copy number gains and Epstein-Barr virus-associated malignancies. Diagn Mol Pathol. 2001;10(4):223–7.
46. Morscio J, Tousseyn T. Recent insights in the pathogenesis of post-transplantation lymphoproliferative disorders. World J Transplant. 2016;6(3):505–16.
47. Ferreiro JF, Morscio J, Dierickx D, Vandenberghe P, Gheysens O, Verhoef G, et al. EBV-positive and EBV-negative posttransplant diffuse large B cell lymphomas have distinct genomic and transcriptomic features. Am J Transplant. 2016;16(2):414–25.
48. Morscio J, Dierickx D, Ferreiro JF, Herreman A, Van Loo P, Bittoun E, et al. Gene expression profiling reveals clear differences between EBV-positive and EBV-negative posttransplant lymphoproliferative disorders. Am J Transplant. 2013;13(5):1305–16.
49. Callan MF, Steven N, Krausa P, Wilson JD, Moss PA, Gillespie GM, et al. Large clonal expansions of CD8+ T cells in acute infectious mononucleosis. Nat Med. 1996;2(8):906–11.
50. Margolskee E, Jobanputra V, Jain P, Chen J, Ganapathi K, Nahum O, et al. Genetic landscape of T- and NK-cell post-transplant lymphoproliferative disorders. Oncotarget. 2016;7(25):37636–48.
51. Ranganathan S, Webber S, Ahuja S, Jaffe R. Hodgkin-like posttransplant lymphoproliferative disorder in children: does it differ from posttransplant Hodgkin lymphoma? Pediatr Dev Pathol. 2004;7(4):348–60.

Olivia M. Martinez

Biology of EBV

Infection

EBV is a double-stranded DNA herpesvirus first identified by Epstein, Achong, and Barr in tissue obtained from a patient with Burkitt lymphoma [1]. Today we know that over 90% of the world's population is infected with EBV. Typically the virus is transmitted through the saliva, and infection is asymptomatic, although infectious mononucleosis can result in adolescents and young adults. In the setting of clinical transplantation, EBV can also be transmitted via an organ from a seropositive donor to a seronegative recipient. The 172 kilobase pair EBV genome is packaged in a nucleocapsid surrounded by a viral tegument and enclosed within a lipid bilayer envelope containing glycoprotein spikes. The major viral envelope glycoprotein is gp350/220, which participates in viral infection by interacting with the CD21 molecule (complement receptor 2) on B cell membranes, thereby mediating the initial attachment of the virion to the cell. The interaction of gp350/220 and CD21 also induces capping of CD21 on the membrane and triggers endocytosis of the virus. Viral entry into the cell requires fusion of the viral envelope with the B cell membrane, a process mediated by interaction between the viral envelope glycoprotein, gp42, and major histocompatibility complex (MHC) class II proteins (HLA-DR, −DQ, or –DP) expressed on the cell membrane. gH, and gL are other viral envelope glycoproteins required for the fusion event [2]. While B cells are the predominant cellular host for EBV, epithelial cells are also susceptible to infection. Whereas gH and gL have been shown to be essential for epithelial cell infection by EBV, gp350/

O. M. Martinez (✉)
Department of Surgery/Division of Transplantation and Stanford Immunology,
Stanford University School of Medicine, Stanford, CA, USA
e-mail: omm@stanford.edu

© Springer Nature Switzerland AG 2021
V. R. Dharnidharka et al. (eds.), *Post-Transplant Lymphoproliferative Disorders*,
https://doi.org/10.1007/978-3-030-65403-0_3

gp220 and gp42, which are necessary for infection of B cells by EBV, are not required for infection of epithelial cells. Recently, the Ephrin receptor A2 (EphA2) was shown to be important for EBV infection of epithelial cells and was found to associate with gH/gL and gB [3]. EphA2 appears to play a role in facilitating the internationalization and fusion of membrane-associated EBV. Interestingly, EphA2 is also a receptor for Kaposi sarcoma-associated herpesvirus (KSHV) that shares a similar cell tropism as EBV.

Other cell types that EBV has been reported to infect include T cells, NK cells, and possibly monocytes, although the mechanisms of viral entry into these cell types are not well understood. Nevertheless, rare cases of EBV-associated T cell or NK cell post-transplant lymphomas have been reported [4].

The Viral Life Cycle

EBV is generally acquired through close contact with oral secretions from a carrier. The virus initially infects epithelial cells in the oropharynx and undergoes productive replication whereby infectious viral particles are produced. These viral particles can be the source of transmission of the virus to another host and can also go on to infect B cells in the vicinity [5]. Ultimately, EBV persists for the lifetime of the host in a subset of circulating memory B cells. As with other herpesviruses, EBV persistence is linked to viral latency, although infected memory B cells that differentiate to plasma cells activate the lytic program to release new viral particles. Thus the EBV life cycle takes two forms: the latent phase in which the virus remains dormant within B lymphocytes and the lytic phase, in which the virus is actively replicated and infectious virions are released that can go on to infect bystander cells or be shed to infect naive individuals. Using this life cycle strategy, EBV is highly successful at achieving widespread infection of the human population while perpetuating viral survival and minimizing the pathologic consequences for the host. An important component of this strategy is that EBV has achieved a seemingly harmonious state with the host immune system though this is likely a delicately balanced co-existence [6]. Indeed, disruption of the viral-host equilibrium predisposes individuals to the development of EBV-associated B cell lymphomas as in immunosuppressed transplant recipients with PTLD or immunocompromised people co-infected with HIV.

How EBV gains access to the memory B cell compartment has been studied extensively [7]. One prominent model is that the virus initially infects a naïve B cell and then exploits the normal B cell differentiation process [8, 9] (Fig. 3.1). During the early stages of infection of B cells, the linear EBV genome circularizes and is subsequently maintained as an extrachromosomal episome. The first of several latent cycle gene programs is triggered within 12–16 hours of infection, and nine key latent cycle genes are expressed that lead to cellular activation and autonomous proliferation of the infected cell. This program of viral gene expression has been termed latency type III (or the growth program) and is characterized by expression of Epstein-Barr nuclear antigens (EBNAs) 1, 2, 3A, 3B, 3C, LP, and latent

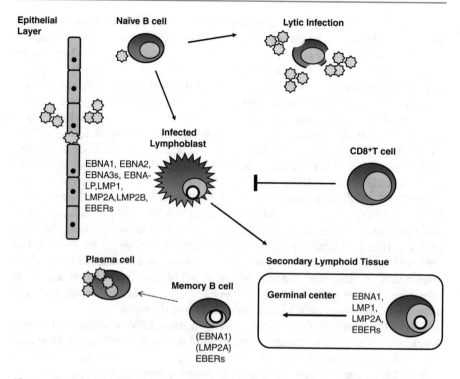

Fig. 3.1 EBV exploits the normal B cell differentiation process to gain access to memory B cells. EBV typically is transferred through oral secretions and then passes through the epithelial layer of the oropharynx. Viral particles infect naïve B cells and can establish a lytic infection where infectious viral particles are produced to subsequently infect other bystander cells or are shed to infect naïve individuals. Infection of naïve B cells can lead to establishment of a latent infection in which B cells take on a lymphoblastic phenotypic, associated with expression of the full complement of latent cycle genes. These infected lymphoblasts can proliferate autonomously but are under stringent control by EBV-specific CD8+ T cells. Infected lymphoblasts can migrate to secondary lymphoid tissue where the viral gene expression shifts to a more restricted group of latent cycle genes that facilitate survival and transit through the germinal center reactions. Once infected cells exit the germinal center and emerge in the memory B cell pool, minimal viral genes are expressed to enhance viral persistence. The differentiation of infected memory B cells to plasma cells can elicit reactivation of the virus and production of infectious particles to perpetuate the viral life cycle

membrane protein (LMP1, LMP2A, LMP2B) in addition to polyadenylated viral RNAs (EBERS 1 and 2) and a group of transcripts from the BamH1A region of the genome whose function is unknown. The resulting infected B cells resemble antigen-activated B lymphoblasts. In immunocompetent individuals the outgrowth of the EBV-activated lymphoblasts is controlled by a robust, anti-viral cytotoxic T lymphocyte (CTL) response. However, disruption of host immunity can lead to development of EBV+ B cell lymphomas, as seen in PTLD, that are also characterized by the latency III program of viral gene expression. Finally, the same viral gene expression program is found in B cells infected with EBV in vitro, resulting in the generation of immortalized lymphoblastoid cell lines (LCL).

In the normal course of EBV infection, the activated lymphoblasts can migrate to the B cell follicles of secondary lymphoid tissue where the growth program is silenced and replaced by latency type II (default program) characterized by expression of EBNA1, LMP1, and LMP2A. In conventional T cell-dependent immune responses, the follicles are sites where activated B cell blasts that have encountered antigen undergo isotype switching and somatic mutation of immunoglobulin genes to differentiate into antibody forming cells or memory cells bearing high-affinity B cell receptors (BCR). This process of differentiation depends upon encounter with antigen-presenting follicular dendritic cells and T helper cells. Cells expressing BCR that do not bind antigen die via apoptosis. In type II latency, the expression of EBNA1, LMP1, and LMP2A provides key signals that ensure survival of the infected cell and drive it through the B cell differentiation process associated with the GC reaction without requirement for interaction with antigen, follicular dendritic cells or T helper cells. Infected memory cells that emerge from GC then switch to type I, or latency program, where either no viral genes are expressed or only EBNA1 is expressed during cell division to ensure maintenance of the EBV episome. At the same time, the viral life cycle can be perpetuated when memory B cells harboring the virus recirculate to the lymphoid tissues in the epithelium and differentiate to plasma cells, eliciting reactivation of the virus.

The virtual absence of viral gene expression when EBV is harbored in resting memory B cells in the periphery promotes viral persistence and escape from host anti-viral immune mechanisms. This scenario suggests that EBV has co-evolved with the host immune system and utilizes its ability to induce autonomous proliferation of infected B cells only transiently as a means to exploit the process of B cell development to transit safely through to the memory B cell compartment [10]. Thus, the development of EBV-associated B cell lymphomas, including PTLD, may be an inadvertent and unintended consequence of this process in the context of impaired immunity or when additional mutations arise.

Latent Cycle Genes of EBV

How do latent cycle proteins shepherd EBV through the process of B cell differentiation? In this section the key properties of the 11 gene products expressed during type III latency and in PTLD-associated B cell lymphomas are summarized (Table 3.1).

(i) EBNA1: a DNA-binding protein that attaches to the origin of plasmid replication (OriP) of EBV and is required for episomal replication of the viral genome. Further, EBNA tethers the viral genome to mitotic chromosomes and is sufficient to ensure passage of the viral genome to daughter cells during cell division. EBNA1 also plays a role in transcription activation of latent viral genes and host cell genes.

(ii) EBNA2: a transcriptional activator that regulates the function of several viral genes including LMP1 and LMP2A as well as numerous cellular genes.

Table 3.1 Latent cycle genes expressed in EBV-associated PTLD B cell lymphomas and in type III latency

Gene	Function/activity
LMP1	Major oncogene of EBV; activates several signal transduction pathways to provide growth and survival signals to B lymphoblasts; constitutively active mimic of CD40
LMP2A	Acts as constitutively active mimic of BCR to provide key survival signals; inhibits BCR signaling by sequestering signaling proteins normally utilized by BCR
LMP2B	Participates in regulation of LMP2A function
EBNA1	Required for maintenance of viral genome as an episome; binds to mitotic chromosomes
EBNA2	Major viral transactivator of EBV; involved in expression of numerous cellular and viral genes
EBNA3A, B, and C	EBNA3A and EBNA3C are required for B cell transformation in vitro; like EBNA3A and EBNA3C, EBNA3B is involved in transcriptional regulation
EBNA-LP	Enhances the function of EBNA2
EBERs	Highly abundant, small nonpolyadenylated RNAs that can modulate apoptosis pathways, induce IL-10 production, and alter the host immune response

EBNA2 does not directly interact with DNA regulatory sequences but instead mimics Notch signaling by interacting with the DNA-binding protein, RBP-Jκ, to prevent B cell differentiation. EBNA2 is required for transformation of human B cells in vitro.

(iii) EBNA3A, 3B, 3C: encoded by genes that lie in tandem within the EBV genome. All three proteins interact with cellular DNA-binding protein RBP-Jκ and modulate transactivation by EBNA2. EBNA3A inhibits differentiation of B cells to plasma cells. EBNA3A and EBNA3C are required for immortalization of B cells in vitro, but EBNA3B is dispensable. EBNA3A and EBNA3C promote tumorigenesis, while EBNA3B can suppress tumorigenesis. EBNA3C, through interaction with cyclin proteins, can disrupt cell cycle checkpoints. EBNA3s are the primary target of the host CD8$^+$ T cell immune response.

(iv) EBNA-LP: the initial latent cycle gene expressed following infection of B cells. Important in transformation of B cells in vitro and enhances the ability of EBNA2 to transactivate cellular and viral genes.

(v) LMP1: the major oncogene of EBV since it is sufficient to transform rodent fibroblasts in vitro and is required for generation of LCL from human B cells. LMP1 is an integral membrane protein with a short intracellular N-terminal tail, six membrane-spanning domains, and a long cytoplasmic C-terminal tail. Within the intracellular tail are three carboxy-terminal activating regions (CTAR) that interact with cellular adaptor proteins to activate multiple cellular signaling pathways. In this way LMP1 mimics a constitutively active member of the tumor necrosis factor receptor (TNFR) superfamily and activates NF-κB; the mitogen-activated protein (MAP) kinases p38, Erk, and JNK; and PI3K/Akt through the use of the cellular adaptor proteins TRAF and TRADD. LMP1 signaling induces expression of cell adhesion molecules, anti-apoptotic proteins including bcl-2, cFLIP, A-20, and the production of the B cell lymphoma autocrine growth factor IL-10 [11, 12]. Thus, LMP1 provides critical growth and survival signals to infected B cells. Indeed, the ability of LMP1 to inhibit apoptosis through death receptors [13] suggests it may play an important role in survival of B cells through the GC in the absence of encounter with antigen by providing signals normally delivered through T cell help. Mice expressing a transgene for LMP1 under the control of the immunoglobulin promoter develop lymphomas at three times the frequency as LMP1-negative, control mice [14], and expression of LMP1 in B cells of mice that are depleted of T cells leads to lymphomagenesis [15].

(vi) LMP2A: expressed in the membrane of infected B cells and contains immunoreceptor tyrosine-based activation motifs (ITAM) similar to the BCR. Like LMP1, LMP2A is aggregated in the membrane and constitutively signals. LMP2A sequesters key tyrosine kinases, including Syk, from the BCR and thus inhibits BCR-mediated cell activation, thereby inhibiting entry into the lytic phase of infection. However, LMP2A supplies the tonic signals normally provided by the BCR for cell survival and can drive cellular proliferation and production of the growth factor IL-10.

(vii) LMP2B: the second isoform of LMP2 and is controlled by a separate promoter from LMP2A. Neither LMP2A nor LMP2B is essential for B cell transformation in vitro. LMP2B has been one of the most enigmatic of the EBV latent cycle proteins. Recent studies suggest the LMP2B can physically associate with LMP2A [16] and negatively regulates the ability of LMP2A to inhibit switching from the latent to the lytic cycle [17].

(viii) EBER: EBERs 1 and 2 are small polyadenylated, non-coding RNAs expressed in each of the three forms of latency. Commonly used as targets for in situ hybridization to establish the presence of EBV in clinical specimens. Abundant in EBV-transformed cells, contribute to oncogenesis, and can modulate the immune response. They have been reported to inhibit apoptosis [18], induce IL-10 production in Burkitt lymphoma cells [19], promote cell cycle transition [20], and activate the PI3K/Akt signaling pathway [21].

EBV Genetics and Oncogenic Mechanisms

PTLD

PTLD represents a heterogeneous group of disorders, the majority of which are B cell proliferations associated with EBV. Within the B cell proliferations, various malignant subtypes have been defined and will be discussed in another chapter. PTLD tumors can arise during primary infection with EBV or as a result of viral reactivation. Further, EBV-*associated* PTLD lymphomas can be polyclonal or monoclonal, with polyclonal tumors arising more often in the early post-transplant period, while tumors that occur more than 1 year post-transplant tend to be of the monoclonal variety but are more biologically heterogeneous. Thus, the factors contributing to the pathogenesis of PTLD are multiple and complex and include an immunosuppressed host, a virus with the ability to confer autonomous growth on infected cells and to invoke clever strategies of immune evasion, and the direct effects of immunosuppressive drugs on virally infected or transformed cells – all in the setting of alloreactivity. Despite these common factors, most transplant recipients do not develop PTLD. How then does PTLD arise?

Transplant recipients generally maintain higher EBV loads than healthy individuals, have increased numbers of latently infected memory B cells, and have increased frequency of viral reactivation [22]. The elevated viral loads and lytic replication could lead to more viral infection events in naïve B cells raising the number of cells that initially express the latency III growth program. If these cells cannot exit the cell cycle or fail to successfully progress through the differentiation program, then lymphomas could arise. Similarly, infection of bystander GC B cells or memory B cells could lead to aberrant expression of the growth program, without the ability to differentiate, and subsequent clonal expansion. Alternately, latently infected GC B cells or memory B cells could inappropriately turn on the growth program, perhaps due to accumulated mutations or as yet unidentified signals [10]. Coupled with the impaired T cell response, the autonomous growth properties of EBV+ lymphoblasts that result in each of these scenarios could culminate in PTLD. In support of this, analysis of immunoglobulin gene sequences shows that PTLD tumors can originate from naïve B cells, GC cells, or memory cells. Extensive molecular and phenotypic studies of EBV+ monoclonal PTLD indicate that the majority appears to be GC-experienced cells that reflect different stages of B cell differentiation [23]. The high rate of proliferation in these cells could lead to additional mutations that further drive oncogenesis, in some cases perhaps independent of EBV. Sporadic alterations in c-Myc [24], p53 [25] and other oncogenes have been described in PTLD lesions; however, it is unclear whether they contribute to enhanced tumor cell growth [26]. Monoclonal forms of PTLD tend to carry a higher frequency of mutations in tumor suppressor genes and altered proto-oncogene expression.

A variety of other factors could influence the development and progression of PTLD-associated B cell lymphomas including viral determinants that drive tumor growth and survival, viral mechanisms of immune evasion or subversion, and EBV genomic diversity and microRNA (miRNA). The following section will highlight some specific examples pertinent to each of these categories.

Viral Determinants That Drive Growth and Survival of PTLD-Associated B Cell Lymphomas

EBV has evolved to effectively co-opt several cellular signaling pathways within the host B cell to promote growth and survival of infected cells. The cellular cytokines IL-6 and IL-10 are both well-described autocrine growth factors in EBV+ B cell lymphomas [12, 27]. In addition, elevated levels of IL-6 and IL-10 are found in the circulation of patients with PTLD [28, 29]. In the case of IL-10, it has been definitively shown that the EBV-encoded protein, LMP1, activates the cellular mitogen-activated protein kinase p38 and the PI3K/Akt pathway to induce production of IL-10 [11]. The latent cycle protein, LMP2A, acts as a constitutively active mimic of the BCR to deliver tonic signals to EBV-infected B cells through activation of the Syk pathway. Furthermore, LMP2A can provide signals for survival and differentiation of B cells in the absence of BCR signaling through constitutive activation of the ERK/MAPK pathway [30, 31]. Other cell signaling pathways including NF-κB are constitutively active in EBV⁺ B cell lymphomas in PTLD. Finally, the EBNA3A and EBNA3C proteins function to promote cell cycle progression in B cells. Together, these virally induced mechanisms likely support ongoing cell survival and proliferation.

Viral Mechanisms of Immune Evasion or Subversion and the Tumor Microenvironment

EBV-encoded proteins that can counter apoptotic signals are a common theme in viral subversion strategies. LMP1 can actively block apoptotic signals delivered through the Fas/Fas ligand and TRAIL death receptor pathways. This function of LMP1 could help ensure survival of infected cells through the process of B cell differentiation and could also prevent elimination of EBV⁺ lymphoblasts by viral-specific CTL. LMP1 is also able to block apoptotic signals in EBV-infected B cells through upregulation of a variety of survival proteins including bcl-2, A20, mcl-1, and bfl-1. The EBV lytic cycle gene, BHRF1, encodes a viral homolog of bcl-2 that can inhibit apoptosis induced by multiple stimuli including anti-Fas antibodies and TNF-α. EBNA1 can block apoptosis induced by p53 expression which may be particularly relevant in Burkitt lymphoma where EBNA1 is the sole latent cycle protein expressed [32]. A second EBV nuclear antigen, EBNA2, interferes with apoptosis induced by some stimuli through the intrinsic pathway by sequestering Nur77 in the nucleus and preventing its translocation to the cytoplasm where it can induce cytochrome C release from the mitochondria [33].

Immunomodulatory cytokines or their receptors, either encoded by EBV or induced by EBV, are also an important tactic utilized by the virus to evade host immunity. The lytic cycle gene BCRF1 encodes viral IL-10 (vIL-10), a functional homolog of cellular IL-10. vIL-10 is expressed early following infection of B cells by EBV and, because of its immunosuppressive properties, may facilitate transformation by impairing T cell and macrophage responses. In particular, vIL-10 can inhibit production of IFN-γ by T cells and production of IL-12 by monocytes. As discussed earlier, LMP1 induces cellular IL-10, which acts as an autocrine growth factor for EBV⁺ B cell lymphomas. Cellular IL-10 can also have potent inhibitory effects on host T cells and monocytes during viral latency as in PTLD-associated lymphomas. The lytic cycle EBV gene, BARF1, encodes a functional, soluble receptor for colony-stimulating factor 1 (CSF-1) that can interfere with the ability of CSF-1 to augment monocyte/macrophage proliferation and produce IL-12. Finally, EBV infection of B cells induces expression of a cellular protein, EB13, that is a functional homolog of the IL-12 p40 subunit. Thus, it has been suggested that EB13 can antagonize IL-12 activity [34]. EB13 can also pair with p28, an IL-12p35-related protein, to form the cytokine IL-27. IL-27 is a complex cytokine with diverse pro- and anti-inflammatory properties, but strong evidence exists to indicate that IL-27 can inhibit a variety of effector functions by T cells [35].

Other immunomodulatory pathways that could alter the tumor microenvironment have been described. LMP1 has been shown to upregulate PD-L1 through an NF-κB-dependent pathway [36, 37]. The expression of PD-L1/2 on B cell lymphomas and identification of amplification of 9p24.1 using comparative genomic hybridization leading to overexpression of PD-L1/2 on EBV⁺ PTLD clinical specimens [38] indicate that immunomodulation of PD-1⁺ T cells in the tumor microenvironment is plausible [38].

Clearly, there are multiple avenues by which EBV can modulate host immunity that could impact on the development and progression of PTLD.

EBV microRNAs and Host Cell microRNAs

In 2004, EBV was the first virus shown to encode microRNA (miRNA), a family of small non-coding single-stranded RNA of ~22 nucleotides that are post-transcriptional regulators of gene expression predominantly via complementary base pairing with mRNA transcripts. Since that time, more than 40 EBV miRNAs have been identified and localized within the BART and BHRF1 clusters of the EBV genome. EBV miRNAs are expressed in the lytic and the latent cycle of infection and can modulate a number of processes relevant to oncogenesis and viral persistence. For example, EBV miRNA can regulate expression of EBV latent cycle genes, inhibit transition to the lytic phase, inhibit cellular apoptosis, inhibit tumor suppressor genes, and modulate the host innate and adaptive immune responses [39]. In addition to the expression of virally encoded miRNA, EBV infection can markedly alter the cellular miRNA profile and disrupt host cell homeostasis. The latent cycle gene LMP1, in particular, has been shown to alter the expression of numerous host cell miRNAs important in processes ranging from production of cytokines [40], activation of signal transduction pathways, to the immunogenicity of the infected cell. Finally, the viral and host cell miRNA can be transported as cargo in exosomes from the EBV-infected cell to other cells, thereby potentially modulating the tumor microenvironment.

EBV Genomic Diversity

There has been ongoing interest in understanding the extent of EBV genome diversity in health and disease with the possibility of identifying specific variants linked to pathogenesis. Targeted sequencing of the cytoplasmic domain of LMP1 identified gain-of-function mutations at amino acids 212 and 366 that were commonly present in EBV isolated from B cell lines derived from patients with EBV+ PTLD [41]. These mutations were shown to elicit sustained ERK MAPK activation and cFOS induction suggesting another potential pathway of signal transduction dysregulation that may contribute to oncogenesis. More broadly, early classification schemes based on genomic sequences of EBNA2, EBNA3s [42], and LMP1 [43] were established, but it has been difficult to demonstrate definitive links between viral subtypes and EBV-driven tumorigenesis.

The advent of next-generation sequencing approaches has rapidly expanded the number of whole genome sequences available for EBV including sequences from FFPE sections of PTLD lesions [44] as well as B cell lines established from PTLD patients [45, 46]. It is likely that additional PTLD-derived whole-genome EBV sequences will become available and, coupled with computational analysis, may reveal PTLD-associated variants of interest that can be exploited as biomarkers for increased risk of PTLD and potential targets of cellular immunotherapy.

Conclusion

EBV is a highly successful virus that has developed effective strategies to persist in memory B cells of healthy individuals with minimal clinical consequences. However, disruption of the delicate balance between EBV and anti-viral immunity, as in transplant recipients, can result in the development of EBV⁺ B cell lymphomas. Host-viral interactions play an important role in the development of EBV-associated PTLD. Elucidating the underlying host-viral mechanisms in the pathogenesis of PTLD could identify new therapeutic opportunities for the treatment of EBV-associated PTLD.

References

1. Epstein MA, Achong BG, Barr YM. Virus particles in cultured lymphoblasts from Burkitt's lymphoma. Lancet. 1964;1:702–3.
2. Sathiyamoorthy K, Longnecker R, Jardetzky TS. The COMPLEXity in herpesvirus entry. Curr Opin Virol. 2017;24:97–104.
3. Zhang H, Wang H-B, Zhang A, Chen M-L, Fang Z-X, Dong X-D, Li S-B, Du Y, Xiong D, He J-Y, Li M-Z, Lui Y-M, Zhou A-J, Zhong Q, Zeng Y-X, Kieff E, Zhang Z, Gewurz BE, Zhao B, Zeng M-S. Ephrin receptor A2 is an epithelial cell receptor for Epstein–Barr virus entry. Nat Microbiol. 2018;3:1–8.
4. Swerdlow SH. T-cell and NK-cell posttransplantation lymphoproliferative disorders. Am J Clin Pathol. 2007;127:887–95.
5. Cohen JI. Epstein Barr virus infection. N Engl J Med. 2000;343:481–92.
6. Snow AL, Martinez OM. Epstein-Barr virus: evasive maneuvers in the development of PTLD. Am J Transplant. 2007;7:271–7.
7. Young LS, Rickinson AB. Epstein-Barr virus: 40 years on. Nat Rev Cancer. 2004;4:757–68.
8. Thorley-Lawson DA. Epstein-Barr virus: exploiting the immune system. Nat Rev Immunol. 2001;1:75–82.
9. Thorley-Lawson DA. EBV persistence-introducing the virus. Curr Top Microbiol Immunol. 2015;390:151–209.
10. Thorley-Lawson DA. EBV the prototypical human tumor virus--just how bad is it? J Allergy Clin Immunol. 2005;116:251–61; quiz 262.
11. Lambert SL, Martinez OM. Latent membrane protein 1 of EBV activates phosphatidylinositol 3-kinase to induce production of IL-10. J Immunol. 2007;179:8225–34.
12. Beatty PR, Krams SM, Martinez OM. Involvement of IL-10 in the autonomous growth of EBV-transformed B cell lines. J Immunol. 1997;158:4045–51.

13. Snow AL, Lambert SL, Natkunam Y, Esquivel CO, Krams SM, Martinez OM. EBV can protect latently infected B cell lymphomas from death receptor-induced apoptosis. J Immunol. 2006;177:3283–93.
14. Thornburg NJ, Kulwichit W, Edwards RH, Shair KH, Bendt KM, Raab-Traub N. LMP1 signaling and activation of NF-kappaB in LMP1 transgenic mice. Oncogene. 2006;25:288–97.
15. Zhang B, Kracker S, Yasuda T, Casola S, Vanneman M, Homig-Holzel C, Wang Z, Derudder E, Shuang L, Chakraborty T, Cotter SE, Koyama S, Currie T, Freeman GJ, Kutok JL, Rodig SJ, Dranoff G, Rajewsky K. Immune surveillance and therapy of lymphomas drive by Epstein-Barr-virus protein LMP1 in a mouse model. Cell. 2012;148:739–51.
16. Rovedo M, Longnecker R. Epstein-Barr virus latent membrane protein 2B (LMP2B) modulates LMP2A activity. J Virol. 2007;81:84–94.
17. Rechsteiner MP, Berger C, Zauner L, Sigrist JA, Weber M, Longnecker R, Bernasconi M, Nadal D. Latent membrane protein 2B regulates susceptibility to induction of lytic Epstein-Barr virus infection. J Virol. 2008;82:1739–47.
18. Ruf IK, Lackey KA, Warudkar S, Sample JT. Protection from interferon-induced apoptosis by Epstein-Barr virus small RNAs is not mediated by inhibition of PKR. J Virol. 2005;79:14562–9.
19. Samanta M, Iwakiri D, Takada K. Epstein-Barr virus-encoded small RNA induces IL-10 through RIG-I-mediated IRF-3 signaling. Oncogene. 2008;27:4150.
20. Yin H, Qu J, Peng Q, Gan R. Molecular mechanisms of EBV-driven cell cycle progression and oncogenesis. Med Microbiol Immunol. 2018;208:573. https://doi.org/10.1007/s00430-018-0570-1.
21. Herbert KM, Pimienta G. Consideration of Epstein-Barr virus-encoded noncoding RNAs EBER1 and EBER2 as a functional backup of viral oncoprotein latent membrane protein 1. MBio. 2016;7:e01926–15.
22. Babcock GJ, Decker LL, Freeman RB, Thorley-Lawson DA. Epstein-Barr virus-infected resting memory B cells, not proliferating lymphoblasts, accumulate in the peripheral blood of immunosuppressed patients. J Exp Med. 1999;190:567–76.
23. Capello D, Cerri M, Muti G, Berra E, Oreste P, Deambrogi C, Rossi D, Dotti G, Conconi A, Vigano M, Magrini U, Ippoliti G, Morra E, Gloghini A, Rambaldi A, Paulli M, Carbone A, Gaidano G. Molecular histogenesis of posttransplantation lymphoproliferative disorders. Blood. 2003;102:3775–85.
24. Polack A, Hortnagel K, Pajic A, Christoph B, Baier B, Falk M, Mautner J, Geltinger C, Bornkamm GW, Kempkes B. c-myc activation renders proliferation of Epstein-Barr virus (EBV)-transformed cells independent of EBV nuclear antigen 2 and latent membrane protein 1. Proc Natl Acad Sci U S A. 1996;93:10411–6.
25. Knowles DM, Cesarman E, Chadburn A, Frizzera G, Chen J, Rose EA, Michler RE. Correlative morphologic and molecular genetic analysis demonstrates three distinct categories of post-transplantation lymphoproliferative disorders. Blood. 1995;85:552–65.
26. Moscio J, Dierickx D, Toursseyn T. Molecular pathogenesis of B-cell posttransplant lymphoproliferative disorder: what do we know so far? Clin Dev Immunol. 2013;2013:1–13.
27. Tosato G, Tanner J, Jones KD, Revel M, Pike SE. Identification of interleukin-6 as an autocrine growth factor for Epstein-Barr virus-immortalized B cells. J Virol. 1990;64:3033–41.
28. Martinez OM, Villanueva JC, Lawrence-Miyasaki L, Quinn MB, Cox K, Krams SM. Viral and immunologic aspects of Epstein-Barr virus infection in pediatric liver transplant recipients. Transplantation. 1995;59:519–24.
29. Tosato G, Jones K, Breinig MK, McWilliams HP, McKnight JL. Interleukin-6 production in posttransplant lymphoproliferative disease. J Clin Invest. 1993;91:2806–14.
30. Caldwell RG, Wilson JB, Anderson SJ, Longnecker R. Epstein-Barr virus LMP2A drives B cell development and survival in the absence of normal B cell receptor signals. Immunity. 1998;9:405–11.
31. Anderson LJ, Longnecker R. EBV LMP2A provides a surrogate pre-B cell receptor signal through constitutive activation of the ERK/MAPK pathway. J Gen Virol. 2008;89:1563–8.

32. Kelly GL, Milner AE, Baldwin GS, Bell AI, Rickinson AB. Three restricted forms of Epstein-Barr virus latency counteracting apoptosis in c-myc-expressing Burkitt lymphoma cells. Proc Natl Acad Sci U S A. 2006;103:14935–40.
33. Lee JM, Lee KH, Weidner M, Osborne BA, Hayward SD. Epstein-Barr virus EBNA2 blocks Nur77- mediated apoptosis. Proc Natl Acad Sci U S A. 2002;99:11878–83.
34. Cohen JI. The biology of Epstein-Barr virus: lessons learned from the virus and the host. Curr Opin Immunol. 1999;11:365–70.
35. Kastelein RA, Hunter CA, Cua DJ. Discovery and biology of IL-23 and IL-27: related but functionally distinct regulators of inflammation. Annu Rev Immunol. 2007;25:221–42.
36. Fang W, Zhang J, HOng S, Zhan J, Chen N, Qin T, Tang Y, Zhang Y, Kang S, Zhou T, Wu X, Liang W, Hu Z, Ma Y, Zhao Y, Tian Y, Yang Y, Xue C, Yan Y, Hous X, Huang P, Huang Y, Zhao H, Zhang L. EBV-driven LMP1 and IFN-γ up-regulate PD-L1 in nasopharyngeal carcinoma: implications for oncotargeted therapy. Oncotarget. 2014;5:12189–202.
37. Bi XW, Wang H, Zhang WW, Wang JH, Liu WJ, Xia ZJ, Huang HQ, Jiang WQ, Zhang YJ, Wang L. PD-L1 is upregulated by EBV-driven LMP1 through NF-κB pathway and correlates with poor prognosis in natural killer/T cell lymphoma. J Hematol Oncol. 2016;9:109–20.
38. Finalet Ferreiro J, Morscio J, Dierickx D, Vandenberghe P, Gheysens O, Verhoef G, Zamani M, Tousseyn T, Wlodarska I. EBV-positive and EBV-negative posttransplant diffuse large B cell lymphomas have distinct genomic and transcriptomic features. Am J Transplant. 2016;16:4514–425.
39. Albanese M, Tagawa T, Buschle A, Hammerschmidt W. MicroRNAs of Epstein-Barr virus control innate and adaptive antiviral immunity. J Virol. 2017;91:e01667.
40. Harris-Arnold A, Arnold CP, Schaffert S, Hatton O, Krams SM, Esquivel CO. Epstein-Barr virus modulates host cell microRNA-194 to promote IL-10 production and B lymphoma survival. Am J Transplant. 2015;15:2814–24.
41. Vaysberg M, Lambert SL, Snow AL, Krams SM, Martinez OM. Tumor variants of Epstein-Barr virus latent membrane protein 1 induce sustained Erk and cFos. J Biol Chem. 2007;283:36573–83.
42. Sample J, Young L, Martin B, Chatman T, Kieff E, Rickinson A, Kieff E. Epstein-Barr virus types 1 and 2 differ in their EBNA-3A, EBNA- 3B, and EBNA-3C genes. J Virol. 1990;64(9):4084–92. http://www.ncbi.nlm.nih.gov/pubmed/2166806.
43. Edwards RH, Seillier-Moiseiwitsch F, Raab-Traub N. Signature amino acid changes in latent membrane protein 1 distinguish Epstein-Barr virus strains. Virology. 1999;261(1):79–95. https://doi.org/10.1006/viro.1999.9855.
44. Dharnidharka VR, Ruzinova MB, Chen CC, Parameswaran P, O'Gorman H, Goss CW, Gu H, Storch GA, Wylie K. Metagenomic analysis of DNA viruses form posttransplant lymphoproliferative disorders. Cancer Med. 2019;8:1013–23.
45. Palser AL, Grayson NE, White RE, Corton C, Correia S, Ba Abdullah MM, Watson SJ, Cotton M, Arrand JR, Murray PG, Allday MJ, Rickinson AB, Young LS, Farrell PJ, Kellam P. Genome diversity of Epstein-Barr virus from multiple tumor types and normal infection. J Virol. 2015;89:5222–37.
46. Maloney EM, Busque VA, Hui ST, Toh J, Fernandez-Vina, Krams S, Esquivel CO, Martinez ON. Genomic variations in EBNA3C of EBV associate with posttransplant lymphoproliferative disorder. JCI Insight. 2020;5:e131644.

Host Genetic Mutations and Expression Analyses in PTLD

4

Charlotte Lees and Maher K. Gandhi

Introduction

In 50–80% of cases, PTLD develop in association with the oncogenic virus EBV [1]. However, the purpose of this chapter is to examine the host genetic and epigenetic mutations of cellular genes in PTLD as well as gene expression profiling, as opposed to the role of EBV in the malignant process which will be covered in other chapters. The majority of EBV-positive and EBV-negative PTLD are of B cell origin, arising from a range of B cells that accumulate genetic mutations. The nature of the B cells is heterogenous. Some cases of PTLD originate from antigen-experienced B cells, with mutations in the variable regions of the immunoglobulin genes (IGV) indicating that they have undergone a germinal centre reaction [2]. Others, however, appear to originate from naïve B cells, as they do not demonstrate mutated immunoglobulin heavy chain (IgH) genes [3]. There is also evidence in PTLD of an atypical post-germinal B cell origin, with random and inactivating mutations of IgH genes [3].

EBV-negative PTLD appear to be clinically, morphologically and genetically distinct from EBV-positive PTLD. They classically present late (defined as >12 months post-transplant) and are more commonly of the monomorphic type, i.e.

C. Lees
Blood Cancer Research Group, Mater Research, University of Queensland, Translational Research Institute, Brisbane, QLD, Australia

Princess Alexandra Hospital Southside Clinical Unit, Faculty of Medicine, University of Queensland, Translational Research Institute, Brisbane, QLD, Australia

M. K. Gandhi (✉)
Blood Cancer Research Group, Mater Research, University of Queensland, Translational Research Institute, Brisbane, QLD, Australia

Department of Haematology, Princess Alexandra Hospital, Brisbane, QLD, Australia
e-mail: Maher.Gandhi@mater.uq.edu.au

representing lymphoma types seen in immunocompetent individuals [4]. There is no definitive evidence of an inferior prognosis to EBV-positive PTLD [4]. Immunohistochemically, EBV-negative PTLD demonstrate higher expression of BCL6 and lower expression of MUM1 compared to EBV-positive cases [5].

Genetic mutations seen in PTLD include defects in DNA mismatch repair mechanisms, aberrant somatic hypermutation and mutations of proto-oncogenes. Other frequently observed abnormalities include dysregulation of transcriptional control including aberrant hypermethylation and altered microRNA expression. The molecular features of different monomorphic PTLD histological subtypes are distinct from each other. However, the genetic aberrations observed in specific monomorphic PTLD subtypes overlap with their respective histological counterparts seen in immunocompetent patients (Table 4.1) [6–8].

Consistent with the known transforming capability of the virus, EBV-positive PTLD harbour some different genetic features to EBV-negative PTLD (Table 4.2). EBV-positive PTLD express viral latency genes such as EBV latent membrane protein (LMP) and EBV nuclear antigen (EBNA) genes which have well characterised oncogenic properties; these will be discussed in depth in other chapters. Further differences are demonstrated by analysis of copy number alterations (CNA) in posttransplant DLBCL; only one recurrent imbalance was found to be shared by EBV-positive and EBV-negative post-transplant DLBCL, gain of 12q21 [6]. In contrast, EBV-negative post-transplant DLBCL shared 11 recurrent CNA with immunocompetent-DLBCL including gain of 3/3q(*FOXP1*) and loss of 6q23(*TNFAIP3*) and 9p21(*CDKN2A*) [6]. *FOXP1*, the most significantly upregulated gene in EBV-negative post-transplant DLBCL and also commonly overexpressed in immunocompetent-DLBCL, encodes an oncogenic transcription factor that represses tumour suppressors such as S1PR2 [9]. Interestingly, *FOXP1* expression in EBV-positive post-transplant DLBCL appears to be low suggesting that it is not an important pathway in its pathogenesis. Loss of the tumour suppressor gene *TNFAIP3* leads to increased NF-κB signalling and subsequent evasion of apoptosis [10]. *CDKN2A* encodes the tumour suppressors p16 and p14, which both have a role in regulating the cell cycle.

The most common genetic aberration seen in EBV-positive post-transplant DLBCL was gain of 9p24.1 (24% cases), with transcriptomic data indicating *PDCD1LG2*(PD-L2) to be the target of this alteration [6]. PD-L2 (programmed death ligand 2) along with PD-L1 engages their receptor PD-1 to deliver coinhibitory signals that modulate effector T cell function. Interestingly the viral latency gene *LMP1* has been shown to upregulate PD-L1 expression, via the JAK-STAT and AP-1 pathways, although LMP1's effect on PD-L2 is not known [11]. As this data is only from one study, further large-scale cohorts profiled by modern high-throughput technologies are required to further clarify the genetic differences between EBV-positive and EBV-negative PTLD.

Table 4.1 The differential genetic features commonly seen in the PTLD subtypes [7]

PTLD type	Genetic features	
Monomorphic PTLD	The majority of cases display clonally rearranged immunoglobulin (Ig) genes, which cause malignant transformation by translocation of proto-oncogenes into the Ig loci. Most also display somatically mutated variable regions of the immunoglobulin genes (IGV), known as somatic hypermutation Proto-oncogene mutations are common, e.g. *BCL6* somatic hypermutation (but not *BCL6* translocation) and chromosomal translocations between *c-MYC* and Ig genes may occur Chromosomal abnormalities are frequent, with varying recurrent lesions reported Dysregulation of transcriptional control is seen, including aberrant promoter hypermethylation of genes such as the DNA repair gene *MGMT*	
	Post-transplant DLBCL	Mutations of proto-oncogenes as found in immunocompetent-DLBCL are often found. These may include *RAS, TP53* and *c-MYC* EBV-negative post-transplant DLBCL frequently displays loss of 6q23.3(TNFAIP3) and 9p21(CDKN2A) and gain of chromosome 3/3q(FOXP1)
	Post-transplant Burkitt lymphoma	Ig/*MYC* translocations are very common
	Post-transplant plasmablastic lymphoma	Ig/*MYC* translocations are common
	T cell PTLD	Clonal T cell receptor gene rearrangements are seen. Chromosomal abnormalities are akin to those found in immunocompetent T cell lymphomas
Polymorphic PTLD	Clonal rearrangement of Ig genes are present, but with less predominant clones than monomorphic PTLD. Somatic hypermutation of IGV is seen in around 75% cases Somatic hypermutation of *BCL6* occurs in around 50% of cases Chromosomal abnormalities are less common than in monomorphic PTLD	

PTLD are subclassified into those that fulfil definitions of immunocompetent lymphoma types (monomorphic PTLD) and those that do not (polymorphic PTLD). PTLD develop from a T or, more commonly, B cell that accumulates genetic mutations, often in an accelerated fashion due to defects in the DNA mismatch repair system, termed the 'mutator phenotype'. Specific genetic mutations that occur in the different subtypes include aberrant somatic hypermutations and mutations of proto-oncogenes such as MYC. There is also evidence of dysregulation of transcriptional control including aberrant hypermethylation and altered microRNA expression

Table 4.2 The distinct genetic and transcriptomic features of EBV-positive versus EBV-negative PTLD, which are in keeping with the known oncogenic properties of the virus

PTLD type	Genetic/transcriptomic features
EBV-positive PTLD	Oncogenic viral latency genes are expressed, e.g. EBV latent membrane protein (LMP) and EBV nuclear antigen (EBNA) genes EBV-positive post-transplant DLBCL upregulates genes associated with immune tolerance, e.g. *CD274(PD-L1)*, *VSIG4* and *IDO1* EBV-positive post-transplant DLBCL upregulates genes involved in the innate antiviral immune response including the interferon pathway, e.g. IFIT2–3, cytokines like CCL4, interleukin receptor IL-1RB and NK cell marker CD94

EBV-negative PTLD	EBV-negative post-transplant DLBCL frequently displays recurrent chromosomal abnormalities as found in immunocompetent-DLBCL including:
	    Loss of *6q23.3(TNFAIP3)* and *9p21(CDKN2A)*, tumour suppressor genes with roles in apoptosis and cell cycle regulation, respectively
	    Gain of chromosome *3/3q(FOXP1)* which encodes an oncogenic transcription factor that represses tumour suppressors such as S1PR2

EBV-positive PTLD upregulate genes involved in immune tolerance and the innate antiviral immune response. EBV-negative PTLD display recurrent chromosomal abnormalities as seen in their immunocompetent counterparts

The Mutator Phenotype

PTLD exhibit defects in DNA mismatch repair mechanisms which accelerate accumulation of mutations, termed the 'mutator phenotype', that are uncommonly seen in immunocompetent hosts. Genes with high mutational frequencies include those involved in apoptosis such as *BAX* and *CASPASE 5* as well as DNA repair gene *RAD50* [12]. In one study 8.1% of PTLD cases were microsatellite instability-high, regardless of EBV status [12]. Why this mutator phenotype is more common in immunodeficiency-related lymphoma compared to immunocompetent hosts is unclear. One theory involves neoantigens, tumour-specific peptide antigens produced as the product of gene mutation, which are displayed via MHC molecules on the cell surface of the mutator phenotype. In immunocompetent hosts, T cells would recognise and destroy these immunogenic cells. Post-transplant immunodeficient hosts however are unable to mount an effective immune response against these cells.

Gene Expression Profiling

The distinct genetic features of EBV-positive and EBV-negative PTLD already discussed are mirrored by differential gene expression profiles. It has been demonstrated that in a cohort of post-transplant DLBCL and immunocompetent-DLBCL, samples clustered by EBV status not immune status [13]. As expected, expression of viral genes distinguished EBV-positive from EBV-negative post-transplant DLBCL [13, 14]. In one study it was noted that very few genes were differentially expressed between EBV-negative post-transplant DLBCL and EBV-negative immunocompetent-DLBCL [13]. Genes upregulated in EBV-negative post-transplant DLBCL were related to B cell development. Genes involved in T cell signalling were however found to be downregulated in EBV-negative post-transplant DLBCL compared to immunocompetent-DLBCL, likely due to immunosuppression [13].

Despite immunosuppression, EBV-positive post-transplant DLBCL demonstrated increased expression of genes involved in the innate immune response, likely directed against EBV [13, 14]. These included proteins from the interferon pathway such as IFIT2–3, cytokines like CCL4, interleukin receptor IL-1RB and the NK cell marker CD94. EBV-positive post-transplant DLBCL also displayed upregulation of genes associated with immune tolerance, such as CD274(PD-L1), VSIG4 and IDO1 [13]. We have already described the action of PD-L1 to inhibit T cell activity and that it is upregulated by EBV [11]. The B7 family-related protein VSIG4 suppresses T cell proliferation as well as the production of IL-2 [15]. IDO1 (indoleamine 2,3-dioxygenase 1) also plays a critical role in immune tolerance by suppressing T cell proliferation and activating suppressive T regulatory cells [16]. It has been suggested that the additional immunosuppressive effect of EBV could account for the earlier development of EBV-positive PTLD.

Host Polymorphisms

It is known that host polymorphisms involving *IFN-gamma*, *IL-10* and *TGF-beta* predispose to PTLD. Many of these polymorphisms relate to the interaction of malignant cells with their surrounding environment, termed the tumour microenvironment. Cytokines such as IL-10 and IL-6 have been shown to be elevated in PTLD, irrespective of EBV status, and the levels correlate with disease progression [17]. Moreover, polymorphisms in *IL-10* and *TGF-beta* promoters have been linked to development of EBV-positive PTLD [18].

Variation in the highly polymorphic *HLA* loci has also been linked to PTLD development, with suggestions that *HLA* genes or others at that loci may predispose or protect from PTLD [19–22], although this is contentious. The theory is that HLA molecule specificity may affect the ability of T cells to detect EBV-infected or malignant cells; this may be exacerbated by immunosuppression. For example, in one study of 106 PTLD patients, EBV-negative patients with HLA-B40 were associated with a higher risk of PTLD [22]. Moreover, both donor and recipient HLA-A26 were linked with PTLD development in a study of 110 PTLD patients, whereas another variant seemed to have protective value attributed to a 'hyperactive immune system' [20]. However, not all studies have accounted for multiple hypothesis testing, which considerably confounds interpretation. A statistically rigorously conducted study of 97 patients found no evidence that HLA Class I molecules were associated with developing EBV-positive PTLD [23].

Aberrant Somatic Hypermutation

Somatic hypermutation (SHM) is a mechanism that enables diversification of the B cell receptor (BCR) so it can recognise novel antigens. It is a process of mutation involving the IGV genes that occurs in the germinal centre. Aberrant SHM is implicated in around half of DLBCL cases in immunocompetent patients, targeting various loci including proto-oncogenes *PIM1*, *PAX5*, *RhoH/TTF* and *c-MYC* and key regulators of B cell differentiation such as *MYC*, *BCL2*, *BCL6* and *CCND1* [24]. In PTLD, aberrant SHM has been demonstrated in donor as well as recipient B cells and in both EBV-positive and EBV-negative cases [25, 26]. Aberrant SHM is seen far more commonly in monomorphic PTLD compared to polymorphic PTLD; for example, it is seen in around 40% of post-transplant DLBCL [2, 25]. Up to half of PTLD originate from B cells lacking in a functional BCR as a consequence of aberrant SHM [27]. Usually a non-functional BCR would lead to apoptosis of the cell in the germinal centre transit; hence development of PTLD suggests evasion of this process as occurs with a transforming virus such as EBV [3].

Proto-oncogenes

c-MYC

Genetic alterations in *c-MYC* are best explained by the paradigm of Burkitt lymphoma (BL), although they have also been demonstrated in post-transplant DLBCL and post-transplant plasmablastic lymphoma. As in BL in the immunocompetent, post-transplant BL displays chromosomal breaks at 8q24, juxtaposing *c-MYC* with immunoglobulin (Ig) enhancer elements and causing *c-MYC* overexpression [7, 8]. The *c-MYC* proto-oncogene upregulates genes for cell growth and downregulates apoptotic genes, culminating in cell proliferation.

Unlike PTLD which occur in an immunosuppressed environment, BL in the immunocompetent should be detected and destroyed by cytotoxic T cells. There are many facets to the immune escape of BL, and it is thought that *c-MYC* plays an important role via differential expression of genes involved in the nuclear factor kappa beta (NF-κB) and interferon pathways [28]. It has been shown that STAT1, a vital component of the type I and II interferon responses, is inhibited both directly and indirectly by c-MYC [28]. Moreover, expression of microRNAs (see microRNA section) involved in c-MYC signalling is affected by EBV infection [29].

BCL6

BCL6 is a repressor of transcription and is key to the formation and survival of germinal centres. Translocation of the *BCL6* locus at 3q27 occurs in around 40% of DLBCL in the immunocompetent but is rarely seen in PTLD [30, 31]. Instead 40–50% PTLD demonstrate *BCL6* mutations in the same non-coding region of the gene; in one study 43% of polymorphic PTLD and 90% of non-Hodgkin lymphoma or myeloma-type PTLD demonstrated *BCL6* mutations and/or deletions, but none of the plasmacytic hyperplasia cases [32]. It is hypothesised that this non-coding region contains a regulatory element, although it is also not clear whether *BCL6* mutation is itself a trigger for malignancy or a general marker of genetic instability. As mutations were not seen in plasmacytic hyperplasia, *BCL6* has been proposed as a marker of malignancy versus hyperplasia and hence a predictor of response to reduction in immunosuppression. This conclusion is controversial, however, as 30% of normal germinal centre B cells have mutated *BCL6* [33].

TP53

Notably, the pan-cancer tumour suppressor gene *TP53* (also known as *p53*) is only occasionally mutated in PTLD, seen in 2 of 28 specimens in one study [34]. TP53 acts in a complex with p21, a cyclin kinase inhibitor, liberating Bax to stimulate apoptosis; this process is interrupted by *TP53* missense mutations [35].

Transcriptional Regulation

Mechanisms that regulate gene expression include epigenetic changes (i.e. that do not involve DNA alterations) such as methylation, acetylation and histone modifications. These particularly affect silencing of genes that are involved in regulating the cell cycle, apoptosis and angiogenesis that serve as tumour suppressors, which are integral to tumour development. Within the context of PTLD, the best studied epigenetic aberration is DNA methylation.

Aberrant DNA Methylation

Aberrant hypermethylation of CpG islands in tumour suppressor gene promoter regions can lead to their inactivation and has been implicated in post-transplant lymphomagenesis. In one study 57% of PTLD samples demonstrated aberrant hypermethylation of the DNA repair gene O^6-methylguanine-DNA methyltransferase (*MGMT*), 72% of the pro-apoptotic death-associated protein kinase (*DAP-K*) gene and 21% of the cell cycle control gene *p73* [36]. MGMT is a dealkylating enzyme that repairs DNA by removing methyl groups from the mutagenic O^6 position of guanine; *MGMT* inactivation promotes lymphomagenesis in knock-out mice [37]. Loss of *MGMT* is thought to promote genetic instability and development of further mutations such as in *p53* [38]. DAP-K is a serine/threonine kinase integral to gamma interferon-induced apoptosis. *DAP-K* is also upregulated following c-MYC activation, thought to be a safeguard against initial tumorigenesis by utilising p53 towards apoptosis [39]. The *p73* gene is in the same family of transcription factors as p53 and functions to suppress growth and induce apoptosis.

MicroRNA (miRNA)

A miRNA is a small non-coding RNA, around 22 nucleotides long, that binds in a sequence-specific manner typically but not exclusively to the 3'UTR of a target mRNA causing translational silencing and/or transcriptome degradation. MiRNAs regulate multiple processes including cell proliferation, differentiation and death. It is therefore unsurprising that miRNA expression profiles differ in malignant versus non-malignant tissues [40]. In malignancies associated with oncogenic viruses such as EBV, both viral and cellular miRNAs affect viral replication and the subsequent malignant process [41].

One study examined the microRNAomes of primary CNS (pCNS) PTLD (89% EBV positivity) as well as both EBV-positive and EBV-negative systemic PTLD [29]. Analysis of viral and cellular microRNA expression patterns revealed three major clusters associated with EBV status (Fig. 4.1): cluster I contained all the EBV-negative PTLD cases, and cluster II and III consisted of EBV-associated lymphomas. Regarding EBV-positive PTLD, the viral miRNA cluster BHRF1, comprising ebv-miR-BHRF1-1 to 3, was expressed in most cluster II (5/6) and cluster III (5/9) cases. Expression of the BHRF1 cluster is thought to potentiate viral persistence in the host via downregulation of viral antigen production and consequent evasion of the immune system. In one study cells infected by an EBV virus engineered to lack the BHRF1 cluster had markedly slower growth than those infected by EBV wild type [42]. All cluster III samples also expressed many of the BamHI-A rightward transcript (BART) miRNAs, a group of miRNAs which have also been shown to play a role in viral replication [43]. When comparing pCNS and systemic PTLD, it was found that pCNS PTLD expressed lower hsa-miR-199a-5p/3p and hsa-miR-143/145 than systemic PTLD. Decreased expression of hsa-miR-143 has been found in other B cell malignancies [44]. One of its gene targets is *ERK5* MAPK, with downstream effects on c-MYC that are thought to increase cell proliferation [44].

Conclusion

Much of the previous research on the genetics of PTLD has focussed on the role of EBV. Aside from the well-documented viral factors, there are multiple host genetic changes that occur to trigger lymphomagenesis. EBV-positive and EBV-negative PTLD display distinct genomic and transcriptomic landscapes, with the potential for disparate tailored treatments. EBV-negative PTLD share many genetic features with their respective immunocompetent lymphoma subtypes. These similarities suggest that EBV-negative PTLD is less likely to be driven by another unknown virus. Larger studies using high-throughput technologies are needed to clearly elucidate the biological differences between EBV-positive and EBV-negative PTLD to inform future therapeutic strategies.

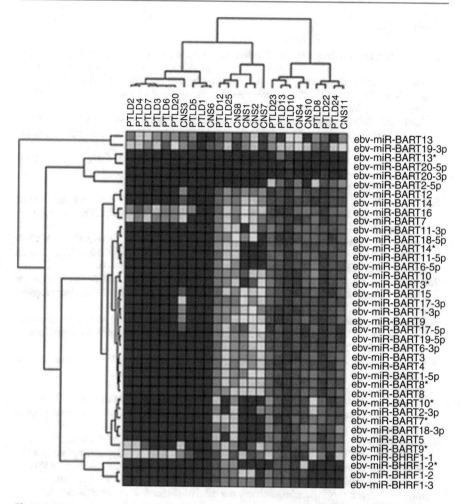

Fig. 4.1 Expression profile of EBV-specific microRNAs in primary central nervous system PTLD and systemic PTLD samples. Blue denotes minimal and red indicates high microRNA expression. Unsupervised nonhierarchical clustering defines three groupings or 'clusters' termed I–III from left to right within the studied PTLD samples. Cluster I includes EBV-negative PTLDs, cluster II consists of PTLD samples that display a globally weak expression of viral microRNAs, and cluster III includes those with a globally strong expression of these genetic elements. Some PTLD samples in groups II and III exhibit a restricted expression pattern of the transforming viral BHRF1 microRNA cluster. EBV Epstein–Barr virus, PTLD post-transplant lymphoproliferative disorder. (From Fink et al. [29]. Reproduced with kind permission from the American Journal of Transplantation)

References

1. Nourse J, Jones K, Gandhi M. Epstein-Barr virus-related post-transplant lymphoproliferative disorders: pathogenetic insights for targeted therapy. Am J Transplant. 2011;11(5):888–95.
2. Vakiani E, Basso K, Klein U, Mansukhani MM, Narayan G, Smith PM, et al. Genetic and phenotypic analysis of B-cell post-transplant lymphoproliferative disorders provides insights into disease biology. Hematol Oncol. 2008;26(4):199–211.
3. Timms JM, Bell A, Flavell JR, Murray PG, Rickinson AB, Traverse-Glehen A, et al. Target cells of Epstein-Barr-virus (EBV)-positive post-transplant lymphoproliferative disease: similarities to EBV-positive Hodgkin's lymphoma. Lancet. 2003;361(9353):217–23.
4. Luskin MR, Heil DS, Tan KS, Choi S, Stadtmauer EA, Schuster SJ, et al. The impact of EBV status on characteristics and outcomes of posttransplantation lymphoproliferative disorder. Am J Transplant. 2015;15(10):2665–73.
5. Johnson LR, Nalesnik MA, Swerdlow SH. Impact of Epstein-Barr virus in monomorphic B-cell posttransplant lymphoproliferative disorders: a histogenetic study. Am J Surg Pathol. 2006;30(12):1604–12.
6. Ferreiro JF, Morscio J, Dierickx D, Vandenberghe P, Gheysens O, Verhoef G, et al. EBV-positive and EBV-negative posttransplant diffuse large B cell lymphomas have distinct genomic and transcriptomic features. Am J Transplant. 2016;16(2):414–25.
7. Swerdlow S, Campo E, Harris N, Jaffe E, Pileri S, Stein H, et al. WHO classification of tumours of haematopoietic and lymphoid tissue. Revised 4th ed. Lyon: International Agency for Research on Cancer (IARC); 2017.
8. Djokic M, Le Beau MM, Swinnen LJ, Smith SM, Rubin CM, Anastasi J, et al. Post-transplant lymphoproliferative disorder subtypes correlate with different recurring chromosomal abnormalities. Genes Chromosomes Cancer. 2006;45(3):313–8.
9. Flori M, Schmid CA, Sumrall ET, Tzankov A, Law CW, Robinson MD, et al. The hematopoietic oncoprotein FOXP1 promotes tumor cell survival in diffuse large B-cell lymphoma by repressing S1PR2 signaling. Blood. 2016;127(11):1438–48.
10. Honma K, Tsuzuki S, Nakagawa M, Tagawa H, Nakamura S, Morishima Y, et al. TNFAIP3/A20 functions as a novel tumor suppressor gene in several subtypes of non-Hodgkin lymphomas. Blood. 2009;114(12):2467–75.
11. Green MR, Rodig S, Juszczynski P, Ouyang J, Sinha P, O'Donnell E, et al. Constitutive AP-1 activity and EBV infection induce PD-L1 in Hodgkin lymphomas and posttransplant lymphoproliferative disorders: implications for targeted therapy. Clin Cancer Res. 2012;18(6):1611–8.
12. Duval A, Raphael M, Brennetot C, Poirel H, Buhard O, Aubry A, et al. The mutator pathway is a feature of immunodeficiency-related lymphomas. Proc Natl Acad Sci U S A. 2004;101(14):5002–7.
13. Morscio J, Dierickx D, Ferreiro JF, Herreman A, Van Loo P, Bittoun E, et al. Gene expression profiling reveals clear differences between EBV-positive and EBV-negative posttransplant lymphoproliferative disorders. Am J Transplant. 2013;13(5):1305–16.
14. Craig FE, Johnson LR, Harvey SA, Nalesnik MA, Luo JH, Bhattacharya SD, et al. Gene expression profiling of Epstein-Barr virus-positive and -negative monomorphic B-cell post-transplant lymphoproliferative disorders. Diagn Mol Pathol. 2007;16(3):158–68.
15. Vogt L, Schmitz N, Kurrer MO, Bauer M, Hinton HI, Behnke S, et al. VSIG4, a B7 family-related protein, is a negative regulator of T cell activation. J Clin Invest. 2006;116(10):2817–26.
16. Munn DH. Blocking IDO activity to enhance anti-tumor immunity. Front Biosci (Elite Ed). 2012;4:734–45.
17. Hinrichs C, Wendland S, Zimmermann H, Eurich D, Neuhaus R, Schlattmann P, et al. IL-6 and IL-10 in post-transplant lymphoproliferative disorders development and maintenance: a longitudinal study of cytokine plasma levels and T-cell subsets in 38 patients undergoing treatment. Transpl Int. 2011;24(9):892–903.
18. Babel N, Vergopoulos A, Trappe RU, Oertel S, Hammer MH, Karaivanov S, et al. Evidence for genetic susceptibility towards development of posttransplant lymphoproliferative disorder in solid organ recipients. Transplantation. 2007;84(3):387–91.

19. Pourfarziani V, Einollahi B, Taheri S, Nemati E, Nafar M, Kalantar E. Associations of Human Leukocyte Antigen (HLA) haplotypes with risk of developing lymphoproliferative disorders after renal transplantation. Ann Transplant. 2007;12(4):16–22.

20. Reshef R, Luskin MR, Kamoun M, Vardhanabhuti S, Tomaszewski JE, Stadtmauer EA, et al. Association of HLA polymorphisms with post-transplant lymphoproliferative disorder in solid-organ transplant recipients. Am J Transplant. 2011;11(4):817–25.

21. Subklewe M, Marquis R, Choquet S, Leblond V, Garnier JL, Hetzer R, et al. Association of human leukocyte antigen haplotypes with posttransplant lymphoproliferative disease after solid organ transplantation. Transplantation. 2006;82(8):1093–100.

22. Lustberg ME, Pelletier RP, Porcu P, Martin SI, Quinion CD, Geyer SM, et al. Human leukocyte antigen type and posttransplant lymphoproliferative disorder. Transplantation. 2015;99(6):1220–5.

23. Jones K, Wockner L, Thornton A, Gottlieb D, Ritchie DS, Seymour JF, et al. HLA class I associations with EBV+ post-transplant lymphoproliferative disorder. Transpl Immunol. 2015;32(2):126–30.

24. Pasqualucci L, Neumeister P, Goossens T, Nanjangud G, Chaganti RS, Küppers R, et al. Hypermutation of multiple proto-oncogenes in B-cell diffuse large-cell lymphomas. Nature. 2001;412(6844):341–6.

25. Morscio J, Tousseyn T. Recent insights in the pathogenesis of post-transplantation lymphoproliferative disorders. World J Transplant. 2016;6(3):505–16.

26. Capello D, Rasi S, Oreste P, Veronese S, Cerri M, Ravelli E, et al. Molecular characterization of post-transplant lymphoproliferative disorders of donor origin occurring in liver transplant recipients. J Pathol. 2009;218(4):478–86.

27. Capello D, Cerri M, Muti G, Lucioni M, Oreste P, Gloghini A, et al. Analysis of immunoglobulin heavy and light chain variable genes in post-transplant lymphoproliferative disorders. Hematol Oncol. 2006;24(4):212–9.

28. Schlee M, Hölzel M, Bernard S, Mailhammer R, Schuhmacher M, Reschke J, et al. C-myc activation impairs the NF-kappaB and the interferon response: implications for the pathogenesis of Burkitt's lymphoma. Int J Cancer. 2007;120(7):1387–95.

29. Fink SE, Gandhi MK, Nourse JP, Keane C, Jones K, Crooks P, et al. A comprehensive analysis of the cellular and EBV-specific microRNAome in primary CNS PTLD identifies different patterns among EBV-associated tumors. Am J Transplant. 2014;14(11):2577–87, First published: 04 August 2014. https://doi.org/10.1111/ajt.12858.

30. Delecluse HJ, Rouault JP, Jeammot B, Kremmer E, Bastard C, Berger F. Bcl6/Laz3 rearrangements in post-transplant lymphoproliferative disorders. Br J Haematol. 1995;91(1):101–3.

31. Lo Coco F, Ye BH, Lista F, Corradini P, Offit K, Knowles DM, et al. Rearrangements of the BCL6 gene in diffuse large cell non-Hodgkin's lymphoma. Blood. 1994;83(7):1757–9.

32. Cesarman E, Chadburn A, Liu YF, Migliazza A, Dalla-Favera R, Knowles DM. BCL-6 gene mutations in posttransplantation lymphoproliferative disorders predict response to therapy and clinical outcome. Blood. 1998;92(7):2294–302.

33. Pasqualucci L, Migliazza A, Fracchiolla N, William C, Neri A, Baldini L, et al. BCL-6 mutations in normal germinal center B cells: evidence of somatic hypermutation acting outside Ig loci. Proc Natl Acad Sci U S A. 1998;95(20):11816–21.

34. Knowles DM, Cesarman E, Chadburn A, Frizzera G, Chen J, Rose EA, et al. Correlative morphologic and molecular genetic analysis demonstrates three distinct categories of posttransplantation lymphoproliferative disorders. Blood. 1995;85(2):552–65.

35. Kim EM, Jung CH, Kim J, Hwang SG, Park JK, Um HD. The p53/p21 complex regulates cancer cell invasion and apoptosis by targeting Bcl-2 family proteins. Cancer Res. 2017;77(11):3092–100.

36. Rossi D, Gaidano G, Gloghini A, Deambrogi C, Franceschetti S, Berra E, et al. Frequent aberrant promoter hypermethylation of O6-methylguanine-DNA methyltransferase and death-associated protein kinase genes in immunodeficiency-related lymphomas. Br J Haematol. 2003;123(3):475–8.

37. Sakumi K, Shiraishi A, Shimizu S, Tsuzuki T, Ishikawa T, Sekiguchi M. Methylnitrosourea-induced tumorigenesis in MGMT gene knockout mice. Cancer Res. 1997;57(12):2415–8.
38. Gerson SL. MGMT: its role in cancer aetiology and cancer therapeutics. Nat Rev Cancer. 2004;4(4):296–307.
39. Raveh T, Kimchi A. DAP kinase-a proapoptotic gene that functions as a tumor suppressor. Exp Cell Res. 2001;264(1):185–92.
40. Lu J, Getz G, Miska EA, Alvarez-Saavedra E, Lamb J, Peck D, et al. MicroRNA expression profiles classify human cancers. Nature. 2005;435(7043):834–8.
41. Gottwein E, Cullen BR. Viral and cellular microRNAs as determinants of viral pathogenesis and immunity. Cell Host Microbe. 2008;3(6):375–87.
42. Feederle R, Linnstaedt SD, Bannert H, Lips H, Bencun M, Cullen BR, et al. A viral microRNA cluster strongly potentiates the transforming properties of a human herpesvirus. PLoS Pathog. 2011;7(2):e1001294.
43. Barth S, Pfuhl T, Mamiani A, Ehses C, Roemer K, Kremmer E, et al. Epstein-Barr virus-encoded microRNA miR-BART2 down-regulates the viral DNA polymerase BALF5. Nucleic Acids Res. 2008;36(2):666–75.
44. Akao Y, Nakagawa Y, Kitade Y, Kinoshita T, Naoe T. Downregulation of microRNAs-143 and -145 in B-cell malignancies. Cancer Sci. 2007;98(12):1914–20.

Immune Responses to EBV in the Immunocompromised Host

Diana M. Metes

Immune Responses to EBV Infection in Immunocompetent Individuals

Innate Immunity

Most data on innate responses to EBV are derived from studies performed on blood samples from young adults with infectious mononucleosis (IM), a self-limiting EBV-triggered symptomatic disease, or from EBV seropositive healthy subjects during EBV established infection entailing virus latency and episodic viral reactivations. Innate immune cells, including monocytes/macrophages, plasmacytoid dendritic cells (pDC), and conventional (c)DC and NK cells, provide the first, non-specific line of defense against EBV infection [1, 2]. A memory-like function for innate effectors (e.g., NK cells and monocytes/macrophages), known as trained immunity, was described to occur upon secondary encounters with pathogens [3, 4]. This confers enhanced immunity to secondary infections and may be relevant to EBV infection as well. Innate cells through their germline-encoded pattern recognition receptors (PRRs), including Toll-like receptors (TLRs), sense pathogen-associated molecular patterns (PAMPs), and in response they trigger the induction of MyD88-dependent phosphorylation of MAPKs and activation of NF-kB and IRFs [5]. As a result, inflammatory cytokines, chemokines, and cytotoxic molecules are directly released and contribute to pathogen neutralization and lysis of pathogen-infected cells. Subsequently these inflammatory mediators promote and shape the generation of potent pathogen-specific CD8+ and CD4+ T cell adaptive immunity. EBV can be sensed mainly by TLR9 and TLR3 expressed by innate cells, although other TLRs were recently identified to play a role in EBV recognition.

D. M. Metes (✉)
University of Pittsburgh School of Medicine, Thomas E. Starzl Transplantation Institute, Pittsburgh, PA, USA
e-mail: metesdm@upmc.edu

© Springer Nature Switzerland AG 2021
V. R. Dharnidharka et al. (eds.), *Post-Transplant Lymphoproliferative Disorders*,
https://doi.org/10.1007/978-3-030-65403-0_5

TLR9 expressed by monocytes and plasmacytoid DC (pDC) senses EBV-derived unmethylated CpG dsDNA motifs and promote production of type-1 interferon (IFN)-α/β and transforming growth factor-β (TGF-β) as well as release of the danger signal molecule HMGB1 [6]. All these mediators contribute to the immediate host defensive inflammatory responses leading to inhibition of EBV reactivation and subsequent lytic replication, as well as priming and activating adaptive immunity. In addition, B cells, who are infected by EBV and thus may function as innate immune cells, can sense EBV and respond to TLR9 stimulation [7]. Conversely, the virus can down-modulate TLR9-triggered signaling in B cells and thus protects itself from innate control [8]. More recent data demonstrated that EBV can directly infect primary human monocytes and subsequently may specifically induce activation of the inflammasome and caspase-dependent IL-1β production [9].

TLR3 expressed by macrophages and conventional (c)DCs may recognize noncoding EBV small interfering RNA (siRNA) and EBERs. These RNA species may be released by EBV-infected cells as exosomes [10] and may be detected free in the sera of patients with active EBV diseases or in the EBV$^+$ tumor tissue [11]. These may trigger TLR3 expressed by macrophages and cDCs to upregulate their Ag cross-presentation capability and release type-1 interferons and inflammatory cytokines such as IL-12p70 and IL-6, leading to further activation of innate and adaptive immune cells [12]. In addition, myeloid antigen-presenting cells via EBV-TLR2 triggering may result in MCP-1 release that may further upregulate TLR2 expression on myeloid cells [13].

NK cell contribution to the innate immune control against EBV is quite significant during primary infection, whether symptomatic IM or asymptomatic infection [14, 15]. NK cells become activated directly following NK cell-TLR3 ligation by (i) small EBV RNA molecules; (ii) pro-inflammatory cytokines IL-12p70 and IL-18 secreted by myeloid innate cells; and (iii) IFN-γ secreted either by CD4$^+$ and CD8$^+$ T cells or by NK cell themselves. As a consequence, the CD56^{bright} NK cell subset produces elevated levels of cytokines (IFN-γ/TNF-α) that interfere with EBV infectivity, while CD56^{dim} subset upregulates activating cytotoxic molecules (NKp30, NKp46, NKG2D) and releases perforin and granzyme B that leads to increased lysis of EBV-infected cells. Moreover, tissue-resident (tonsillar) NK cells were shown to be more effective at controlling B cell transformation than blood NK cells, a process depending on IFN-γ release in response to IL-12p70 stimulation [16].

Altogether, the magnitude of the innate responses and the combination of effector mediators released at one time may directly correlate with the immunopathologic and clinical manifestations caused by active EBV infection [17, 18].

Adaptive Immunity

EBV-specific T cell responses in healthy individuals reflect EBV life cycle that entails expression of both latent and lytic viral proteins. Both provide good Ag sources for priming effectors of adaptive immunity that control primary EBV infection and for memory generation and maintenance to survey EBV latent state and its lytic replication during established infection. There are six EBV nuclear Ag (EBNA1, 2, 3A, 3B, 3C, LP) and three EBV membrane proteins (LMP1, 2A, 2B) expressed by infected B lymphocytes within lymphoid tissues (tonsils and lymph nodes). In addition, there are numerous EBV lytic Ag. The immediate early (IE) genes ($n = 2$) are critical for inducing the switch from latency to EBV production, whereas the early (E) ($n > 30$) and late (L) ($n > 30$) genes contribute to viral replication and may be expressed in both B cells and epithelial cells of the nasopharynx [19, 20]. The different locations and sources of EBV Ags impact the EBV Ag-specific CD4+ and CD8+ T cell responses in terms of their phenotypic profiles, function, and trafficking capabilities. More importantly, monitoring of EBV-specific CD4+ and CD8+ T cells in the peripheral circulation by flow cytometry using fluorochrome-tagged EBV Ag-loaded HLA tetramers in conjunction with fluorochrome-tagged mAbs allows for an accurate assessment of Ag-specific T cell phenotype, differentiation state, and function at any given time.

T Cell Responses During Primary EBV Infection

During infectious mononucleosis (IM), literature describes a significant expansion of EBV lytic-specific type-1 CD8+ T cells (IFN-γ/GzB/Perf), whose frequencies may represent up to 50% of the expanded CD8+ T cell repertoire in the peripheral circulation of patients [21, 22]. The immunodominance hierarchy of these Ag-specific CD8+ T cells consists of IE>E>L and most likely reflected EBV antigen availability and differential accessibility to the HLA class I processing pathway for CD8+ T cell priming [23]. EBV-latent-specific CD8+ T cell responses were also detected, but at significant lower levels, with individual epitope specificities directed mostly against immunodominant EBNA3A, 3B, and 3C epitopes and the subdominant LMP2A epitope and with frequencies representing approximately 5% of the peripheral CD8+ T cell population [23, 24]. EBNA1 CD8+ T cell responses may not be detected, since the glycine/alanine repeat domain within EBNA1 protects it from the MHC class I processing pathway [25]. In addition, circulating EBV-specific CD8+ T cells during IM are phenotypically activated (CD38+, CD69+, HLA-DR+), proliferating (Ki67+), in an effector memory (CD45RO+CD62L−) (EM) phase. They also express CXCR3+ and were highly functionally (IFN-γ+) active [21, 26, 27]. Moreover, the CD8+ T cell responses to some of the immunodominant epitopes involve highly conserved T cell receptor (TCR) usage, with possible consequences for cross-reactive recognition of other target antigen structures.

Upon IM resolution, EBV-specific CD8+ T cell frequencies decline, and their phenotype and function display resting profiles [28]. Interestingly, EBV-latent- but not EBV-lytic-specific CD8+ T cells gain CD45RO+CD62L+ expression, indicative of central memory (CM) phenotypes. These may be recruited to the B cell follicles of the tonsils, to control local EBV latent B cell transformation. EBV-lytic-specific CD8+ T cells remain in the EM phase or re-express CD45RA and are poorly represented in the tonsils, consistent with the continued high-level shedding of virus in saliva [28].

EBV-specific CD4+ T cell responses during IM are minimal compared to CD8+ T cell responses, are dominated by latent-specific responses over lytic-specific responses, and present also activated phenotypes [29]. During IM resolution, the % of EBV-specific CD4+ T cell responses diminish as well. Interestingly, EBNA1-specific CD4+ T cell responses could be detected in peripheral circulation at later times. EBNA1-specific CD4+ T cells are fully functional and can recognize and lyse EBNA1+ lymphoma cells in vitro [30]. This is important since EBNA1-specific CD8+ T cell responses are minimal due to poor accessibility of EBNA1 to be processed and presented via MHC class I pathway.

There are few studies that monitored healthy children or young adults undergoing asymptomatic primary EBV infection. These individuals presented with elevated activated EBV-specific CD8+ and CD4+ T cells, similar to those from IM cases, but at much lower level of expansion and activation as those from IM patients [31].

Memory T Cell Responses During Established Infection

EBV-specific CD8+ T cell memory responses could be easily detected in peripheral circulation of EBV-positive individuals and are directed against same lytic Ag and latent Ag specificities as seen in IM patients, but here EBV-lytic-specific CD8+ T cells do not exceed on average more than 2% of the total CD8+ T cells. The levels of latent Ag-specific CD8+ T cells are even smaller, up to 1% of the total CD8+ T cells [32]. EBV-latent-specific responses are directed primarily to EBNA3A/C and LMP2a, and the epitope choices for each Ag are HLA allele specific. In most healthy individuals, over time, EBV appears to establish a stable balance with the host's immune response, although occasional fluctuations in the size and function of the EBV-specific CD8+ T cell compartment are seen, possibly due to subclinical occasional EBV lytic and latent reactivation [33].

EBV Ag-specific memory CD4+ T cell phenotype and size differ significantly from those of EBV Ag-specific memory CD8+ T cell in the circulation of healthy EBV-positive individuals [34]. While the memory CD8+ T cell repertoire against EBV lytic and EBV latent Ags is broad and encompasses immunodominant and subdominant responses [23], the memory CD4+ T cell repertoire is more focused and dominated by EBNA1-specific responses [35], due to its accessibility to the MHC-II pathway within the infected cell itself via autophagy [36]. EBV-specific CD4+ T cell responses directed against other lytic and latent Ag specificities have been also reported and are minimally represented in circulation. Of note, in addition to their principal helper role (e.g., co-stimulatory molecules and cytokine production), EBV-specific memory CD4+ T cells still can recognize and kill infected B cells or established EBV+ tumors [30].

EBV Evasion from Innate and Adaptive Immunity

EBV exploits innate immune control through multiple mechanisms [37]. Several EBV gene products (e.g., BCRF1 or vIL-10, BNLF2, BGLF5, LMP1) may interfere with MHC class I peptide loading and presentation or may trigger down-modulation of TLR expression, resulting in downstream intracellular signaling inhibition of

NFkB and IRFs, with subsequent decreased transcription and expression of pro-inflammatory cytokines and chemokines and diminished cell proliferation [8, 38, 39]. The untranslated EBERs and siRNAs released from EBV-infected cells may also contribute to EBV immune evasion through multiple mechanisms by concomitantly conveying subtle inhibitory signals that are sensed by regulatory networks, allowing EBV to protect itself from host immunity [39, 40]. In addition, EBV may confer EBV-infected cell resistance to cell death signals by allowing the upregulation of several anti-apoptotic genes (including bcl-2, bfl-1, mcl-1, A20, and cIAP2) or by activation of the Ras/PI3K/Akt signaling axis in B cells [41, 42].

EBV evasion from adaptive immunity was also described and may interfere at several levels. It may reduce immunogenicity of antigen-presenting cells (APC) by hindering MHC class I and II loading with EBV peptides or by down-modulating MHC expression. It can also diminish the ability of APC to secrete anti-viral type-1 pro-inflammatory cytokines such as IL-12p70 while enhancing production of anti-inflammatory cytokines IL-10 and TGFβ and therefore rendering the microenvironment tolerogenic.

All these events allow EBV to establish latency or to undergo lytic reactivations and thus to survive, co-exist, and persist with the host rather than be eliminated by host immunity. In addition, these events may contribute to EBV-associated malignancies due to the failure of the immune system to eliminate EBV-transformed cells.

Immune Responses to EBV Infection in Immunocompromised Solid Organ Transplantation Recipients

While EBV infection in healthy individuals is dominated by its latent phase with protracted viral antigen exposure, and interrupted by occasional EBV reactivation, both well controlled by a functional type-1 innate and adaptive immunity, EBV infection after organ transplantation may become at times uncontrolled due to the iatrogenic immunosuppression burden on host immunity. In addition, EBV evasion mechanisms may become prevalent in individuals with impaired cellular immunity and can easily tip the balance toward favoring EBV-triggered B cell oncogenesis and development of post-transplant lymphoproliferative disorders (PTLD) [43].

The vast majority of patients undergoing transplantation are EBV positive, display memory responses to EBV, and are at low risk of PTLD. For those patients who EBV seroconvert post-transplant in the presence of high levels of immunosuppressive drugs, or for those with less mature immunity (e.g., mixed type 1/type 2), EBV can easily switch its latency phenotypes from the expected, benign latency 0/I (no Ag or EBNA1 expression) to the dangerous latency III (EBNA1–6, LMP1, LMP2a and LMP2b) or latency II (EBNA1, LMP1, and LMP2a) [44]. These latency phenotypes are indicative of the stages where B cell lymphoproliferation occurred, where EBV latent Ag-specific immune control failed, and whether the immunodominance hierarchy of these responses is perturbed or not [45]. Impaired immunity against EBV lytic Ags can also develop to allow EBV to undergo frequent productive reactivations, translated in part by increased immune evasion and accumulation of high

EBV loads in peripheral circulation. Together, these concur to the development of progressive immune functional exhaustion of innate and adaptive immune responses and to an increased risk for EBV[+] PTLD.

Specifically, EBV-negative pediatric patients receiving an EBV-positive transplant are at highest risk of developing chronic high EBV load (HVL) carrier status and PTLD [46, 47]. Indeed, clinically asymptomatic chronic HVL status in pediatric transplant carriers, specifically heart recipients, was proven not to be a benign state, but a strong predictor for PTLD [48]. Understanding the defects in innate and adaptive immune control against EBV after transplantation and identifying the concomitant occurrence of immune regulatory and exhausted networks paralleled by EBV immune evasion mechanisms are important elements in predicting the risk of EBV-associated PTLD and in determining how to harness immunity for therapy of this complication [49].

Perturbations of Innate Immunity

A longitudinal study conducted on peripheral blood mononuclear cell (PBMC) samples from 45 adult kidney recipients during the first 24 months post-transplant showed impaired inflammatory cytokine secretion by CD14[+]CD16[+] monocytes in response to EBV peptide stimulation and retrospectively identified patients at increased risk of infectious complications [50]. In another longitudinal study, significant elevated levels of IL-10 and IL-6 were detected in plasma of 38 adult transplant recipients undergoing treatment for PTLD. Interestingly, IL-6 levels, but not IL-10, correlated with disease progression, highlighting the role of IL-6 as a B cell growth factor to enhance B cell proliferation, a phenomenon seen with PTLD [51, 52]. In a model of lymphoproliferative disease using humanized NOD-SCID mice, Lim et al. showed that EBV-stimulated pDCs produced IFN-α that promoted activation of NK cells and of IFN-γ producing CD3[+]T cells, a phenomenon dependent on cell-to-cell contact, in part mediated by TLR-9 signaling. When pDC function was preserved, mice EBV-related mortality was delayed, whereas when pDC were impaired, EBV-driven mortality was significantly increased, highlighting the importance of pro-inflammatory IFN-α for PTLD control [53]. All these suggest that perturbations in the pro-inflammatory/anti-inflammatory milieu may be permissive for impaired EBV antigen presentation and T cell immune control, leading to increased risk for complications.

The importance of NK cells in EBV control after organ transplantation was emphasized by several groups. A cohort of pediatric liver transplant recipients displayed a significant decrease in the percentage of circulating NK cells immediately post-transplant, while the expression of NK natural cytotoxicity triggering receptor NKp30 was significantly increased. NKp46 and NKG2D levels remained stable through follow-up [54]. In a cohort of six pediatric heart transplant recipients with PTLD, our group has identified decreased circulating CD56[bright] and CD56[dim]CD16[+] NK cell subset levels that downregulated NKp46 and NKG2D and significantly upregulated inhibitory molecule PD-1. These phenotypic changes were paralleled by NK functional impairment, resembling cellular exhaustion. Interfering with PD-1/PD-L1 pathway resulted in increased NK cytotoxic function [55]. A decrease in NK cell number accompanied by a reversed CD4:CD8 ratio with increased CD8$^+$ T cells was shown to predispose to recalcitrant EBV-PTLD in 14 pediatric PTLD cases [56].

Defects in T Cell Immune Responses

To assess the functional polarization and potency of EBV-specific memory T cells after transplantation, our group has investigated a cohort of adult kidney transplant recipients. We reported that patients exhibited similar circulating EBV-specific CD8$^+$ T cell frequencies and EBV-epitope specificities as compared to those of healthy controls. In contrast, they displayed significantly elevated EM phenotypes, decreased IFN-γ production, and elevated IL-10 in response to EBV peptide stimulation in vitro. These cells suppressed noncognate CD4$^+$ T cell proliferation via cell-cell contact, suggesting their induced Tr1 polarization. These changes were induced at least in part by chronic immunosuppression that altered cDC phenotype and function, in a NFkB-dependent manner [57–59]. Moreover, our results suggested that even in EBV-positive, stable immunosuppressed transplant patients, regulatory pathways in the myeloid compartment are elevated and trigger alternative activation (re-programing) of EBV-specific CD8+ T cells with potential clinical consequences for certain patients that carry genetic or epigenetic alterations.

T Cell Responses During Primary EBV Infection After Transplantation

Given that EBV-negative patients receiving an EBV-positive organ are at higher risk of EBV complications post-transplantation, the issue of EBV seroconversion after solid organ transplantation was investigated by several groups. Longitudinal monitoring of EBV-specific T cell response in an adult EBV seronegative recipient following cardiac transplantation determined that effective EBV-specific immune response can be initiated quickly after primary EBV infection post-transplantation [60]. EBV-specific CD8$^+$ T cell frequency and IFN-γ production increased upon each subsequent viral reactivation. Falco et al. have investigated circulating EBV-lytic- and EBV-latent-specific CD8$^+$ T cells in a cohort of EBV-negative pediatric liver transplant recipients after EBV seroconversion [61]. These immune cells were easily detected in a few weeks post-EBV seroconversion and displayed activated/EM phenotype. These studies support that an EBV-specific T cell response capable of adequate control of a primary EBV infection and of subsequent viral reactivations can develop in EBV-seronegative adult and pediatric transplant recipients in the presence of severe immunosuppression. However, IL-10 production by CD8$^+$ T cells was not measured in these studies.

Memory T Cell Responses and EBV Load After Transplantation

EBV pediatric patients that develop chronic high EBV load in peripheral circulation have a 45% risk for PTLD [48]. To address this clinical observation, our group has focused on analyzing EBV CD8+ T cell immunity in a cohort of EBV asymptomatic pediatric heart transplant recipients. As compared to the EBV asymptomatic adult kidney recipients, pediatric recipients displayed a subverted EBV-specific CD8+ T cell immunity from the Tr1 (IFN-γ/IL-10) seen in adult kidney recipients to a mixed "Type-0" (IFN-γ/IL-5/IL-10) polarization in pediatric heart transplant recipients [62]. Pediatric patients that carried an EBV load (either low viral load, LVL, or high viral load, HVL) displayed significant increased levels of EBV-lytic-specific CD8+ T cells over EBV-latent-specific CD8+ T cells, with activated phenotypes (CD38+ and EM). Moreover, EBV-specific CD8+ T cells from HVL patients concomitantly displayed exhausted phenotypes (PD-1+CD127−) and function (low IFN-γ), unlike LVL patients whose EBV-specific CD8+ T cells were functional (high IFN-γ) and lacked phenotypic features of exhaustion [62]. Moreover, approximately 1/3 of LVL patients displayed EBV-specific CD8+ T cells that co-expressed CXCR5, a chemokine receptor that may localize them in CXCL13-rich areas, and IL-7Rα that may confer a potential for self-renewal. These findings provide a potential mechanistic explanation for differences in outcomes between LVL and HVL carriers in this cohort [63] . Anti-viral CXCR5+CD8+ T cells, termed follicular cytotoxic T (T_{FC}) cells, were previously described during persistent viral infections [64]. They seem to co-localize with B cells in the B cell follicles and have a significant role in viral control; and therefore may represent valuable therapeutic targets to explore, specifically since B lymphocytes in the follicles are the reservoire of EBV. We have also evaluated global and EBV-specific CD4+ T cell immunity in this cohort and identified a selective CD4+ T cell immunosuppression in HVL patients [65]. While these heterogeneous states of EBV-specific T cells have been identified in different categories of EBV load transplant carriers, the complex molecular and cellular mechanisms contributing to such diverse outcomes after transplantation still need further elucidation.

Memory T Cell Responses During PTLD
T cell immune monitoring of patients undergoing PTLD is of great interest as it may provide mechanistic understanding of the immunopathogenesis of this heterogeneous entity. Hinrichs et al. studied lymphocyte subsets of 38 adult transplant recipients with PTLD. They identified HLA-DR+CD8+ T cells significantly elevated in PTLD cases that correlated with impaired cytotoxic T lymphocytes in PTLD [51]. Smets et al. reported that while the numbers of EBV-specific CD8+ T cells were maintained, CD4+ T cell levels were lower in a cohort of pediatric transplant recipients with PTLD. The overall capacity of T cells to secrete IFN-γ in response to EBV peptides was progressively lost and coincided with the significant increase in circulating EBV load. Therefore, the ratio between IFN-γ and EBV load may be used as a marker for PTLD risk [66]. In contrast, in a cohort of 16 patients with PTLD, there were no changes in the numbers of EBV-specific CD4+ and CD8+ T cells or levels of IFN-γ when compared to control groups. EBV-specific T cells tended to be lower in early PTLD compared with late PTLD cases, and CD4+ and CD8+ EBV-specific

T cells increased in most patients treated with rituximab [67]. Interestingly, in a separate study, peripheral blood lymphocytes from two PTLD patients stimulated with an EBV peptide mix resulted in decreased polyfunctional EBV-specific T cells, expressing TNF-α and CD107 release but no IFN-γ production [68]. While these results obtained on peripheral blood from patients with PTLD generated by different groups are somewhat contradictory, this is expectable, due to the (i) heterogeneity of PTLD (early vs late; monomorphic vs polymorphic, etc.), (ii) timing of the samples (at diagnosis; before or after treatment), and (iii) differences in technical approaches.

Due to the possible contribution of PD-1/PD-L1 pathway to the failed EBV-specific T cell and NK cell immune control during PTLD [55, 62], this pathway may be considered a tempting target for PTLD treatment. However, this therapeutic approach for transplant patients with PTLD may represent a double-edged sword. On the one hand, exhausted EBV-specific T cells may be unleashed functional against the EBV$^+$ PTLD; on the other hand, allo-reactive T cells may become revigorated as well and may inflict graft injury and graft loss. Therefore, personalized immune monitoring to assess the presence of EBV-specific vs allo-specific CD8$^+$ T cells with phenotypes of Tbet^{hi}PD-1^{int} exhausted progeny (rescuable by checkpoint inhibitor blockade) and Eomes^{hi}PD-1^{hi} terminally exhausted progenitors (non-responsive to checkpoint inhibitor blockade) may identify significantly variability between patients and may indicate those patients likely to benefit from this treatment [69]. In addition, the same PD-1/PD-L1 checkpoint inhibitor blockade may also target EBV-specific CXCR5$^+$CD8$^+$ T$_{FC}$ cells when present. These may respond with a proliferative burst of functional cells and replenish the exhausted EBV-specific CXCR5$^-$CD8$^+$ T cells. Alternatively, EBV-specific CXCR5$^-$CD8$^+$ T cells may be turned into EBV-specific CXCR5$^+$CD8$^+$ T$_{FC}$ cells-like by (i) culturing them in a T$_{FC}$-inducing cytokine milieu; (ii) using vectors to generate CXCR5$^+$ CAR T cells; or (iii) expressing T$_{FC}$-promoting transcription factors [64]. In addition, monitoring for the recently described soluble PD-L1 decoy that hinders the success of PD-1/PD-L1 checkpoint inhibitor blockade therapeutic approach in some patients may also prove of value [70].

In conclusion, the dominant expression of regulatory cytokines (IL-10, IL-6) and of inhibitory molecules (PD-1) triggered by chronic immunosuppression and the multiple EBV evasion mechanisms encountered after transplantation and during PTLD [43, 71, 72] together contribute to the attenuation of anti-viral innate and adaptive immune control and allow for autocrine growth of EBV in its target cells. Unfortunately, till date there is no consensus on what marker or combination of markers may be of value to monitor in order to predict EBV complications/PTLD after transplantation. However, accumulation of improved technologies, of personalized monitoring and diagnosis, coupled with the prospect of novel immunotherapies that may target the complex and heterogeneous mechanistic interplay between EBV biology and human immune responses to EBV after organ transplantation, may soon allow for significant improved PTLD outcomes.

References

1. Chijioke O, Azzi T, Nadal D, Munz C. Innate immune responses against Epstein Barr virus infection. J Leukoc Biol. 2013;94(6):1185–90.
2. Lunemann A, Rowe M, Nadal D. Innate immune recognition of EBV. Curr Top Microbiol Immunol. 2015;391:265–87.
3. Netea MG. Training innate immunity: the changing concept of immunological memory in innate host defence. Eur J Clin Investig. 2013;43(8):881–4.
4. Sun JC, Lanier LL. Is there natural killer cell memory and can it be harnessed by vaccination? NK cell memory and immunization strategies against infectious diseases and cancer. Cold Spring Harb Perspect Biol. 2018;10(10):a029538.
5. Kawasaki T, Kawai T. Toll-like receptor signaling pathways. Front Immunol. 2014;5:461.
6. Fiola S, Gosselin D, Takada K, Gosselin J. TLR9 contributes to the recognition of EBV by primary monocytes and plasmacytoid dendritic cells. J Immunol. 2010;185(6):3620–31.
7. Zauner L, Melroe GT, Sigrist JA, Rechsteiner MP, Dorner M, Arnold M, et al. TLR9 triggering in Burkitt's lymphoma cell lines suppresses the EBV BZLF1 transcription via histone modification. Oncogene. 2010;29(32):4588–98.
8. van Gent M, Griffin BD, Berkhoff EG, van Leeuwen D, Boer IG, Buisson M, et al. EBV lytic-phase protein BGLF5 contributes to TLR9 downregulation during productive infection. J Immunol. 2011;186(3):1694–702.
9. Torii Y, Kawada JI, Murata T, Yoshiyama H, Kimura H, Ito Y. Epstein-Barr virus infection-induced inflammasome activation in human monocytes. PLoS One. 2017;12(4):e0175053.
10. Meckes DG Jr. Exosomal communication goes viral. J Virol. 2015;89(10):5200–3.
11. Iwakiri D, Zhou L, Samanta M, Matsumoto M, Ebihara T, Seya T, et al. Epstein-Barr virus (EBV)-encoded small RNA is released from EBV-infected cells and activates signaling from Toll-like receptor 3. J Exp Med. 2009;206(10):2091–9.
12. Iwakiri D. Epstein-Barr virus-encoded RNAs: key molecules in viral pathogenesis. Cancers (Basel). 2014;6(3):1615–30.
13. Gaudreault E, Fiola S, Olivier M, Gosselin J. Epstein-Barr virus induces MCP-1 secretion by human monocytes via TLR2. J Virol. 2007;81(15):8016–24.
14. Azzi T, Lunemann A, Murer A, Ueda S, Beziat V, Malmberg KJ, et al. Role for early-differentiated natural killer cells in infectious mononucleosis. Blood. 2014;124(16):2533–43.
15. Chijioke O, Muller A, Feederle R, Barros MH, Krieg C, Emmel V, et al. Human natural killer cells prevent infectious mononucleosis features by targeting lytic Epstein-Barr virus infection. Cell Rep. 2013;5(6):1489–98.
16. Freud AG, Yu J, Caligiuri MA. Human natural killer cell development in secondary lymphoid tissues. Semin Immunol. 2014;26(2):132–7.
17. Dunmire SK, Odumade OA, Porter JL, Reyes-Genere J, Schmeling DO, Bilgic H, et al. Primary EBV infection induces an expression profile distinct from other viruses but similar to hemophagocytic syndromes. PLoS One. 2014;9(1):e85422.
18. Balfour HH Jr, Verghese P. Primary Epstein-Barr virus infection: impact of age at acquisition, coinfection, and viral load. J Infect Dis. 2013;207(12):1787–9.
19. Hadinoto V, Shapiro M, Sun CC, Thorley-Lawson DA. The dynamics of EBV shedding implicate a central role for epithelial cells in amplifying viral output. PLoS Pathog. 2009;5(7):e1000496.
20. Thorley-Lawson DA. EBV the prototypical human tumor virus--just how bad is it? J Allergy Clin Immunol. 2005;116(2):251–61; quiz 62.
21. Callan MF, Tan L, Annels N, Ogg GS, Wilson JD, O'Callaghan CA, et al. Direct visualization of antigen-specific CD8+ T cells during the primary immune response to Epstein-Barr virus in vivo. J Exp Med. 1998;187(9):1395–402.
22. Hislop AD, Kuo M, Drake-Lee AB, Akbar AN, Bergler W, Hammerschmitt N, et al. Tonsillar homing of Epstein-Barr virus-specific CD8+ T cells and the virus-host balance. J Clin Invest. 2005;115(9):2546–55.

23. Rickinson AB, Moss DJ. Human cytotoxic T lymphocyte responses to Epstein-Barr virus infection. Annu Rev Immunol. 1997;15:405–31.
24. Catalina MD, Sullivan JL, Bak KR, Luzuriaga K. Differential evolution and stability of epitope-specific CD8(+) T cell responses in EBV infection. J Immunol. 2001;167(8):4450–7.
25. Tellam J, Connolly G, Green KJ, Miles JJ, Moss DJ, Burrows SR, et al. Endogenous presentation of CD8+ T cell epitopes from Epstein-Barr virus-encoded nuclear antigen 1. J Exp Med. 2004;199(10):1421–31.
26. Catalina MD, Sullivan JL, Brody RM, Luzuriaga K. Phenotypic and functional heterogeneity of EBV epitope-specific CD8+ T cells. J Immunol. 2002;168(8):4184–91.
27. Hislop AD, Annels NE, Gudgeon NH, Leese AM, Rickinson AB. Epitope-specific evolution of human CD8(+) T cell responses from primary to persistent phases of Epstein-Barr virus infection. J Exp Med. 2002;195(7):893–905.
28. Dunne PJ, Faint JM, Gudgeon NH, Fletcher JM, Plunkett FJ, Soares MV, et al. Epstein-Barr virus-specific CD8(+) T cells that re-express CD45RA are apoptosis-resistant memory cells that retain replicative potential. Blood. 2002;100(3):933–40.
29. Balfour HH Jr, Odumade OA, Schmeling DO, Mullan BD, Ed JA, Knight JA, et al. Behavioral, virologic, and immunologic factors associated with acquisition and severity of primary Epstein-Barr virus infection in university students. J Infect Dis. 2013;207(1):80–8.
30. Paludan C, Bickham K, Nikiforow S, Tsang ML, Goodman K, Hanekom WA, et al. Epstein-Barr nuclear antigen 1-specific CD4(+) Th1 cells kill Burkitt's lymphoma cells. J Immunol. 2002;169(3):1593–603.
31. Jayasooriya S, de Silva TI, Njie-jobe J, Sanyang C, Leese AM, Bell AI, et al. Early virological and immunological events in asymptomatic Epstein-Barr virus infection in African children. PLoS Pathog. 2015;11(3):e1004746.
32. Abbott RJ, Quinn LL, Leese AM, Scholes HM, Pachnio A, Rickinson AB. CD8+ T cell responses to lytic EBV infection: late antigen specificities as subdominant components of the total response. J Immunol. 2013;191(11):5398–409.
33. Crough T, Burrows JM, Fazou C, Walker S, Davenport MP, Khanna R. Contemporaneous fluctuations in T cell responses to persistent herpes virus infections. Eur J Immunol. 2005;35(1):139–49.
34. Long HM, Chagoury OL, Leese AM, Ryan GB, James E, Morton LT, et al. MHC II tetramers visualize human CD4+ T cell responses to Epstein-Barr virus infection and demonstrate atypical kinetics of the nuclear antigen EBNA1 response. J Exp Med. 2013;210(5):933–49.
35. Khanna R, Burrows SR, Steigerwald-Mullen PM, Thomson SA, Kurilla MG, Moss DJ. Isolation of cytotoxic T lymphocytes from healthy seropositive individuals specific for peptide epitopes from Epstein-Barr virus nuclear antigen 1: implications for viral persistence and tumor surveillance. Virology. 1995;214(2):633–7.
36. Paludan C, Schmid D, Landthaler M, Vockerodt M, Kube D, Tuschl T, et al. Endogenous MHC class II processing of a viral nuclear antigen after autophagy. Science. 2005;307(5709):593–6.
37. Ressing ME, van Gent M, Gram AM, Hooykaas MJG, Piersma SJ, Wiertz EJHJ. Immune evasion by Epstein-Barr virus. In: Münz C, editor. Epstein Barr virus volume 2: one herpes virus: many diseases. Cham: Springer International Publishing; 2015. p. 355–81.
38. Salek-Ardakani S, Arrand JR, Mackett M. Epstein-Barr virus encoded interleukin-10 inhibits HLA-class I, ICAM-1, and B7 expression on human monocytes: implications for immune evasion by EBV. Virology. 2002;304(2):342–51.
39. Horst D, Favaloro V, Vilardi F, van Leeuwen HC, Garstka MA, Hislop AD, et al. EBV protein BNLF2a exploits host tail-anchored protein integration machinery to inhibit TAP. J Immunol. 2011;186(6):3594–605.
40. Albanese M, Tagawa T, Bouvet M, Maliqi L, Lutter D, Hoser J, et al. Epstein-Barr virus microRNAs reduce immune surveillance by virus-specific CD8+ T cells. Proc Natl Acad Sci U S A. 2016;113(42):E6467–E75.
41. Young LS, Dawson CW, Eliopoulos AG. Epstein-Barr virus and apoptosis: viral mimicry of cellular pathways. Biochem Soc Trans. 1999;27(6):807–12.

42. Portis T, Longnecker R. Epstein-Barr virus (EBV) LMP2A mediates B-lymphocyte survival through constitutive activation of the Ras/PI3K/Akt pathway. Oncogene. 2004;23(53):8619–28.
43. Dharnidharka VR, Webster AC, Martinez OM, Preiksaitis JK, Leblond V, Choquet S. Posttransplant lymphoproliferative disorders. Nat Rev Dis Primers. 2016;2:15088.
44. Thorley-Lawson DA, Hawkins JB, Tracy SI, Shapiro M. The pathogenesis of Epstein-Barr virus persistent infection. Curr Opin Virol. 2013;3(3):227–32.
45. Martinez OM. Biomarkers for PTLD diagnosis and therapies. Pediatr Nephrol. 2020;35(7):1173–81.
46. L'Huillier AG, Dipchand AI, Ng VL, Hebert D, Avitzur Y, Solomon M, et al. Posttransplant lymphoproliferative disorder in pediatric patients: characteristics of disease in EBV-seropositive recipients. Transplantation. 2019;103:e369.
47. Francis A, Johnson DW, Teixeira-Pinto A, Craig JC, Wong G. Incidence and predictors of post-transplant lymphoproliferative disease after kidney transplantation during adulthood and childhood: a registry study. Nephrol Dial Transplant. 2018;33(5):881–9.
48. Bingler MA, Feingold B, Miller SA, Quivers E, Michaels MG, Green M, et al. Chronic high Epstein-Barr viral load state and risk for late-onset posttransplant lymphoproliferative disease/lymphoma in children. Am J Transplant. 2008;8(2):442–5.
49. Hislop AD, Taylor GS. T-cell responses to EBV. Curr Top Microbiol Immunol. 2015;391:325–53.
50. Vallin P, Desy O, Beland S, Bouchard-Boivin F, Houde I, De Serres SA. Impaired secretion of TNF-alpha by monocytes stimulated with EBV peptides associates with infectious complications after kidney transplantation. Transplantation. 2018;102(6):1005–13.
51. Hinrichs C, Wendland S, Zimmermann H, Eurich D, Neuhaus R, Schlattmann P, et al. IL-6 and IL-10 in post-transplant lymphoproliferative disorders development and maintenance: a longitudinal study of cytokine plasma levels and T-cell subsets in 38 patients undergoing treatment. Transpl Int. 2011;24(9):892–903.
52. Tosato G, Jones K, Breinig MK, McWilliams HP, McKnight JL. Interleukin-6 production in posttransplant lymphoproliferative disease. J Clin Invest. 1993;91(6):2806–14.
53. Lim WH, Kireta S, Russ GR, Coates PT. Human plasmacytoid dendritic cells regulate immune responses to Epstein-Barr virus (EBV) infection and delay EBV-related mortality in humanized NOD-SCID mice. Blood. 2007;109(3):1043–50.
54. Pham B, Piard-Ruster K, Silva R, Gallo A, Esquivel CO, Martinez OM, et al. Changes in natural killer cell subsets in pediatric liver transplant recipients. Pediatr Transplant. 2012;16(2):176–82.
55. Wiesmayr S, Webber SA, Macedo C, Popescu I, Smith L, Luce J, et al. Decreased NKp46 and NKG2D and elevated PD-1 are associated with altered NK-cell function in pediatric transplant patients with PTLD. Eur J Immunol. 2012;42(2):541–50.
56. LeVasseur R, Ganjoo J, Green M, Janosky J, Reyes J, Mazariegos G, et al. Lymphocyte subsets may discern treatment effects in children and young adults with post-transplant lymphoproliferative disorder. Pediatr Transplant. 2003;7(5):370–5.
57. Macedo C, Donnenberg A, Popescu I, Reyes J, Abu-Elmagd K, Shapiro R, et al. EBV-specific memory CD8+ T cell phenotype and function in stable solid organ transplant patients. Transpl Immunol. 2005;14(2):109–16.
58. Macedo C, Popescu I, Abu-Elmagd K, Reyes J, Shapiro R, Zeevi A, et al. Augmentation of type-1 polarizing ability of monocyte-derived dendritic cells from chronically immunosuppressed organ-transplant recipients. Transplantation. 2005;79(4):451–9.
59. Popescu I, Macedo C, Abu-Elmagd K, Shapiro R, Hua Y, Thomson AW, et al. EBV-specific CD8+ T cell reactivation in transplant patients results in expansion of CD8+ type-1 regulatory T cells. Am J Transplant. 2007;7(5):1215–23.
60. Pietersma FL, van Oosterom A, Ran L, Schuurman R, Meijer E, de Jonge N, et al. Adequate control of primary EBV infection and subsequent reactivations after cardiac transplantation in an EBV seronegative patient. Transpl Immunol. 2012;27(1):48–51.
61. Falco DA, Nepomuceno RR, Krams SM, Lee PP, Davis MM, Salvatierra O, et al. Identification of Epstein-Barr virus-specific CD8+ T lymphocytes in the circulation of pediatric transplant recipients. Transplantation. 2002;74(4):501–10.

62. Macedo C, Webber SA, Donnenberg AD, Popescu I, Hua Y, Green M, et al. EBV-specific CD8+ T cells from asymptomatic pediatric thoracic transplant patients carrying chronic high EBV loads display contrasting features: activated phenotype and exhausted function. J Immunol. 2011;186(10):5854–62.
63. Macedo CHK, Rowe D, Luce J, Webber S, Feingold B, Metes D. Identification of CXCR5+EBV-specific CD8+ T cells in peripheral blood of pediatric heart transplant recipients correlates with IL-21 production and EBV reactivation. Am J Transplant. 2015;15(3):D225.
64. Yu D, Ye L. A portrait of CXCR5(+) follicular cytotoxic CD8(+) T cells. Trends Immunol. 2018;39(12):965–79.
65. Macedo C, Zeevi A, Bentlejewski C, Popescu I, Green M, Rowe D, et al. The impact of EBV load on T-cell immunity in pediatric thoracic transplant recipients. Transplantation. 2009;88(1):123–8.
66. Smets F, Latinne D, Bazin H, Reding R, Otte JB, Buts JP, et al. Ratio between Epstein-Barr viral load and anti-Epstein-Barr virus specific T-cell response as a predictive marker of post-transplant lymphoproliferative disease. Transplantation. 2002;73(10):1603–10.
67. Wilsdorf N, Eiz-Vesper B, Henke-Gendo C, Diestelhorst J, Oschlies I, Hussein K, et al. EBV-specific T-cell immunity in pediatric solid organ graft recipients with posttransplantation lymphoproliferative disease. Transplantation. 2013;95(1):247–55.
68. Ning RJ, Xu XQ, Chan KH, Chiang AK. Long-term carriers generate Epstein-Barr virus (EBV)-specific CD4(+) and CD8(+) polyfunctional T-cell responses which show immuno-dominance hierarchies of EBV proteins. Immunology. 2011;134(2):161–71.
69. Paley MA, Kroy DC, Odorizzi PM, Johnnidis JB, Dolfi DV, Barnett BE, et al. Progenitor and terminal subsets of CD8+ T cells cooperate to contain chronic viral infection. Science. 2012;338(6111):1220–5.
70. Gong B, Kiyotani K, Sakata S, Nagano S, Kumehara S, Baba S, et al. Secreted PD-L1 variants mediate resistance to PD-L1 blockade therapy in non-small cell lung cancer. J Exp Med. 2019;216(4):982–1000.
71. Ohga S, Nomura A, Takada H, Tanaka T, Furuno K, Takahata Y, et al. Dominant expression of interleukin-10 and transforming growth factor-beta genes in activated T-cells of chronic active Epstein-Barr virus infection. J Med Virol. 2004;74(3):449–58.
72. Prockop SE, Vatsayan A. Epstein-Barr virus lymphoproliferative disease after solid organ transplantation. Cytotherapy. 2017;19(11):1270–83.

Technical Aspects of Epstein-Barr Viral Load Assays

6

Jutta K. Preiksaitis and Catherine Burton

Introduction

Quantitative measurement of Epstein-Barr virus (EBV) DNA in peripheral blood, most often using assays employing nucleic acid amplification technology, has significantly impacted the management of both solid organ (SOT) and hematopoietic stem cell (HSCT) recipients at high risk for or with post-transplant lymphoproliferative disorders (PTLDs). Since the introduction of these assays two and a half decades ago, our understanding of the biology of acute and persistent EBV infection and its pathophysiologic role in the development of EBV-positive (+) PTLD has increased significantly [1, 2]. In addition, technologic advancements have made EBV viral load (VL) assays more sensitive and precise, and the development of a World Health Organization (WHO) International Standard (IS) has impacted result harmonization among assays [3]. Peripheral blood EBV VL assays have been extensively used by transplant clinicians for surveillance of patients at high risk for PTLD as part of preemptive programs for PTLD prevention, for PTLD and EBV disease diagnosis in symptomatic patients, and to monitor response to PTLD therapy [4]. They have also been used for safety monitoring in clinical trials of new immunosuppressive agents [5] and for tailoring immunosuppression in individual patients [6, 7]. However, result interpretation and the optimal matrix for testing (plasma vs peripheral blood mononuclear cells (PBMC) vs whole blood (WB)) remain uncertain.

J. K. Preiksaitis (✉)
Division of Infectious Diseases, Department of Medicine, University of Alberta, Edmonton, AB, Canada
e-mail: jutta@ualberta.ca

C. Burton
Division of Infectious Diseases, Department of Pediatrics, University of Alberta, Edmonton, AB, Canada
e-mail: cburton@ualberta.ca

© Springer Nature Switzerland AG 2021
V. R. Dharnidharka et al. (eds.), *Post-Transplant Lymphoproliferative Disorders*,
https://doi.org/10.1007/978-3-030-65403-0_6

This chapter summarizes current knowledge regarding EBV cell tropism, EBV DNA dynamics, and the biologic forms of EBV DNA in the cellular and acellular fractions of peripheral blood during acute and persistent EBV infection and in EBV+ PTLD. We highlight how this information influences choice of testing matrix, EBV DNA assay design, and result interpretation when using quantitative EBV DNA assays in specific clinical settings. The current status of result harmonization among assays is reviewed along with the impact of standards and calibrators, nucleic acid extraction methods, target and probe design, and other factors. Testing of non-peripheral blood samples and possible future enhancements to EBV VL measurement are also discussed.

What Are We Measuring When Quantifying EBV DNA in Peripheral Blood? Biological Form and Cell Tropism

How Are Biological Forms of EBV DNA and Cell Tropism Assessed?

The phenotype of EBV-infected cells has most commonly been studied by sorting cell subsets based on surface markers using fluorescence-activated cell sorting (FACS) followed by detection of EBV DNA in each subset [8]. More recently, some investigators have used ImmunoFISH techniques with infected cells detected by either flow cytometry [9] or cell counting on slides by fluorescent microscopy [10]. EBV DNA in latently infected cells exists in an extrachromosal episome (~170 kb) with a nucleosome structure similar to that of the host genome [11]. In addition, integration of subgenomic fragments of EBV into specific sites of the cancer genome has been observed in a subset of malignant cells in some EBV-associated malignancies [11]. Lytically infected cells also contain concatemeric DNA molecules as well as monomeric EBV DNA encapsidated in virions. EBV DNA in virions is free of nucleosomes. EBV-infected cells may have long half-lives depending on their rate of generation, homeostatic cell division, and cell death as well as immune-mediated killing (see Section "EBV VL Kinetics: Implications for Monitoring Algorithms").

EBV DNA in plasma could exist as naked free DNA released by apoptosis or necrosis of EBV-infected cells, encapsidated in virions or in exosomes. Naked EBV DNA in plasma has a very short half-life of ~2 hours [12], making dynamic changes in its measurement more rapidly responsive to treatment interventions than changes in cellular EBV DNA. Two primary techniques have been used to determine whether EBV DNA in plasma is encapsidated virion DNA or is "naked" EBV DNA released from cells. The first exploits the property that virions, but not free DNA, will be protected from DNase digestion; the second examines the proportion of EBV DNA in pellets versus supernatant after pelleting virions by ultracentrifugation [13]. The distribution of EBV DNA fragment sizes in plasma has historically been estimated using quantitative polymerase chain reaction (PCR) using different sized amplicons [13].

Circulating cell-free DNA (ccf DNA) is present at low levels in all human plasma and is composed of mono-nucleosomal DNA fragments originating from apoptotic and necrotic normal hematopoietic cells; ccf DNA levels rise in inflammatory states. During apoptosis, DNA is fragmented by caspase-activated DNase resulting in fragment lengths that are multiples of nucleosomal intervals (166 bps) forming a characteristic ladder on sizing gels. DNA fragment length is impacted by cause of cell death (necrosis longer fragments than apoptosis [14]) and varies by cell source resulting in a "nucleosome footprint" pattern that allows identification of very small amounts of non-hematopoietic tumor cell DNA in the background of normal DNA in plasma [15, 16]. Recently, target-capture deep sequencing to both count and profile EBV DNA fragment lengths in plasma has been used to study their origin, exploiting the non-nucleosomal profile that would be observed in EBV DNA originating from virions/lytically infected cells versus the nucleosomal pattern of latently infected cells [17].

Biologic Form of EBV DNA and EBV-Infected Cell Type Varies with Host Immune Status and Clinical Context

The number and type of cells either lytically or latently EBV infected in peripheral blood and the presence and biologic form of EBV DNA in plasma (naked vs. encapsidated in virions) vary and depend on clinical context. Because data in transplant populations are limited, we also extrapolate and glean important information from studies in immunocompetent hosts and other immunocompromised populations such as HIV-infected subjects; these data are summarized below and in Table 6.1.

Table 6.1 What biologic forms of Epstein- Barr virus (EBV) DNA are we measuring in the whole blood of immunocompetent subjects and immunocompromised patients?

Clinical setting	EBV DNA in plasma	EBV-infected cells
Immunocompetent		
Asymptomatic seropositive subjects with remote infection	Very small fragments of naked ccf** EBV DNA (predominantly <110 bp) Not encapsidated in virions May originate from apoptotic lytically infected cells in tissues [17] *Rarely detected and when present only transient [17, 26]* *Increased detection during critical illness and sepsis [26]*	Predominantly:* resting memory B cell IgG genes hypermutated, class-switched (CD10+, CD20+, CD3−, CD23−, CD80−, Ki67−, CD27+ IgD− CD5−) [18–21]; 2–5 genomes/cell (episomal form) [20]; latency 0 [22, 23] Fewer: other memory B cells CD27+ IgD+ IgM+ or CD27− IgA+ [24, 25] *Individual-specific stable "set point" VL [66, 153, 198] (estimates: in US 5–3000/10⁷ B cells [1], in UK median 79/10⁶ PBMC infected)* [181]

(continued)

Table 6.1 (continued)

Clinical setting	EBV DNA in plasma	EBV-infected cells
Primary infection symptomatic subjects with infectious mononucleosis (IM) and asymptomatic subjects	ccf naked EBV DNA, not further characterized Presence of EBV DNA encapsidated in virions uncertain [30] *Almost always detected at symptom onset; duration 15–31 days* [29–33]	Predominantly: as above* [22] Fewer: other memory B cells CD27+ IgD+ [25] EBV-infected T cells in EBV-2-infected African infants [28]
EBV-HLH	Not available *Always detected (numbers studied small)* [32]	As in seropositive healthy adult plus EBV infection of activated CD8 T cell [39]
CAEBV	ccf naked EBV DNA, not further characterized Not encapsidated in virions [38] *Detected in 86% of patients* [37, 38]	As in seropositive healthy adult plus EBV infects a lymphoid progenitor cell with clonal evolution of a specific cell lineage or multiple lineages detectable in peripheral blood, predominantly T cell (CD4 or CD8) or NK cell in Japan [35, 38], B cell (CD20+ or CD20−) in North America [36]
EBV-associated malignancy	Very small fragments of naked EBV DNA, 87% fragments<181 bp, unique fragment length peak (150 bp in NPC) Not encapsidated in virions [13, 17, 41] *Tumor marker in this matrix*	Not available
HIV-infected patients		
Children with primary infection Adults with persistent high load/ set point	Not available *Infants: detected >3 months in most infants* [34] *Adults: variably detected with prevalence significantly lower than in WB* [51]	Children with primary EBV infection: B cells (not further phenotyped) plus small number of CD4 and CD8 T cells [52] Adults: B cells (not further phenotyped), EBV also detected in plasmablasts and plasma cells, monocyte cells not carrying B, T, or monocyte markers in some patients [10]
EBV+ lymphoma	ccf naked EBV DNA, not further characterized [30]	Not available
Transplant recipients		
SOT early <1 year post-transplant	ccf naked EBV DNA, not further characterized [30] *Pediatric primary infection: always detected, duration may be >1 year* [67, 75] *Adults seropositive pre-transplant: variably detected, prevalence proportional to quantitative levels in WB or PBMC* [60, 66, 68]	Adult population (presumably seropositive pre-Tx): as in seropositive healthy adult* [18] *Pediatric population experiencing primary EBV infection has not been studied during this phase*

Table 6.1 (continued)

Clinical setting	EBV DNA in plasma	EBV-infected cells
SOT >1 year post-transplant with persistent viral load/high set point	Not available *Rarely detected and when present only transiently; prevalence proportional to quantitative levels in WB or PBMC* [8, 42, 47, 75]	Pediatric with persistent low viral load: as in healthy seropositive adult (disproportionately IgM+) [42, 43] Pediatric with persistent high viral load: As in low load recipient plus up to 30% of infected cells highly atypical predominantly Ig null cells with 30–60 genome copies/cell (CD19+, CD5−, CD10−, CD27− CD23− CD38− and CD69− with variable expression of CD20 and CD40, often HLA class I and class II negative); may be transient and fall with decreasing viral load [43, 45] Predominantly CD20+ IgM+, IgD+CD27+ memory B cells, with~ 16.7 genome copies/cell [9] Some patients also have EBV-infected T cells and monocytes and EBV-infected cells lacking B, T, and monocyte markers [10, 47]
HSCT with early high-level reactivation	Not available *Variably detected, prevalence proportional to quantitative levels in WB or PBMC* [74]	Isotype-switched memory B cells (CD19+CD27+) of donor origin (median 19 genome copies/cell); significant proportion proliferating (Ki67+) rather than resting and express a plasmablastic (CD24− CD38^{hi}) phenotype and have latency III EBV gene expression [50]
EBV+ PTLD	ccf naked EBV DNA, not further characterized *Almost always positive (exception CNS PTLD and EBV+ mucocutaneous ulcer)* [48, 49, 68, 82]	Not available (patients not studied immediately before or at the time of PTLD diagnosis)

Abbreviations: *CAEBV* chronic active EBV infection, *ccf* circulating cell free, *HLH* hemophagocytic lymphohistiocytosis, *NPC* nasopharyngeal carcinoma

Immunocompetent Patients

Asymptomatic EBV Seropositive with Remote Infection When ultra-sensitive assays are used, EBV DNA can be found in the peripheral blood of all EBV-seropositive patients, predominately in long-lived resting B cells with the phenotypic hallmark of classical antigen-selected memory B cells (CD10+, CD20+, CD3−, CD23−, CD80−, Ki67−, CD27+ IgD− CD5−); Ig genes are hypermutated and class switched [18–21]. They are latently infected, express no EBV proteins (latency 0) [22, 23], and contain two to five genomes/cell [20]. Some investigators have also observed EBV DNA in a smaller number of CD27+, IgD+ IgM+, and CD27− IgA+ memory B cells, suggesting EBV can enter memory B cells without germinal center transit [24, 25]. The number of infected cells among individuals varies significantly from 5 to 3000 /10^7 memory B cells, but each individual appears to have a unique relatively stable "set point" with respect to infected cell number. It is estimated that only ~1% of the systemic EBV VL in an individual is in peripheral blood [1].

EBV DNA is highly cell associated in healthy adult patients almost all of whom are EBV seropositive and is only rarely detected in plasma (0.6–5.5%); when detected it is usually transiently present (<4 weeks) [17, 26]. EBV detection prevalence increases significantly relative to similarly aged immunocompetent subjects in the setting of critical illness with rates higher in WB vs plasma as follows (15/127 (11.8%) vs. 3/55 (5.4%)); even higher rates are observed in immunocompetent critically ill patients with sepsis (275/522 (52.7%) vs. 75/235 (31.9%) [26].

Children and Adults with Primary EBV Infection (Symptomatic or Asymptomatic) The limited available data comes from studies of adolescents and young adults presenting with symptoms of infectious mononucleosis (IM). As in EBV-seropositive patients with remote infection, EBV DNA is found in a latent form in memory B cells (CD27+ IgD−) exclusively [22] or predominantly, with some CD27+, IgD+ cells also infected [25]. However, in IM, up to 50% of all memory B cells can carry EBV DNA [22]. Whether infectious virions are being produced is uncertain; limiting dilution RT-PCR studies of IM peripheral blood demonstrated the presence of a very low frequency of cells expressing lytic cycle gene BZLF in only two of five IM patients [22, 23].

Non-B cells can be infected during primary EBV infection, even in immunocompetent hosts. A recent study of the tonsils of IM patients suggests that approximately 9% of EBV-infected cells in this tissue express T cell antigens [27]. In a Kenyan study of HIV-uninfected mother/infant pairs, Coleman et al. observed that young infants infected with EBV-2 had EBV DNA in T cells while those infected with EBV-1 did not. Interestingly, T cell EBV infection was not observed in the EBV-2-infected mothers [28].

Using real-time PCR assays, EBV DNA is detected in plasma in almost all symptomatic adult and pediatric patients with IM at lower levels and for a significantly shorter period (<30 days from symptom onset) than in PBMCs [29–33]. Using a DNase assay to study the plasma of 20 IM patients, Ryan et al. [34] found 60% had only naked EBV DNA present. The remainder had incomplete degradation of the control β-globulin DNA as well as EBV DNA making the interpretation of results as demonstrating the presence of virion-associated EBV DNA uncertain (see discussion of this confounder by Chan et al. [13]). These results have not been validated by others. While the plasma of asymptomatic adults with primary EBV infection has not been studied, Slyker et al. studied EBV infection in Kenyan infants and found that 55% of EBV-infected, HIV-uninfected infants and 83.6% of HIV-infected EBV-infected infants had EBV DNA detected in plasma; EBV DNA remained detectable in the plasma for >3 months in 62% of the HIV-infected infants but not in any of the HIV-uninfected infants [34].

Chronic Active EBV Infection (CAEBV)/Hemophagocytic Lymphohistiocytosis (HLH) This rare disorder appears to be a pre-malignant condition initiated by infection of a lymphoid progenitor cell from which malignant cells evolve by acquiring DDX3X and other driver mutations leading to monoclonal and less often oligoclonal evolution of EBV-infected T, NK, or B cells [35]. Patients exhibit persistent/recurrent IM-like symptoms as well as atypical symptoms and a high predilection for progression to lymphoma or leukemia; B cell depletion and hypogammaglobulinemia have been described in B cell CAEBV [36, 37]. EBV DNA in the form of naked EBV DNA, not encapsidated in virions, was detected in the plasma of 95/108 (86%) patients in a T/NK CAEBV cohort [37, 38]. In EBV-associated HLH, a hyper-inflammatory syndrome characterized by uncontrolled activation of T cells as well as macrophages, the EBV-infected cell appears to be an activated CD8 T cell [39]. EBV-associated HLH has been described in the transplant setting [40].

EBV-Associated Malignancies in Immunocompetent Patients EBV DNA detection in plasma appears to be preferred when compared to its detection in WB as a tumor marker. It has been evaluated as a screening tool for malignancy, as a prognostic marker, and to monitor response to therapy in settings such as NPC, diffuse large B cell lymphoma, extranodal T/NK lymphoma, and Hodgkin lymphoma [41]. In these settings, plasma EBV DNA appears to be naked DNA, not virion-associated, and fragments are very short (majority <180 bp) [13]. Recent studies using target capture sequencing and fragment length profiling of EBV DNA in plasma have demonstrated that NPC patients have a characteristic 150 bp peak unique to tumor cells and a nucleosome-bound fingerprint pattern suggesting latently infected cells as the source of plasma EBV DNA [17]. The size of the fragment length peak proposed as a tumor marker of NPC cells of epithelial origin cannot be extrapolated to PTLD which is of hematopoietic origin. However, this approach could be explored to determine whether EBV-associated smooth muscle tumors that occur after transplant also have a characteristic fragment length predominance.

Immunosuppressed Patients
Pediatric and adult SOT: Most studies examining the phenotype of infected cells in transplant recipients have studied patients with persistent VL elevation, usually later than 1 year after transplant, sometimes without reference to pre-transplant EBV serostatus (Table 6.1). While little is known about the type of cells infected in early primary EBV infection post-transplant, studies of adult kidney recipients and pediatric allograft recipients with persistent EBV VL, most of whom had experienced primary EBV infection with or without PTLD, suggest EBV is present primarily in resting memory B cells as in immunocompetent adults [18, 42, 43]. Schauer et al. [43] found that in pediatric SOT >1 year post-transplant with low persistent VLs, infected memory B cells contained one to two genomes/infected cells that were

disproportionately IgM+. In contrast, high EBV VL load carriers have a mixed population of EBV infected cells including the cell type found in low load carriers and EBV-infected cells containing 30–60 genome copies/cell which disproportionately contributed to total VL [43]. While the significance of this finding is not totally clear, the genome copy number/cell is known to reflect the number of replication cycles the EBV-infected cell has undergone [44]. These highly atypical cells were predominantly Ig-null. Surface immunoglobulin (sIg), when expressed, was disproportionately IgA+. These atypical cells appear transient, decreasing in number as VL falls in serially followed patients [45]. The observations related to these atypical high copy number cells have not been confirmed by others. As non-EBV-infected cells of this type are also found in pediatric transplant patients with undetectable VL, they are not solely the result of EBV infection [45]. Despite these observations, several investigators have found a reasonable correlation between total VL measured directly in peripheral blood of patients with persistent high loads and the number of EBV-infected cells detected by in situ hybridization [9, 10, 46]. An ImmunoFISH study of the peripheral blood of four pediatric Japanese liver transplant recipients with elevated VL found that the EBV-infected cells were predominantly CD20+ IgM+, IgD+CD27+ memory B cells, with an estimated 16.7 genome copies/cell [9]; this cell subset is usually only a minor infected population in the immunocompetent host [25].

Most investigators have found that in adult and pediatric SOT patients with elevated persistent VL, EBV infection is restricted to B cells. However, Greijer et al. [47] found EBV DNA in T cells and monocytes in two of six SOT recipients, and Calattini et al. [10] found EBV DNA in cells lacking B, T, and monocyte markers in two of three transplant recipients. The phenotype of EBV-infected cells in the blood of SOT patients at the time of or immediately prior to PTLD diagnosis has not been studied; whether they have circulating cells with any unique phenotypic features is unknown.

Most SOT transplant patients with chronic elevated EBV load studied late after transplant do not have detectable EBV DNA in plasma. When present, it is generally found in patients with higher VL in PMBC, is present in small amounts, and is transient [8, 42, 47]. EBV DNA is known to be present in the plasma of almost all cases of EBV+ PTLD in adult transplant patients, although it is not detected in EBV-negative PTLD and may miss EBV+ CNS disease and EBV+ mucocutaneous ulcers [48, 49]. Ryan et al. [30] studied the plasma of two transplant patients without PTLD and five with PTLD using a DNase 1 assay and found EBV DNA to be free DNA, not virion-associated in six, with uninterpretable results because of incomplete digestion of control DNA in one PTLD patient.

HSCT Recipients Burns et al. [50] recently studied the cellular tropism of EBV in HSCT recipients with high EBV load detected by WB monitoring within 3 months of transplant. They found that EBV resides almost exclusively in supranormal numbers of isotype-switched memory B cells (CD19+CD27+) of donor origin, prior to a time when memory B cell reconstitution is expected to occur, suggesting the appearance of these cells is EBV-driven. Moreover, the EBV infection is latent (median, 19 genome copies/cell), but a significant proportion of infected cells are proliferating rather than resting and express a plasmablastic (CD24– CD38^{hi}) phenotype and have latency III EBV gene expression.

HIV-Infected Patients   Adult EBV-infected HIV positive patients frequently have persistent high levels of EBV DNA detected in whole blood (65.5%) even on HAART therapy; detection in plasma is less frequent (4.8%) [51]. In addition to infected B cells, non-B cells of variable phenotype may be infected [10, 52] (Table 6.1). Using a DNase assay, Ryan et al. [30] found the EBV DNA in the plasma of 11 HIV-related lymphoma patients was free DNA, not encapsidated in virions in 10; in one results are uninterpretable because of failure to digest control DNA.

Conclusions Re: Biologic Form of EBV in Plasma and Phenotype of EBV-Infected Cells in WB
There is no clear evidence that the EBV DNA in plasma is encapsidated in virions at any time during acute or persistent infection or in EBV-associated malignancies in either immunocompetent or immunocompromised hosts. EBV DNA in plasma likely exists as fragmented free DNA, released predominantly from latently or lytically infected cells outside the circulation. Fragment length profiling of EBV DNA in plasma during different phases of infection and malignancy may be a useful tool to confirm this. EBV DNA appears in plasma only during a specific period during the course of primary EBV infection and only rarely after viral "set point" is reached in a stable patient. Whether the presence of EBV DNA in plasma could be used as a surrogate marker of immune control of EBV is unknown.

EBV DNA in the peripheral blood of transplant patients exists as complex mixtures of forms in the cellular and plasma fractions that may vary during stages of acute and persistent infection, inter-current illness, as well as evolving malignancy. There is evidence that EBV DNA may be found surprisingly often in atypical B cells as well as non-B cells in the peripheral blood, particularly in the immunocompromised host. In transplant patients with persistent viral elevated load detectable in WB, it may be important to differentiate patients who have only an altered viral set point from patients who carry clonally abnormal B, T, or NK EBV-infected cells in their circulation as is seen in CAEBV in the immunocompetent host.

Choosing Peripheral Blood Specimen Type and Reporting Units

Although there is general consensus that peripheral blood is the preferred sampling site for EBV VL assessments in transplant patients, the optimal sample type remains unresolved. Cellular specimen types including WB, leukocytes, PBMC, and isolated B cells (BC), as well as acellular fractions (plasma and serum), have been evaluated [47–49, 53–69]. In both SOT and HSCT recipients, high correlations have been observed between quantitative EBV DNA measurements in different cellular specimen types (WB, PBMC, isolated B cells) when using the same assay [56, 61, 70, 71]. Moreover, normalization of results in cellular sample types to cell number or genomic DNA using either total DNA or housekeeping genes did not significantly change this correlation or alter dynamic trending in serially followed patients compared to the simpler method of reporting the results/volume (ml) [53, 56, 61]. However, the presence of severe lymphocytosis or leukopenia should be reviewed in interpreting dynamic changes in results [53, 72]. Because of reduced processing steps and lower blood volumes required, WB has become the preferred cellular specimen with VL reported in IU/ml, without normalization. Approximate conversion factors among historical reporting units are summarized in Table 6.2.

Serum is sometimes used as an alternative to plasma [49, 58–60, 64]. Although these acellular sample types have not been directly compared for EBV DNA detection, levels of genomic cell-free DNA in serum are known to be significantly higher than in plasma because white blood cells lyse during clotting [73]. On a theoretical basis, to avoid plasma contamination from EBV DNA in circulating cells, particularly when cellular VL is high, plasma is preferred over serum as the non-cellular fraction of choice.

Although, generally, EBV DNA becomes detectable in plasma or serum as EBV VL rises in matched WB or PBMC samples and a linear correlation exists for results in the two matrices [47, 56, 64], the correlation coefficient between quantitative EBV VL measured in WB or lymphocytes versus plasma is relatively low [54, 56, 60, 63, 64, 74]. When detection is discordant, the pattern most commonly observed is EBV DNA detection in WB or PBMC, while plasma is negative, particularly when VL in cellular sample types is low. Quantitative differences between WB and plasma may be $>2 \log_{10}$ copies/ml; differences appear smaller in symptomatic than asymptomatic patients [75]. However, extreme quantitative discordance in both directions has been described, particularly in the HSCT setting [47]. The relatively poor quantitative correlation between WB and plasma is not unexpected. Most

Table 6.2 Approximate conversion factors for historical reporting units of EBV viral load relative to copies/ml of whole blood

Units	Assumption	Conversion factor
IU/ml	Assay calibrated to WHO IS for EBV DNA	Assay specific
Copies/10^5 PBMC[a]		1
Copies /10^6 PMBC		10
Copies/10^7 B cells	3–15% of PBMC, age dependent	667–3333
Copies/µg DNA	16–135 µg /whole blood, white cell count dependent, 2×10^6 PBMC/ml of whole blood	1.5–12.5
Copies/ml	Cell counts including B lymphocyte counts are stable over time, $1.5–2.0 \times 10^6$ PBMC /ml of whole blood	15–20

[a]*PBMC* peripheral blood mononuclear cells

studies comparing peripheral blood fractions were cross-sectional single-center studies of samples submitted to the laboratory and pooled for analyses. Transplant populations studied were in various stages of EBV infection and malignancy and included asymptomatic subjects experiencing primary infection or reactivation infection with or without inter-current illness as well as those diagnosed and being treated for PTLD; asymptomatic patients with persistent high VL are also often included. The biologic forms present and distribution of EBV DNA in the cellular component vs plasma differs over time in individual patients and in different clinical settings, likely explaining these observations. Available studies of longitudinally monitored patients comparing contemporaneous results in different sample types have limitations that make it difficult to determine the preferred sample type in specific clinical settings. These limitations include small patient numbers and few or no PTLD cases studied [56, 57, 60, 66, 74], monitoring of groups at very low risk of PTLD (seropositive adult SOT recipients) [60, 66], or sampling not starting at the time of transplant in patients in whom PTLD was documented [56].

Choice of Peripheral Blood Specimen Type in Transplant Recipients

The choice of specimen type may depend on the purpose for EBV DNA measurement; one size may not fit all settings. If the goal is to detect EBV infection/reactivation as early as possible in transplant populations at high risk for developing PTLD, with the goal of intervening to re-establish control of the infection assuming this will lower future PTLD risk, then the more sensitive WB sample may be preferred. EBV VL is most often significantly higher, usually by more than a $\log_{10}$ in cellular peripheral blood fractions than in acellular fractions [54, 55, 60, 64, 66, 74] and higher during primary infection than reactivation infection in both fractions after SOT [60, 76, 77]. Earlier temporal detection after transplant has been documented in WB compared to plasma in HSCT recipients [74] and seropositive lung transplant recipients [60]. In the small number of EBV-mismatched SOT for whom longitudinal contemporaneous monitoring in both specimen types was reported, EBV DNA was first detected in WB in only three of ten patients studied [57, 60, 67]. In a recent study of EBV-mismatched pediatric liver transplant recipients, all first detection of EBV DNAemia in WB was concordant with its detection in serum [75]. In HSCT recipients plasma monitoring alone has been used successfully in preemptive programs for PTLD prevention [78, 79]. Some investigators found results of testing in both WB and plasma/serum may be additive and increasing levels of EBV DNA in plasma/serum but not WB occur just before PTLD diagnosis; patient numbers however are small [56, 64]. Using an assay not calibrated to the WHO IS, Ruf et al. found 20,000 genome copies/ml of WB and 1000 genome copies in plasma had optimal sensitivity and specificity for PTLD prediction [56]. Using these values they found that the sensitivity, specificity, negative predictive value (NPV), and positive predictive value (PPV) were 100%, 87%, 19%, and 100% for WB; 88%,98%, 54%, and 100% for plasma; and 100%, 94%, 50%, and 100% when WB and plasma values were combined for predicting PTLD in pediatric SOT and HSCT patients; this is not true in adult SOT populations where >50% of PTLD after the first year is EBV negative [48, 80]. Although either specimen type could be used in preemptive PTLD prevention programs, monitoring both would be optimal although associated with increased cost and more complex laboratory logistics. If the goal of EBV DNA testing is early EBV+PTLD diagnosis, treatment monitoring, or prediction of relapse, plasma may be the preferred specimen type, although this requires further validation. This would be in keeping with role of EBV DNA detection in these settings as a tumor marker in a naked cell-free form with a very short half-life.

The advocacy for WB over plasma as the preferred sample type in the transplant setting dates back to early studies that failed to detect EBV DNA in the plasma of a significant number of PTLD cases, despite detection in WB samples cases [58, 59]. However, these studies were performed using less sensitive pre- real-time PCR technology with large amplicons and older nucleic acid extraction methods that may have failed to identify the small EBV DNA fragments in plasma [81]. Studies using RT-PCR found detectable plasma EBV DNA in almost all cases of EBV+PTLD with the exception of CNS PTLD and EBV+ mucocutaneous ulcer [48, 49, 68, 82]. EBV DNA detection in plasma is also a more specific marker of EBV disease, including PTLD than WB or PBMC detection, when used as a diagnostic test in patients with signs or symptoms of PTLD [48, 54, 56, 68] and also discriminates EBV+PTLD from EBV- negative PTLD better [48, 68].

In the HSCT population, Kalra et al. [83] reported that persistently detectable EBV DNAemia in WB after rituximab treatment of PTLD in HSCT recipients had a 71% PPV and a 100% NPV for progression/relapse, though most of the PTLD in that study was not biopsy-proven. Similarly, in a multicenter study of 144 cases of rituximab-treated PTLD in HSCT recipients, Styczynski et al. [84] observed that persistent or increasing EBV DNAemia, from WB or plasma samples (in equal frequency with results pooled for analyses), after 1–2 weeks of therapy was a predictor of poor response and increased mortality. However, in both SOT and HSCT populations, the bulk of data suggest that plasma may be preferred over samples with cellular fractions for monitoring response to therapy and predicting relapse as VL correlations with clinical response appear better [48, 56, 68, 85–87].

The high prevalence of EBV DNA detection after transplant, particularly in WB in low-risk asymptomatic adult patients who are seropositive pre-transplant, raises questions regarding the cost- benefit and risks associated with routine screening of this patient group using either WB or plasma [80, 88]. EBV DNA detection in WB appears to increase with time after transplant and to be a poor marker of future PTLD risk in this low-risk setting [76]. Elevated and often sustained elevation in EBV loads in WB has been observed in many of these patients although peak loads are usually lower than those observed in primary infection and many EBV+ PTLD cases. Investigators have detected EBV DNA in 67–72% of adult liver [89, 90], 31–29% of adult kidney [76, 91], and 13–42% (assay dependent) [48] of adult lung transplant recipients almost all of whom were EBV-seropositive pre-transplant. EBV DNA prevalence appears to be lower when plasma is monitored as illustrated by the 13% prevalence in a longitudinal study of adult liver transplant patients [62].

In a recent cross-sectional study of 808 transplant patients without either EBV disease or PTLD, Kanakry et al. [68] detected EBV DNA in 24% and 7% when testing PBMC and plasma, respectively. Data regarding the prevalence of EBV DNA detection in the peripheral blood of EBV-seropositive pediatric transplant recipients are more limited. In two cohort studies of pediatric kidney transplant patients, EBV DNA was detected in WB above a "significant level (3,000 copies/ml)" in 19.9% [92] and at any level in 44.4% [77]. Children with non-intestinal transplants seropositive pre-transplant are at lower risk of PTLD than those who are seronegative, although the difference may be less marked in pediatric populations than in their adult counterparts [92, 93].

Result Harmonization

Calibration Standards, Traceability, and Commutability

Currently, most clinical laboratories use real-time PCR amplification and detection methods (RT-PCR) for the measurement of EBV DNA in peripheral blood after nucleic acid extraction [94]. RT-PCR assays, used extensively in the last decade, are more precise and less prone to effects of inhibitors and have a broader linear range (6–7 orders of magnitude) compared to earlier generations of competitive endpoint PCR assays, factors that should be considered when reviewing older literature reporting EBV VL results [94].

Even when RT-PCR assays are used, there can be extreme variability in results reported when the same sample is tested using different assays. In 2009, Preiksaitis et al. [95] found the variation of reported results on individual positive samples ranged from a minimum of 2.3 $\log_{10}$ to a maximum of 4.1 $\log_{10}$ with only 47% of all results falling within ±0.5 $\log_{10}$ of the expected results when 28 international transplant center laboratories tested a panel of 12 EBV DNA samples. Inter-laboratory variation was significantly higher than intra-laboratory variation suggesting that the use of an International Standard (IS) for calibration might improve result harmonization. This variability was concordant with observations in the period prior to 2011 using laboratory developed test (LDT) and commercial assays in both the transplant and NPC settings and was observed regardless of peripheral blood matrix tested, plasma [96, 97], PBMC [98], and WB [99–102]. It is not clear how much result variability using RT-PCR assays is achievable or clinically acceptable, but variation of ±0.5 $\log_{10}$ is often used, extrapolated from data in HIV [103].

In October 2011 the WHO Expert Committee on Biological Standardization approved a lyophilized whole virus preparation of the EBV B95-8 strain produced by the National Institutes for Biological Standards and Control (UK) as the first WHO IS for EBV DNA to be used in all nucleic acid testing as a calibrator [3]. The preparation was assigned a potency value in international units (IU), a consensus value not precisely related to genome copies. IS-calibrated assays report results in IU/ml rather than copies or genome copies/ml; the conversion factor from copies to IU will be specific for each assay. In order to improve result agreement, an IS must be "commutable," a concept derived from clinical chemistry which is defined as "the equivalence of the mathematical relationships between the results of different measurement procedures for a reference material and for representative samples from health and diseased individuals" [104]. Commutability of a reference material is both assay and matrix specific [104–106], and when the IS is used and is non-commutable for the assays being tested, result agreement between assays can become worse [107]. The IS may be commutable for assays measuring EBV DNA in WB but not when the same assays are used in plasma [108]. Assays may demonstrate excellent result harmonization when proficiency panels created using whole virus preparations are tested but still show significant result variation when testing clinical samples, perhaps because the biologic form of EBV DNA in the tested samples is different [107, 108]. Therefore, to definitively determine the impact of WHO IS calibration on result harmonization among assays, clinical samples must be studied.

Laboratories have been slowly introducing EBV VL assays calibrated to the IS. When testing the 2013 College of American Pathologists (CAP) EBV DNA proficiency panel, only 9.4% of 319 laboratories reported results in IU [109], and in a survey of 71 transplant programs in 15 European countries in 2013, only 57.1% of virologists supporting these programs were aware of and had accessed information regarding the IS [110]. Most information regarding the impact of the WHO IS on result agreement comes from analysis of EBV DNA testing results of national or international proficiency panels that do not include clinical samples [109, 111, 112]. These studies all concluded that use of the IS for assay calibration significantly reduced result variability, with >80% results reported by multiple laboratories falling within $\pm 0.5 \log_{10}$ IU/ml, for WB and plasma samples [111, 112]. However, when four US laboratories participating in a clinical trial reported results for the WHO IS serially diluted in plasma, only 62% of values for dilutions above 4 log $_{10}$ were within $\pm 0.5 \log_{10}$ IU/ml of expected values [113]. Data using clinical samples tested using assays calibrated to the WHO IS are limited and provide variable results, with studies often demonstrating excellent result agreement when only two assays are compared and others showing significant variability between specific assay pairs when a larger number of assays were studied [107, 117–120]. Other potential sources of variation summarized in Table 6.3 likely contribute to ongoing suboptimal result harmonization. Based on impact validation available to date, use of WHO IS-calibrated EBV DNA assays may have improved result harmonization and should be widely adopted to eliminate this source of variability at a global level.

Assays typically use secondary or tertiary standards often from commercial sources, rather than the primary WHO IS material for calibration. Variable results with different magnitudes of bias compared to nominal assigned values have been observed when commercial secondary CMV standards were tested by different RT-PCR and digital PCR assays, highlighting that these secondary or tertiary standards must also not only be traceable to the WHO material but also be commutable. Similar issues may be at play for EBV, and until the impact of the WHO IS and

Table 6.3 Factors that may need to be addressed to reduce variability of quantitative results of EBV DNA measurement using real-time RT-PCR assays

Calibration
Use of secondary and tertiary calibrators traceable to the WHO IS for EBV DNA is recommended
Commutability should be demonstrated for each assay/standard system
Method for nucleic acid extraction
If plasma tested, cell –stabilizing collection tubes that prevent contamination of plasma with cellular DNA may be warranted to increase purity and yield
Methods that reduce further fragmentation of DNA during the extraction process
Methods that improve isolation of small fragments <100 bp that may be significant component of plasma cell free EBV DNA
Primer and probe design
Target conserved sequence regions
Use of small amplicons <100 bp is recommended to allow quantitation of small fragments of cell –free EBV DNA likely present in plasma
Use of two gene sequences as targets may be beneficial
Other
Use of specific reagents
Probe chemistry
Instrument and software
Automated versus manual pipetting
General
Automation and standardization of all steps in the measurement procedure
Use of commercial versus laboratory developed tests would reduce number of assays used. Reduction in overall number of assays available would make global result harmonization easier

traceable commutable secondary standards on result harmonization among a wider array of assays is validated using clinical samples, inter-institutional result comparison requires formal cross-referencing of measurement results obtained from testing of the same clinical samples between institutions. In the interim, patients should be monitored using the same sample type and the same assay in a single laboratory. The precision of RT-PCR assays should be considered when interpreting results, recognizing that poorest precision occurs at low VLs. Changes in values should differ by at least threefold ($0.5 \log_{10}$) and as much as fivefold ($0.7 \log_{10}$) near the assay's limit of detection to be considered biologically important changes [103, 114].

Digital PCR (dPCR) has been proposed as alternate and perhaps better reference technology for EBV VL measurement as it provides absolute quantification without need for a standard curve [114]. This technology is more precise when quantifying low copy numbers. Other advantages and disadvantages of dPCR relative to RT-PCR have been reviewed [114]. Although it removes the calibrator as a source of result variability, dPCR does require nucleic acid extraction and design of primers and probes which may contribute to variability.

Nucleic Acid Extraction

Nucleic acid extraction procedures are a known source of variation in VL measurement with impact depending on the number and type of extraction systems and PCR systems studied [70, 81, 100, 115, 116]. An understanding of EBV DNA fragment length profiles, in plasma and WB, is important to inform the choice of DNA extraction system. As we have no information regarding EBV DNA fragment length profiles in the plasma and WB of transplant patients, we extrapolate from studies of plasma EBV DNA in NPC population-based screening, where EBV DNA fragments appear to be very short, often <110 bp [13, 17]. Cook et al. [81] recently studied the extraction yields of 11 commercial extraction methods commonly used in viral diagnostic laboratories and 4 new methods designed to isolate the shorter fragments of ccf DNA. Not only were a wide range of extraction yields observed across methods, but yields were especially inconsistent and poorer (<20%) for 50–100 bp fragments, even with two of the ccf extraction methods. If similar very short EBV DNA fragments (<110 bp) are also seen in plasma in the transplant setting, the specific extraction system yield of these very short fragments could significantly impact quantitation and result variability among systems. The DNA fragments in the cellular compartment of WB are likely predominantly episomal in origin and may be significantly longer. WB extraction systems are therefore challenged to extract longer fragments from the cellular fraction along with very small fragments from the plasma compartment. How well they do this is uncertain.

Gene Targets

Since most testing will occur in the setting of transplant PTLD prevention, diagnosis, and monitoring and in NPC screening (in some geographic locations), if possible, a single clinical assay that could be used in both clinical settings should be our goal [117]. Because of the impact of target amplicon size on both the sensitivity of the assay and measurement of VL, participants in a 2015 National Cancer Institute (NCI USA) workshop on harmonization of EBV testing for NPC recommended that the amplicon size for plasma EBV DNA assays should be <100 bp [117].

Advantages and disadvantages of targeting a multi-copy versus a single-copy gene in specific clinical situations should also be considered. Historically, in the NPC setting, plasma assays have amplified the BamHI-W (Bam W) fragment, a sequence found in the EBV nuclear antigen leader protein (EBNA-LP) region of the genome which has a variable tandem reiteration frequency of 5–11 copies in clinical isolates; the WHO IS has 11 copies. Assays using these targets have greater sensitivity than single-copy PCR target but may have more imprecision in quantifying EBV DNA [118, 119]. Although a "more sensitive" assay may be useful for plasma EBV DNA detection, it could prove too sensitive when WB testing is performed if it detects viral latency in healthy seropositive immunocompetent subjects with high viral set points. Current commercial WB assays have levels of detection (LOD) in the range of 1.6–2.5 $\log_{10}$ IU/ml and levels of quantitation (LOQ) in the range of 2.2–3.0 $\log_{10}$ IU/ml [120].

Theoretically, assays targeting highly conserved single-copy EBV genes should have comparable sensitivity and quantitation. However, Ryan et al. [121] and Tsai et al. [48] observed better performance with an EBNA-1 targeted assay with respect to sensitivity or quantitation compared to other single-gene targeted assays. However, it is difficult to attribute the sensitivity differences to gene targets alone as differences in amplification efficiency, amplicon size, calibrators, and polymorphisms in specific genes among clinical isolates may all have contributed.

Since 2013, EBV whole-genome sequences (WGS) available in GenBank have increased from <10 strains to more than 200, significantly increasing information regarding genome heterogeneity [122]. Historically, EBV strains are divided into two major groups that vary geographically, type 1 (type A) and type 2 (type B), based predominantly on polymorphisms in the EBNA-2 and EBNA-3 genes [123–125]. The EBV B95-8 WHO IS a type 1 isolate. Recent EBV WGS data analysis found large numbers of single nucleotide polymorphisms (SNPs) [124, 125], which were more common in latent than viral lytic genes [123, 126]. Although definitive links between specific gene polymorphisms and risk of EBV disease or EBV-associated cancer risk have not been definitively established, several variants are being further studied in this regard [122]. Mutations in lytic EBV genes, such as thymidine kinase, protein kinase, and DNA polymerase, have not been definitively demonstrated. However, these genes are involved in the mechanism of action of drugs with anti-EBV activity such as acyclovir and ganciclovir used frequently after transplant and known to induce resistance in other herpesviruses making it prudent to avoid these genes as targets for EBV DNA assays. Manufacturers of EBV DNA assays should regularly review EBV GenBank data to confirm that the gene sequences targeted remain conserved among clinical isolates. An approach currently commonly used to mitigate the problem of false-negative results due to genetic polymorphisms is to include two gene targets in the assay [117].

Toward Reducing Variability in EBV DNA Measurement Using Real-Time RT-PCR Assays

Factors such as the use of commercial products, specific commercial reagents, probe chemistry, automation, and robotics that have not been extensively evaluated to date [97, 116, 127] may also contribute to result variability and are summarized in Table 6.3. The problem of lack of quantitative nucleic result harmonization is not unique to EBV, and we should extrapolate lessons learned from viruses such as hepatitis B virus, hepatitis C virus, and human immunodeficiency virus infection. Assay result harmonization has significantly improved for these other viruses because a very few commercially produced and highly automated assays are in use and all have been cleared or approved by regulators. International quantitative standards have also been in place for these viruses for long periods of time, allowing continuous quality improvement in the assays [109]. While acknowledging that some redundancy is required with respect to available tests, significantly reducing the number of assays being used for quantitative EBV DNA testing would facilitate global result harmonization.

Measurements of EBV Gene Expression in Peripheral Blood

Several investigators have evaluated EBV gene expression of latent and lytic genes in the peripheral blood of patients as alternative or adjunct biomarkers of PTLD risk or for PTLD diagnosis in both the SOT [8, 18, 47, 128–133] and HSCT settings [47, 50, 129, 130, 134]. Results have been variable, likely due to a combination of factors. Reverse transcriptase-PCR assays are not standardized, and assays for individual genes may have variable sensitivity both within and among studies. Gene expression assays are often performed on pooled cells so the prevalence and distribution of specific expression patterns among individual cells in the pool are unknown [1]. Some investigators studied adult SOT recipients likely seropositive pre-transplant [18, 47, 50, 130, 132, 134], while others studied pediatric populations, a significant proportion of whom are likely experiencing primary infections [8, 128, 129, 131, 133]. Studies are both cross-sectional and longitudinal with variable sampling intervals post-transplant and sometimes included or were restricted to patients with persistent elevated loads late after transplant [8, 47, 128, 129, 131]; data from SOT and HSCT populations are sometimes pooled for analysis [130].

Initial gene expression profiling in the peripheral blood of a limited number of adult, likely seropositive, SOT patients without PTLD suggested that lymphoblasts were not seen, and latency 0 EBV gene expression was observed (EBER, BARTs, and sometimes LMP2) [18]. Although this latency 0 pattern has also been observed by others [8], many investigators also report less restricted latency expression patterns including latency III in some patients with both gene expression levels and latency levels varying significantly over time in individual patients [47, 128, 129, 132, 133]. Lytic gene expression has been observed with variable prevalence in conjunction with different latency expression patterns. No specific latency pattern has been clearly associated with quantitative EBV DNA measurement, although expression levels of LMP2 have been correlated with levels of EBV DNAemia by some investigators [129, 133]. No consistent peripheral blood EBV gene expression patterns have been found that are predictive for or diagnostic of PTLD although only small numbers of patients have been studied [47, 129, 130, 132]. Currently there is no evidence to support any additional benefit of EBV gene expression profiling over measurement of EBV DNAemia alone in transplant recipients.

Measurement of Host and Viral Micro-RNAs (miRNA) in Peripheral Blood

miRNAs are a family of small (18–25 nt) non-coding RNAs, with sequence complementarity to mRNAs that act as negative regulators of gene expression involved in the regulation of cellular differentiation, proliferation, and apoptosis. EBV infection not only impacts host miRNA expression, but EBV encodes ~44 miRNAs almost exclusively from two regions: BHRFI, expressed during latency III and lytic infection, and BART miRNAs expressed in all forms of latency. These viral miRNAs repress expression of both host and viral genes [135]. Because miRNAs are highly stable and easily detected and quantified in either PBMC or plasma/serum using either commercial miRNA microarray analysis or reverse transcriptase-PCR techniques, miRNA profiling is attractive for study as a potential biomarker for PTLD. Kawano et al. [136] identified the plasma EBV miRNAs miBART2-5p, 13, and 15 as potentially more useful biomarkers than plasma EBV DNAemia for differentiating active from inactive CAEBV and for monitoring response to therapy in immunocompetent patients. Recently, investigators have also identified 215 differentially regulated host and viral miRNAs in the PMBC of college-aged immunocompetent students at presentation with IM that regressed to levels seen in age-matched controls over the subsequent 7 months [137]. Similar studies have not yet been performed in transplant recipients with primary EBV infection. However, preliminary studies have identified miR- BART22 in serum as a potential biomarker of EBV reactivation in pediatric liver transplant recipients [138] and plasma miBART2-5p, which targets the stress-induced immune ligand MICB to escape recognition and elimination by NK cells as possibly having a role in sustaining persistent high set points in pediatric kidney transplant recipients [139]. These interesting observations suggest further study of host and EBV miRNA profiling in peripheral blood is warranted as an alternative or adjunct marker for PTLD or PTLD risk.

Testing of Non-peripheral Blood Sample Types

Despite very limited data to inform result interpretation, in clinical transplant practice, CSF and bronchoalveolar lavage fluid (BAL) are often tested to diagnose EBV disease or PTLD in the CNS and lungs, respectively. EBV DNA assays have not been validated for these matrices.

CSF

Testing for EBV VL in the CSF of transplant recipients is used to assist in the diagnosis of CNS PTLD or EBV encephalitis, hoping to avoid the need for invasive biopsy procedures. Because CSF VL studies of SOT and HSCT recipients are extremely limited, data are extrapolated from the HIV-infected population where qualitative detection of EBV DNA in CSF is common in a wide variety of HIV neurological diseases and has poor PPV but good NPV for diagnosis of EBV+ CNS lymphoma [140–142]. Although assays were not calibrated to the WHO IS, quantitative cut-offs in the range of 3.3–4.0 $\log_{10}$ copies/ml in CSF improved both the specificity and PPV of the result for both primary CNS lymphoma and CNS involvement in systemic AIDS-related lymphoma when compared to qualitative results alone [140, 142, 143]. In a study that included five SOT recipients, Weinberg et al. [144] observed that patients with primary CNS lymphoma had high CSF VLs associated with low CSF leukocyte counts. In contrast patients with high leukocyte counts were more likely to be diagnosed with EBV encephalitis in the presence of high VL or post-infectious complications, when VLs were low. In HSCT recipients,

Liu et al. [145] found levels of EBV DNA were higher in CSF than in blood, in which EBV DNA was sometimes undetectable. CSF VL was also better at predicting CNS disease, and declining CSF VL correlated with clinical response.

BAL

In lung and heart-lung transplant patients, the lung is often the primary site of PTLD. Investigators initially suggested that high quantitative levels of EBV load in BAL fluid may be a more sensitive predictor of PTLD than EBV DNA measurement in peripheral blood [146]. However, EBV load in BAL was not predictive of PTLD in a larger multicenter study of pediatric lung transplant recipients [147]. Moreover, EBV DNA was detected in BAL fluid, often at high levels, of adult lung [148] and other transplant recipients [149] in the absence of PTLD.

Saliva

Studies of EBV DNA in saliva use a variety of techniques for specimen collection and assays of variable sensitivity making results difficult to compare. The most common collection method is an oral wash or gargle [150–153], but oral swabs [154] and chewing on cotton plugs [155] have also been used. A consistent observation is that there is more EBV DNA in the cell pellet than in the supernatant, suggesting EBV DNA is predominantly cell associated in saliva, presumably in epithelial cells [150–153, 156–158].

In adult EBV-seropositive healthy subjects with remote infection, the prevalence of EBV DNA saliva detection varies significantly from 24% to 90% tested using PCR technology either in cross-sectional [156, 157] or longitudinal studies [151, 153–155]. In longitudinal studies with follow-up varying from 18 weeks to 18 months, 96% to 100% of patients had detectable EBV DNA at least once [151, 153–155]. Historically, EBV-seropositive individuals have been classified as low-, intermediate-, and high-level saliva EBV shedders. However, Hadinoto et al. found seropositive individuals continuously shed virus in saliva and this reservoir is completely replaced approximately every 2 minutes. Although shedding levels in individuals appear stable over short periods of time, when studied over months to a year, the level of EBV DNA shedding by a given individual varies by 3.5 to 5.5 logs [153]. This rate of virus production in saliva could not be attributed to virus production by B cells alone, and the authors suggested virus must be amplified by epithelial cells.

Saliva excretion studies during acute primary infection are largely limited to patients with IM. EBV DNA appears in the saliva explosively at high levels approximately a week before onset of IM symptoms, peaks at 2 months after onset of illness, and remains markedly elevated over the first year after infection, levels that may persist for as long as 3.1 years [31, 158–160], Levels then decline over time to lower persistent levels seen in all EBV-seropositive subjects [151, 153]. In SOT recipients not receiving anti-viral agents with anti- EBV activity, both the detection prevalence (83–96%) and quantity of EBV DNA in saliva increase significantly beginning in the second month post-transplant with persistence and then decline in the 6–12-month period [150, 161]. Saliva EBV DNA levels were higher with increasing immunosuppression, in primary infection and in patients with PTLD, demonstrating similar patterns to those described in peripheral blood as a predictor of PTLD [150]. In a recent study pre-transplant EBV DNA detection in either saliva or blood did not predict post-transplant EBV DNAemia [162].

The known *in vitro* effects of anti-herpesvirus drugs including IV ganciclovir, IV acyclovir, valacyclovir and valganciclovir have been confirmed *in vivo* by measuring saliva EBV DNA. Clearance or a significant reduction in VL is observed on treatment even in immunocompromised hosts, but rapid rebound occurs on drug withdrawal [150, 152, 154]. Lytic infection appears to be the major source of EBV DNA in saliva supported by the observation that 59–62% of EBV DNA in saliva is DNase resistant suggesting it is present in encapsidated virions [153].

Although, using older tissue culture techniques, Yao et al. [161] found a correlation between virus in saliva and peripheral blood in healthy seropositive subjects with remote infection, no correlation has been observed by others [153, 155, 156]. Patterns and quantitative levels of EBV DNA detection in saliva and peripheral blood have not been directly compared using current NAT technology as predictors of PTLD in transplant patients. Given the variability in sample collection and the frequent post-transplant use of anti-virals with EBV activity, saliva is not recommended as a matrix for VL surveillance in preemptive PTLD prevention programs. EBV VL detection in saliva may, however, prove to be a useful adjunct to serology in clarification of pre-transplant EBV infection status in patients with passive antibody and as an ongoing surveillance tool for community-acquired primary infection in children who remain EBV seronegative after the early post-transplant period, but this requires further study.

EBV VL Kinetics: Implications for Monitoring Algorithms

PTLD guidelines in SOT and HSCT suggest that dynamic changes in peripheral blood EBV VL may be as important as absolute quantitative levels of EBV DNA to inform implementation of preemptive PTLD prevention strategies and to monitor response to prevention and treatment interventions [4, 163]. Defining "abnormal" EBV VL kinetic patterns in transplant recipients requires an understanding of "normal" EBV VL dynamics in different fractions of peripheral blood during acute and persistent infection in immunocompetent people of varying ages. Comparing VL patterns in transplant versus immunocompetent populations is critical to inform optimal monitoring algorithms, interpret responses to interventions in PTLD prevention strategies, and identify possible predictors of PTLD. Since historically serology rather than EBV DNA measurement has been used for the diagnosis of acute EBV infection, data regarding VL dynamics in immunocompetent hosts are recent and limited. Primary EBV infection, assessed by EBV DNA measurements in peripheral blood, is characterized by an incubation or "eclipse phase," an acute and convalescent phase during which EBV VL accelerates to a peak characterized

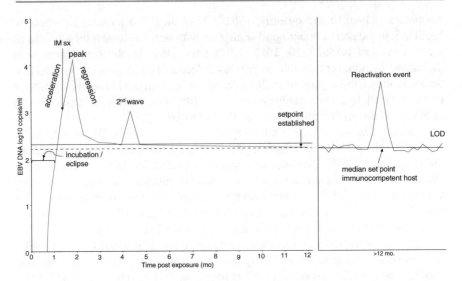

Fig. 6.1 A schematic of quantitative Epstein-Barr virus (EBV) DNAemia measured in whole blood in an immunocompetent subject experiencing primary EBV infection. Symptoms, if present, begin 32–49 days after exposure [158, 159, 164, 165]. EBV DNA can be detected approximately 3 weeks before symptoms using very sensitive research assays [160] becoming detectable by diagnostic assays 7–10 days before symptom onset and rising rapidly to peak over the next 2 weeks [158–160, 179]. EBV DNAemia then regresses in an exponential [166] or biphasic [178] pattern, with a rapid decline over the first 2 weeks and a much slower subsequent decline. EBV DNA is detected for a median of 17 days in adolescents and young adults [159] but may be detected for as long as 5–6 months in infants [192]. Recurrent episodes of EBV DNAemia with or without symptoms can occur [31, 158, 192], documented at 60–90 days after first symptom onset in young adults. EBV DNAemia does not approach a specific individual "set point" until approximately 1 year after symptom onset [22, 166, 180]. Reactivation events can occur after the set point is established in both asymptomatic subjects [17] and during critical illness and sepsis [26]. LOD = lower limit of EBV DNA detection by diagnostic assay [159] [dotted line]; set point [solid line] identified as median EBV viral load in healthy seropositive UK adults (79 copies/1 × 10⁶ peripheral blood mononuclear cells or approximately 158 copies/ml whole blood)

by a doubling time and then regresses, followed by an equilibrium state with an individual "set point" marking persistent infection (Fig. 6.1). Time to first detection, time from first detection to peak, time from peak to set point, and area under the VL time curve (AUC) are additional parameters that might be important to study. Although it is challenging to compare studies because of differences in VL assays and the matrix used for testing, available data are summarized below.

Incubation or "Eclipse" Phase

Patients are asymptomatic and therefore rarely identified during the 32–49-day incubation period prior to development of IM symptoms determined using known or suspected expected exposure to EBV-infected saliva [158, 159, 164, 165]. In a prospective study of 40 EBV-seronegative university students, Dunmire et al. [160] were able to detect very low levels of EBV DNA in WB as early as 22 days prior to IM symptom onset in the absence of both saliva EBV DNA detection and evidence of an adaptive immune response using a very sensitive nested PCR assay. This level of EBV DNA would not be detected by clinical diagnostic assays; investigators attribute the low level EBV DNA detection to relatively slow expansion of latently infected (latency 0) B cells in tonsillar tissues with spillover of these cells into the circulation. Lytic virus replication appears to have no role during this eclipse period aside from the initial transmission of infectious virus by saliva from another host to naïve B cells in the oropharynx of the recipient. There is an explosive increase in EBV DNA detection in both saliva (7 days) and peripheral blood (7–10 days) before IM symptom onset. These observations, particularly the late onset of oral viral shedding, contradict the model of acute IM proposed by Hadinoto et al. [166] who suggested that the VL increase in peripheral blood results from EBV reactivation in latently infected memory B cells that return to the oropharynx and infect new naïve B cells, a repetitive cycle that continues until a cytotoxic T lymphocyte (CTL) response is triggered.

The most comprehensive EBV VL data during primary EBV infection in infants is derived from two longitudinal studies in Africa where infection is almost universal before age 2. One studied EBV DNA in PBMC of infants (14–18 months) in Gambia over 6 months during a period of low malaria prevalence [167]. The other compared EBV VLs in WB in Kenyan infants (serially followed from 1 month to 2 years of age) from two regions, one with high and the other with low rates of both holoendemic malaria and Burkitt lymphoma [168]. While historical evidence suggested that infants may be protected from EBV infection during the first 6 months of life [169–171], mathematical modeling using data from the Kenyan infant study has made two interesting observations regarding the incubation/eclipse phase of primary EBV infection [172]. First, detection of early de novo EBV-specific serologic responses in the infant suggests that "infection" may occur as early as 1–2 months of life, but EBV DNAemia is not detected until maternal antibodies wane. The second is that the timing of EBV DNAemia is dependent on the initial level of maternal antibody and the rate of its decay. A recent Canadian study suggests that infant seropositive donors less than 6 months of age do not appear to transmit EBV to seronegative recipients (i.e., only have passive maternal antibody) and could be considered seronegative when risk stratifying for preemptive strategies [173].

SOT offers a unique opportunity to study the biology of primary EBV infection as the exact timing of EBV exposure is known, in the EBV donor positive/recipient negative scenario (EBV mismatch), and we are often monitoring VL during the eclipse phase. In an era prior to the routine use of anti-virals for CMV prophylaxis after SOT, the median time to EBV detection in saliva during primary donor-derived EBV infection after SOT was 6 weeks [150], similar to the IM incubation period. More recent studies in EBV-mismatched SOT patients monitored serially using RT-PCR EBV DNA assays noted later initial detection of EBV DNAemia at a median of 84 days with only rare detection in the first post-transplant month [173]. The use of anti-viral prophylaxis appeared to delay the onset of EBV DNAemia in a cohort of adult kidney transplant recipients [174], but not in a similar pediatric cohort [175]. In the SOT setting, it is not known whether duration of the eclipse period is influenced by anti-viral therapy or by passive maternal or transfusion-derived antibody in the recipient given the mode of transmission. The low-level early EBV DNAemia described by Dunmire et al. [160] in IM has not been described in SOT recipients: the LOD of clinical assays may not be sensitive enough to detect this, even in immunocompromised hosts.

In three HSCT monitoring studies, the median time to EBV DNAemia post-transplant was 50 days (range 19–368 days) using plasma [176], 99 days (IQR 84–119 days) using WB [50], and 34 days (range 18–60 days) using either plasma or PBMC [54]. It may therefore be reasonable to delay the onset on post-transplant monitoring for preemptive interventions until after the first transplant month, particularly in SOT, to minimize costs; however, from a logistics and compliance perspective, this may increase the complexity of implementation.

Acute and Convalescent Infection Phase

Acceleration phase and peak: Several investigators found that EBV VL in WB or PBMC may already be falling when immunocompetent adolescents and young adults first present with IM symptoms [22, 166, 177, 178]. However, in prospectively followed seroconverting university students undergoing frequent sampling, EBV VL continues to rise and peaks quickly within 2 weeks of symptom onset (median 8 days) [158, 159]. Median peak loads in WB reported in studies of IM patients were 3.0 $\log_{10}$ copies/ml [158], 3.9 $\log_{10}$ copies/ml [179], 7350 copies/10^6 PBMC or ~4.2 $\log_{10}$ copies/ml [180], and 6280 copies/10^6 PBMC or ~4.1 $\log_{10}$ copies/ml [181]. Peak VL is similar in both IM patients and asymptomatic patients [180, 182] supporting the concept that IM symptoms result from an exaggerated immune response rather than a higher VL. In the Kenyan infant study, infants in holoendemic vs. sporadic malaria areas were infected with EBV earlier in life (mean 7.28 months). Earlier infection was associated with higher and more persistent WB EBV VLs, suggesting infants infected earlier in life had poorer control of infection [168]. Mathematical modeling of the data from this study found very short EBV VL doubling times, 1.6 and 2.1 days in high and low malaria transmission regions, respectively [172]. Limited study of plasma EBV DNA in IM suggests that EBV DNA is detectable in the plasma of most patients at symptom onset at lower levels than in WB/PBMC and declines rapidly to undetectable levels 15–30 days later [29, 31–33].

Although there is overlap, transplant recipients with PTLD appear to have higher VLs measured in both plasma [68, 82] and PBMC [46, 68, 183, 184] than those observed in immunocompetent IM patients. The majority of historical studies suggest that high peak VL is a sensitive but not specific marker of EBV+ PTLD occurring early, usually in the first year after transplant, with VL most often peaking before the onset of symptoms (reviewed by [185]). This is the basis of preemptive prevention strategies. Unfortunately, these studies have significant limitations. Most transplant studies are not natural history studies, as clinicians are implementing interventions based on available results. Almost all longitudinal studies attempting to determine EBV DNAemia levels predictive of PTLD are single-center studies, most often involving only pediatric SOT populations. In addition, result interpretation is complicated by the heterogeneity of the populations studied, with high- and low-risk populations and SOT and HSCT populations often pooled for analysis. The use of non-standardized assays and sample types precludes making recommendations regarding quantitative levels of EBV DNA that might be used as trigger points for interventions. The small numbers of PTLD cases limit the statistical analyses performed.

More recent studies of the association between high WB peak load and PTLD have been conflicting in both SOT and HSCT populations. No association was found in German pediatric kidney transplant recipients [77] or a Korean SOT population (predominantly pediatric liver recipients) [186]. However, Colombini et al. [92] identified peak VL as an independent predictor of PTLD, in a multivariate analysis of a multicenter study of pediatric kidney transplant recipients. Similarly early peak load, in univariate analysis, was a risk factor for PTLD in a single-center study of pediatric heart transplant recipients [187]. "EBV exposure" measured as area under the EBV viral load concentration-time curve (AUC) is an alternate potential biomarker of PTLD risk, although in a study of pediatric kidney transplant recipients, AUC of EBV VL during the first post-transplant year was not predictive of symptomatic EBV infection that included PTLD [77]. Although peak load was associated with increased PTLD risk in a HSCT cohort in the Cho et al. study [186], in a recent multicenter UK study of 69 PTLD cases, 45% and 23% of cases had VLs at diagnosis measured predominantly in WB that were lower than 40,0000 copies/ml and 10,000 copies/ml, respectively, commonly used as preemptive triggers in the HSCT setting [188]. Peak VL appears to be temporally concordant in plasma and WB in HSCT recipients [74]. Salano et al. [189] studying a mixed population of HSCT recipients at high and low risk for PTLD using plasma EBV DNA monitoring found that neither initial positive result nor doubling time predicted clinical features associated with high PTLD risk; these parameters also did not predict the need for preemptive rituximab therapy.

As observed during acute infection in immunocompetent hosts, in primary EBV infection after SOT and high-level reactivation of EBV in HSCT, the initial rise in EBV VL is explosive [50, 54, 58, 186]. In high-risk HSCT patients, Burns et al. [50] found the median time from first EBV DNA detection in WB to high-level DNAemia (median load 2.2×10^5 genomes/ml) was 7 days (IQR 0–14 days). Although doubling times as rapid as 56 hours have been described in the lung transplant setting [58], the time to peak has been less well described in the SOT setting. This very rapid initial VL rise makes the logistics of preemptive therapy challenging. Frequent monitoring of at least weekly for at least the 4 first post-transplant months is recommended in guidelines for high-risk HSCT recipients [163]. In SOT recipients, it can be argued that any detectable peripheral EBV VL in the setting of a primary EBV infection should trigger review and minimization of immunosuppression when possible, to optimize opportunities for development of EBV-specific adaptive immune responses. Weekly post-transplant monitoring during the highest risk period for donor-derived infection (1–4 months) [173] is recommended for EBV-mismatched SOT recipients. However, there are no data to suggest that less frequent monitoring (i.e., biweekly or even longer intervals later in the first year after transplant) negatively impacts preemptive strategies [4]. In evaluating interventions during the acceleration phase of primary infection, reduction in doubling time or lower peak or set point may be positive endpoints; short-term absolute quantitative reduction in load may not be an appropriate measurement.

Regression from peak load: VL regression patterns in IM are variable among patients and may be dependent on patient age and the "immunosuppressive environment" in which primary infection occurs. In a study of adolescents and young adults, the median duration of WB EBV DNAemia was 17 days [159], but EBV DNA was detected as long as 202 days in individual patients. EBV DNA in PBMC studied by Fafi-Kremer in 20 IM patients progressively declined over 180 days with levels approaching those in EBV-seropositive patients by 30 days [31]. Investigators have observed that WB/PBMC viral load falls as adaptive immune responses develop in a biphasic pattern, with a rapid decline lasting 2–6 weeks (estimated half-life 1.5 days) followed by a more gradual decline thereafter (mean half-life 38.7 +/− 15 days) [177, 178]. After studying 24 children with IM (age 1–16 years), Nakai et al. [178] found two-thirds were slow regressors with PBMC EBV DNAemia still detectable at last follow-up (up to 90 days after onset of symptoms). VLs generally approach but do not achieve "set point" observed in EBV-seropositive asymptomatic children and adults until approximately 1 year after IM [22, 166, 180]. EBV sero-conversion rates due to community-acquired infection in infants and children are high [190, 191]. Some children awaiting transplant are likely recently infected (i.e., less than 1 year ago); this is particularly true for seropositive infants between 1 and 2 years of age. Although not been specifically studied, these children may be at intermediate PTLD risk, falling between high-risk seronegative and lower-risk seropositive children with remote infection. More extensive pre-transplant and wait-list serology profiling and WB EBV VL testing may be warranted to allow better risk stratification of children as seronegative, acutely (recently) infected, or remotely infected to inform monitoring algorithms for preventive measures. Viral kinetic data in infant EBV infection from a Kenyan study revealed a median duration of WB EBV DNAemia of 6.3 months and 4.9 months for infants in holoendemic and sporadic malaria areas, respectively [192]. The AUC of the first episode of EBV DNA detection, determined by both doubling time and duration, was greater in the high malaria exposure region but was not influenced by age. Malaria is thought to increase VLs either through promoting B cell proliferation [193], altering T cell responses [194], and/or decreasing maternal antibody transfer [195]. Potential analogies in the transplant setting include graft-associated chronic or recurrent B cell stimulation, even in the absence of observed acute rejection, and recurrent infection episodes, exogenous immunosuppression, and possibly more rapid passive maternal antibody elimination because of bleeding and transfusion.

In the transplant setting, observations regarding EBV VL regression kinetics in the absence of interventions are extremely limited. The half-life of the biologic form of EBV DNA being measured, in the order of hours for ccf EBV DNA in plasma versus weeks for latently infected cells, should be considered in interpreting dynamic changes observed. In HSCT patients who spontaneously resolved plasma EBV DNAemia, Solano et al. observed a median half-life of 4 days (range 0.04–123.7 days) and several patterns that included zero-order and first-order elimination kinetics as well as a biphasic "humped" pattern [189]. Unlike IM patients and asymptomatic non-HIV-infected African infants, EBV DNA detection in plasma in asymptomatic pediatric liver transplant recipients experiencing primary infection was prolonged, as long as a year after first detection [67, 75]. It is very difficult to assess the impact of interventions using viral kinetic data in the absence of a control group not receiving the intervention or controlling for the timing of the intervention relative to the onset of EBV DNA detection. When evaluating interventions implemented during the regression phase of acute primary infection after SOT, the regression half-life or time to clearance (for diagnostic assays) may be a better measurement of efficacy than an absolute quantitative reduction in VL. Kumar et al. [196] observed a decline in WB VL in 90.3% of 31 SOT patients experiencing primary EBV infection with median reductions of -0.49 $\log_{10}$ copies/ml and -0.87 $\log_{10}$ copies/ml 14 and 30 days, respectively, after either RIS or anti-viral therapy. The timing of the interventions relative to first EBV DNAemia or phase of infection was not specified in this study.

Recurrent episodes of EBV DNAemia: Acute primary EBV infection may include recurrent episodes or waves of EBV DNAemia that are not necessarily associated with short-term adverse events in either the immunocompetent subject or transplant recipient. In 20 IM patients, Fafi-Kremer et al. [31] observed rebound PBMC EBV DNAemia after initial regression between day 60 and 90 after symptom onset associated with recurrent symptoms in 20%. In Kenyan infants, patterns of WB EBV DNAemia varied with some infants demonstrating a single peak and others having multiple waves of detection [192]. However, a shorter time to subsequent waves that were characterized by both a slower doubling time and shorter duration of EBV DNAemia was seen when infection occurred at a younger age. Repeated waves of infection were more likely in high malaria exposure regions but were less likely with higher AUC with the first episode. Reinfection episodes could not be ruled out as a cause of multiple waves/episodes of infection in this environment. Rebound events after initial regression have also been observed in the SOT setting after primary infection managed by RIS or antiviral therapy [196, 197] with no apparent adverse effects [197].

Equilibrium or Set Point VL

All EBV-seropositive patients have persistent EBV infection in peripheral blood even though it is often below the level of detection of RT-PCR assays in specimen types used in clinical labs in the transplant setting. This host-virus equilibrium or set point is estimated to take up to a year to achieve after acute infection [22, 166, 180] and is unique to an individual and relatively stable for at least 3.5 years [66, 153, 198]. There is some stochastic variation in values around the set point over time estimated at $\pm 25\%$, and this should be considered when defining clinically meaningful VL kinetic outcomes if interventions in transplant patients are initiated after set points are established [153]. Peripheral blood VL may increase with aging in adults [199, 200] although results are not consistent [201]. Whether age-related increases represent more EBV reactivation events or altered "set point" associated with immunosenescence is uncertain. "Set point" VL may also be geographically variable. Healthy children and adults in Gambia have a set point (median 850 copies/ 10^6 PBMC) >10-fold higher than adults in the UK (median 79 copies/10^6 PBMC); some had VLs similar to those seen in UK IM patients [181]. It has been suggested that early age of infection may raise set point; recurrent exposure to malaria may further contribute [167]. It may be important to evaluate interventions occurring after set point has been established separately from those occurring earlier during acute primary infection after SOT as their impact may be significantly different in these settings that likely represent very different stages of host-EBV immune response development.

In the SOT setting, the time required to develop adaptive immune responses and EBV viral set point after donor-derived primary infection may be prolonged compared to the immunocompetent patient because of exogenous immunosuppression. Colombini et al. [92] observed that in the 38% of patients experiencing primary infection after kidney transplantation who "cleared" their EBV DNAemia during a median 5.4 years of follow-up, clearance occurred at a median of 22.1 months after detection. Similar protracted regression was observed by Kullberg-Lindh et al. [75] on withdrawal of all immunosuppression in pediatric liver transplant recipients with "set point" WB VLs sometimes not observed until 2 years after initial detection, often concordant with clearance of EBV DNAemia in serum. A significant proportion of SOT recipients experiencing primary EBV infection have detectable WB EBV DNA, sometimes at very high levels, that is sustained for many years and appears to represent an "abnormally high" viral set point; this is observed less frequently in SOT patients seropositive pre-transplant and has not been described in the HSCT setting [8, 77, 92, 128, 175, 202–206]. The immunopathogenesis and factors that influence setting and sustaining EBV viral set point after primary infection are unknown [207, 208]. Young age at infection, immunodeficiency, and intercurrent infections such as malaria are believed to elevate set points in African infants [209]; warm ischemia time and high graft to recipient weight ratio have been identified as factors in pediatric liver transplant recipients [205]. High EBV set point may be a form of neonatal tolerance also seen with other viral infections such as hepatitis B, CMV, and rubella acquired in utero or the early post-partum period. Examples of variable EBV set points after donor-derived primary EBV infection in three pediatric SOT recipients are illustrated in Fig. 6.2a–c.

Investigators have often defined SOT patients as having a chronic high VL phenotype (CHVLP) when having sustained (>50%) WB EBV VLs in the range of 5000–16,000 copies/ml for >6 months [8, 77, 92, 128, 175, 202–206]. High EBV

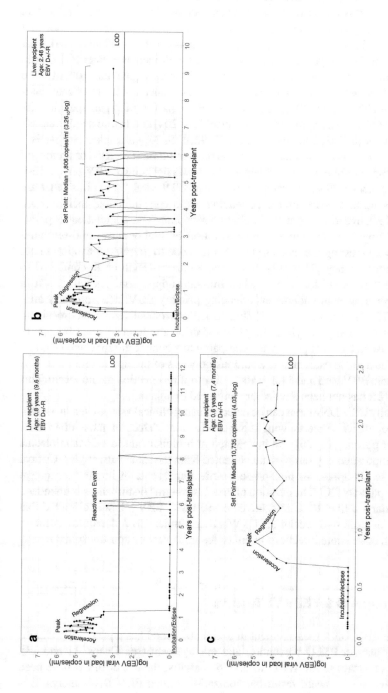

Fig. 6.2 (**a–c**) Kinetics of EBV DNAemia measured in the whole blood of solid organ transplant recipients with primary EBV infection. Post-transplant serial EBV DNAemia measurements in three EBV mismatched (donor seropositive/recipient seronegative) infants who developed an EBV viral load set point that was "undetectable" by the diagnostic assay (**a**), a set point at low detectable EBV DNAemia levels (**b**), and a set point at high detectable EBV DNAemia levels (**c**). None developed PTLD during follow-up. LOD = lower limit of EBV DNA detection by diagnostic assay [solid line]. A conversion of 0.5 can be used to convert from copies/ml to IU/ml (e.g., 2 copies/ml = 1 IU/ml)

viral set point may be a preferred terminology rather than CHVLP to describe this biologic state as it is the terminology that has been used to describe a similar state in the HIV setting [210]. However, it is not known whether 6 months after first detection is sufficient time for equilibrium or set point to be achieved and what specific quantitative set point, if any, is associated with increased later PTLD risk. Although studies of pediatric heart transplant recipients suggest that patients who are chronic high VL carriers may be at significantly increased risk of late-onset EBV-positive PTLD [202, 203], this risk appears in part to be organ-specific with intermediate risks observed in intestinal transplants [204] and low to negligible risk in pediatric liver [8, 205, 206] and kidney [77, 92, 175, 208] transplant recipients.

Whether any intervention such as immune reconstitution (i.e., RIS) or prolonged antiviral therapy can alter set point when established is not known. EBV-seropositive immunocompetent subjects develop increases in EBV viral "set points" that are sustained for up to 5 years after experiencing acute HIV infection; increases are proportional relative to their pre-HIV infection set points. These increased set points remain unchanged despite immune reconstitution by highly active anti-retroviral HIV therapy suggesting the increased set point is due to immune activation rather than immunodeficiency [210–212]. Similarly, Kullberg-Lindh et al. continued to see elevated "set point" loads even when immunosuppression was withdrawn in pediatric liver transplant patients experiencing primary EBV infection early after transplant [75]. Hoshino et al. [213] studied EBV-seropositive subjects receiving 1 year of valacyclovir prophylaxis for HSV infection and found a small but appreciable decrease in EBV set point when compared to a control group where no effect was seen. The authors estimated it would take 6 years of therapy to eliminate 99% of the systemic EBV load and 11.3 years to clear it if re-infection did not occur. This anti-viral effect has not been studied or confirmed by others.

Periodically EBV DNAemia can be detected using clinical assays even in asymptomatic seropositive subjects with remote infection; detection most often lasts <4 weeks in plasma [17, 26] and is detected at a higher rate in WB than plasma when contemporaneously samples are collected from the same patient [26]. Critical illness and sepsis appear to precipitate reactivation events in immunocompetent seropositive patients [26]. The duration of these "set point" disturbances is unknown. In acute malaria a five- to sixfold increase in PBMC EBV VL was observed that persists for at least 4–6 weeks [181]. Whether similar EBV dynamics occur in patients with other acute infections in either the transplant or non-transplant setting is not known.

Future Prospects for EBV VL Testing

Quantitative EBV DNA measurement in peripheral blood has a potentially significant role to play in PTLD prevention and management (see Chaps. 11 and 18). Calibration of assays to the WHO IS and, potentially, the use of dPCR have been important first steps toward result harmonization among EBV DNA assays. It is important that test manufacturers, national regulators, clinical virologists, transplant physicians, and oncologists work collaboratively to continue to improve result harmonization through optimization of the commutability of secondary calibrators, nucleic acid extraction procedures, target design, and other factors that contribute to ongoing result variability. Clinical trials will be required to both validate result harmonization and evaluate the benefit of these assays in specific clinical settings. We must understand what we are measuring. This includes the biologic forms of EBV DNA and host and viral EBV miRNAs in plasma and the cellular blood fraction as well as the phenotype of infected cells and how these change during primary and reactivation infection after transplant and throughout the subsequent stages of PTLD development. This information is critical for assay improvement and identification of new biomarkers. New tools such as target-capture deep sequencing for EBV DNA fragment length profiling [17] in plasma and ImmunoFISH assays [9] that might allow analysis of EBV-infected cells at a single-cell level are potentially useful in that regard.

A high priority for research would be a multicenter trial comparing EBV DNA measurements in both plasma and WB to more definitively determine the optimal specimen type to use in specific clinical settings after transplant. Analyzing EBV DNA kinetics in both WB and plasma, including mathematical modeling of these dynamics [172], would increase our understanding of the biology of EBV transmission and infection in the transplant setting and also improve the definition of "abnormal" relative to natural community-acquired infection in the immunocompetent host. When EBV DNA dynamics in peripheral blood are used as surrogate markers of response to clinical interventions for prevention and treatment of PTLD, modeling of EBV VL data after transplant could also inform identification of VL parameters that could be used as better clinically relevant outcome measures.

References

1. Thorley-Lawson DA. EBV persistence—introducing the virus. Epstein Barr Virus. Curr Top Microbiol Immunol. 2015;390:151–209.
2. Shannon-Lowe C, Rickinson A. The global landscape of EBV-associated tumors. Front Oncol. 2019;9:1–23.
3. Fryer JF, Heath AB, Wilkinson DE, Minor PD. A collaborative study to establish the 1st WHO International Standard for Epstein–Barr virus for nucleic acid amplification techniques. Biologicals. 2016;44:423–33.
4. Allen UD, Preiksaitis JK. Post-transplant lymphoproliferative disorders, Epstein-Barr virus infection, and disease in solid organ transplantation: guidelines from the American Society of Transplantation Infectious Diseases Community of Practice. Clin Transpl. 2019;33:e13652.
5. Humar A, Michaels M. American Society of Transplantation recommendations for screening, monitoring and reporting of infectious complications in immunosuppression trials in recipients of organ transplantation. Am J Transplant. 2006;6:262–74.
6. Ahya VN, Douglas LP, Andreadis C, Arnoldi S, Svoboda J, Kotloff RM, et al. Association between elevated whole blood Epstein–Barr Virus (EBV)-encoded RNA EBV polymerase chain reaction and reduced incidence of acute lung allograft rejection. J Hear Lung Transpl. 2007;26:839–44.
7. Bakker NA, Verschuuren EAM, Erasmus ME, Hepkema BG, Veeger NJGM, Kallenberg CGM, et al. Epstein-Barr virus-DNA load monitoring late after lung transplantation: a sur-

rogate marker of the degree of immunosuppression and a safe guide to reduce immunosuppression. Transplantation. 2007;83:433–8.

8. Gotoh K, Ito Y, Ohta R, Iwata S, Nishiyama Y, Nakamura T, et al. Immunologic and virologic analyses in pediatric liver transplant recipients with chronic high Epstein-Barr Virus loads. J Infect Dis. 2010;202:461–9.

9. Ito Y, Kawabe S, Kojima S, Nakamura F, Nishiyama Y, Kaneko K, et al. Identification of Epstein-Barr virus-infected CD27+ memory B-cells in liver or stem cell transplant patients. J Gen Virol. 2011;92:2590–5.

10. Calattini S, Sereti I, Scheinberg P, Kimura H, Childs RW, Cohen JI. Detection of EBV genomes in plasmablasts/plasma cells and non-B cells in the blood of most patients with EBV lymphoproliferative disorders by using Immuno-FISH. Blood. 2010;116:4546–59.

11. Lieberman PM. Chromatin structure of Epstein-Barr virus latent episomes. Epstein Barr Virus: Springer International Publishing; 2015. p. 71–102.

12. To EWH, Chan KCA, Leung SF, Chan LYS, To KF, Chan ATC, et al. Rapid clearance of plasma Epstein-Barr virus DNA after surgical treatment of nasopharyngeal carcinoma. Clin Cancer Res. 2003;9:3254–9.

13. Chan KCA, Zhang J, Chan ATC, Lei KIK, Leung S-F, Chan LYS, et al. Molecular characterization of circulating EBV DNA in the plasma of nasopharyngeal carcinoma and lymphoma patients. Cancer Res. 2003;63:2028–32.

14. Jahr S, Hentze H, Englisch S, Hardt D, Fackelmayer FO, Hesch RD, et al. DNA fragments in the blood plasma of cancer patients: quantitations and evidence for their origin from apoptotic and necrotic cells. Cancer Res. 2001;61:1659–65.

15. Underhill HR, Kitzman JO, Hellwig S, Welker NC, Daza R, Baker DN, et al. Fragment length of circulating tumor DNA. Kwiatkowski DJ, editor. PLoS Genet. 2016;12:e1006162.

16. Snyder MW, Kircher M, Hill AJ, Daza RM, Shendure J. Cell-free DNA comprises an in vivo nucleosome footprint that informs its tissues-of-origin. Cell. 2016;164:57–68.

17. Lam WKJ, Jiang P, Chan KCA, Cheng SH, Zhang H, Peng W, et al. Sequencing-based counting and size profiling of plasma Epstein–Barr virus DNA enhance population screening of nasopharyngeal carcinoma. Proc Natl Acad Sci. 2018;115:E5115–24.

18. Babcock GJ, Decker LL, Freeman RB, Thorley-Lawson DA. Epstein-Barr Virus–infected resting memory B cells, not proliferating lymphoblasts, accumulate in the peripheral blood of immunosuppressed patients. J Exp Med. 1999;190:567–76.

19. Souza TA, Stollar BD, Sullivan JL, Luzuriaga K, Thorley-Lawson DA. Peripheral B cells latently infected with Epstein-Barr virus display molecular hallmarks of classical antigen-selected memory B cells. Proc Natl Acad Sci. 2005;102:18093–8.

20. Miyashita EM, Yang B, Babcock GJ, Thorley-Lawson DA. Identification of the site of Epstein-Barr virus persistence in vivo as a resting B cell. J Virol. 1997;71:4882–91.

21. Joseph AM, Babcock GJ, Thorley-Lawson DA. EBV persistence involves strict selection of latently infected B cells. J Immunol. 2000;165:2975–81.

22. Hochberg D, Souza T, Catalina M, Sullivan JL, Luzuriaga K, Thorley-Lawson DA. Acute infection with Epstein-Barr virus targets and overwhelms the peripheral memory B-cell compartment with resting. Latently infected cells. J Virol. 2004;78:5194–204.

23. Hochberg DR, Thorley-Lawson DA. Quantitative detection of viral gene expression in populations of Epstein-Barr Virus-infected cells in vivo. DNA viruses. New Jersey: Humana Press; 2005. p. 039–56.

24. van den Heuvel D, Jansen MAE, Bell AI, Rickinson AB, Jaddoe VWV, van Dongen JJM, et al. Transient reduction in IgA + and IgG + memory B cell numbers in young EBV-seropositive children: the generation R study. J Leukoc Biol. 2017;101:949–56.

25. Chaganti S, Heath EM, Bergler W, Kuo M, Buettner M, Niedobitek G, et al. Epstein-Barr virus colonization of tonsillar and peripheral blood B-cell subsets in primary infection and persistence. Blood. 2009;113:6372–81.

26. Walton AH, Muenzer JT, Rasche D, Boomer JS, Sato B, Brownstein BH, et al. Reactivation of multiple viruses in patients with Sepsis. Moldawer LL, editor. PLoS One. 2014;9:e98819.

27. Barros MHM, Vera-Lozada G, Segges P, Hassan R, Niedobitek G. Revisiting the tissue microenvironment of infectious mononucleosis: identification of EBV infection in T cells and deep characterization of immune profiles. Front Immunol. 2019;10:146.
28. Coleman CB, Daud II, Ogolla SO, Ritchie JA, Smith NA, Sumba PO, et al. Epstein-Barr Virus type 2 infects T cells in healthy Kenyan children. J Infect Dis. 2017;216:670–7.
29. Bauer CC, Aberle SW, Popow-Kraupp T, Kapitan M, Hofmann H, Puchhammer-Stöckl E. Serum Epstein-Barr virus DNA load in primary Epstein-Barr virus infection. J Med Virol. 2005;75:54–8.
30. Ryan JL, Fan H, Swinnen LJ, Schichman SA, Raab-Traub N, Covington M, et al. Epstein-Barr Virus (EBV) DNA in plasma is not encapsidated in patients with EBV-related malignancies. Diagn Mol Pathol. 2004;13:61–8.
31. Fafi-Kremer S, Morand P, Brion J, Pavese P, Baccard M, Germi R, et al. Long-term shedding of infectious Epstein-Barr Virus after infectious mononucleosis. J Infect Dis. 2005;191:985–9.
32. Kimura H, Nishikawa K, Hoshino Y, Sofue A, Nishiyama Y, Morishima T. Monitoring of cell-free viral DNA in primary Epstein-Barr virus infection. Med Microbiol Immunol. 2000;188:197–202.
33. Berger C, Day P, Meier G, Zingg W, Bossart W, Nadal D. Dynamics of Epstein-Barr virus DNA levels in serum during EBV-associated disease. J Med Virol. 2001;64:505–12.
34. Slyker JA, Casper C, Tapia K, Richardson B, Bunts L, Huang M-L, et al. Clinical and virologic manifestations of primary Epstein-Barr Virus (EBV) infection in Kenyan infants born to HIV-infected women. J Infect Dis. 2013;207:1798–806.
35. Okuno Y, Murata T, Sato Y, Muramatsu H, Ito Y, Watanabe T, et al. Defective Epstein–Barr virus in chronic active infection and haematological malignancy. Nat Microbiol Springer US. 2019;4:404–13.
36. Cohen JI, Jaffe ES, Dale JK, Pittaluga S, Heslop HE, Rooney CM, et al. Characterization and treatment of chronic active Epstein-Barr virus disease: a 28-year experience in the United States. Blood. 2011;117:5835–49.
37. Kimura H, Ito Y, Kawabe S, Gotoh K, Takahashi Y, Kojima S, et al. EBV-associated T/NK–cell lymphoproliferative diseases in nonimmunocompromised hosts: prospective analysis of 108 cases. Blood. 2012;119:673–86.
38. Kimura H, Hoshino Y, Hara S, Sugaya N, Kawada J, Shibata Y, et al. Differences between T cell–type and natural killer cell–type chronic active Epstein-Barr Virus infection. J Infect Dis. 2005;191:531–9.
39. Kasahara Y, Yachie A, Takei K, Kanegane C, Okada K, Ohta K, et al. Differential cellular targets of Epstein-Barr virus (EBV) infection between acute EBV-associated hemophagocytic lymphohistiocytosis and chronic active EBV infection. Blood. 2001;98:1882–8.
40. Weber T, Wickenhauser C, Monecke A, Gläser C, Stadler M, Desole M, et al. Treatment of rare co-occurrence of Epstein-Barr virus-driven post-transplant lymphoproliferative disorder and hemophagocytic lymphohistiocytosis after allogeneic stem cell transplantation. Transpl Infect Dis. 2014;16:988–92.
41. Kanakry J, Ambinder R. The biology and clinical utility of EBV monitoring in blood. Curr Top Microbiol Immunol. 2015;391:475–99.
42. Rose C, Green M, Webber S, Ellis D, Reyes J, Rowe D. Pediatric solid-organ transplant recipients carry chronic loads of Epstein-Barr Virus exclusively in the immunoglobulin D-negative B-cell compartment. J Clin Microbiol. 2001;39:1407–15.
43. Schauer E, Webber S, Green M, Rowe D. Surface immunoglobulin-deficient Epstein-Barr Virus-infected B cells in the peripheral blood of pediatric solid-organ transplant recipients. J Clin Microbiol. 2004;42:5802–10.
44. Roughan JE, Torgbor C, Thorley-Lawson DA. Germinal center B cells latently infected with Epstein-Barr Virus proliferate extensively but do not increase in number. J Virol. American Society for Microbiology. 2010;84:1158–68.
45. Schauer E, Webber S, Kingsley L, Green M, Rowe D. Increased Ig-null B lymphocytes in the peripheral blood of pediatric solid organ transplant recipients with elevated Epstein-Barr viral loads. Pediatr Transplant. 2009;13:311–8.

46. Kimura H, Morita M, Yabuta Y, Kuzushima K, Kato K, Kojima S, et al. Quantitative analysis of Epstein-Barr virus load by using a real-time PCR assay. J Clin Microbiol. 1999;37:132–6.
47. Greijer AE, Stevens SJ, Verkuijlen SA, Juwana H, Fleig SC, Verschuuren EA, et al. Variable EBV DNA load distributions and heterogeneous EBV mRNA expression patterns in the circulation of solid organ versus stem cell transplant recipients. Clin Dev Immunol. 2012;2012:1–10.
48. Tsai DE, Douglas L, Andreadis C, Vogl DT, Arnoldi S, Kotloff R, et al. EBV PCR in the diagnosis and monitoring of posttransplant lymphoproliferative disorder: results of a two-arm prospective trial. Am J Transplant. 2008;8:1016–24.
49. Limaye AP, Huang ML, Atienza EE, Ferrenberg JM, Corey L. Detection of Epstein-Barr virus DNA in sera from transplant recipients with lymphoproliferative disorders. J Clin Microbiol. 1999;37:1113–6.
50. Burns DM, Tierney R, Shannon-Lowe C, Croudace J, Inman C, Abbotts B, et al. Memory B-cell reconstitution following allogeneic hematopoietic stem cell transplantation is an EBV-associated transformation event. Blood. 2015;126:2665–75.
51. Amiel C, LeGoff J, Lescure FX, Coste-Burel M, Deback C, Fafi-Kremer S, et al. Epstein-Barr Virus load in whole blood correlates with HIV surrogate markers and lymphoma: a French National Cross-Sectional Study. JAIDS J Acquir Immune Defic Syndr. 2009;50:427–9.
52. Bekker V, Scherpbier H, Beld M, Piriou E, van Breda A, Lange J, et al. Epstein-Barr Virus infects B and non-B lymphocytes in HIV-1–infected children and adolescents. J Infect Dis. 2006;194:1323–30.
53. Bressollette-Bodin C, Coste-Burel M, Besse B, André-Garnier E, Ferre V, Imbert-Marcille B-M. Cellular normalization of viral DNA loads on whole blood improves the clinical management of cytomegalovirus or Epstein Barr virus infections in the setting of pre-emptive therapy. J Med Virol. 2009;81:90–8.
54. Kinch A, Öberg G, Arvidson J, Falk KI, Linde A, Pauksens K. Post-transplant lymphoproliferative disease and other Epstein-Barr virus diseases in allogeneic haematopoietic stem cell transplantation after introduction of monitoring of viral load by polymerase chain reaction. Scand J Infect Dis. 2007;39:235–44.
55. Wada K, Kubota N, Ito Y, Yagasaki H, Kato K, Yoshikawa T, et al. Simultaneous quantification of Epstein-Barr Virus, cytomegalovirus, and human herpesvirus 6 DNA in samples from transplant recipients by multiplex real-time PCR assay. J Clin Microbiol. 2007;45:1426–32.
56. Ruf S, Behnke-Hall K, Gruhn B, Bauer J, Horn M, Beck J, et al. Comparison of six different specimen types for Epstein-Barr viral load quantification in peripheral blood of pediatric patients after heart transplantation or after allogeneic hematopoietic stem cell transplantation. J Clin Virol. Elsevier B.V. 2012;53:186–94.
57. Ishihara M, Tanaka E, Sato T, Chikamoto H, Hisano M, Akioka Y, et al. Epstein-Barr virus load for early detection of lymphoproliferative disorder in pediatric renal transplant recipients. Clin Nephrol. 2011;76:40–8.
58. Stevens SJC, Verschuuren EAM, Pronk I, van der Bij W, Harmsen MC, The TH, et al. Frequent monitoring of Epstein-Barr virus DNA load in unfractionated whole blood is essential for early detection of posttransplant lymphoproliferative disease in high-risk patients. Blood. 2001;97:1165–71.
59. Stevens SJC, Pronk I, Middeldorp JM. Toward standardization of Epstein-Barr virus DNA load monitoring: unfractionated whole blood as preferred clinical specimen. J Clin Microbiol. 2001;39:1211–6.
60. Bakker NA, Verschuuren EA, Veeger NJ, van der Bij W, van Imhoff GW, Kallenberg CG, et al. Quantification of Epstein-Barr Virus–DNA load in lung transplant recipients: a comparison of plasma versus whole blood. J Hear Lung Transpl. 2008;27:7–10.
61. Hakim H, Gibson C, Pan J, Srivastava K, Gu Z, Bankowski MJ, et al. Comparison of various blood compartments and reporting units for the detection and quantification of Epstein-Barr Virus in peripheral blood. J Clin Microbiol. 2007;45:2151–5.

62. Loginov R, Aalto S, Piiparinen H, Halme L, Arola J, Hedman K, et al. Monitoring of EBV-DNAemia by quantitative real-time PCR after adult liver transplantation. J Clin Virol. 2006;37:104–8.
63. Wadowsky RM, Laus S, Green M, Webber SA, Rowe D. Measurement of Epstein-Barr Virus DNA loads in whole blood and plasma by TaqMan PCR and in peripheral blood lymphocytes by competitive PCR. J Clin Microbiol. 2003;41:5245–9.
64. Kullberg-Lindh C, Olofsson S, Brune M, Lindh M. Comparison of serum and whole blood levels of cytomegalovirus and Epstein-Barr virus DNA. Transpl Infect Dis. 2008;10:308–15.
65. Wagner HJ, Wessel M, Jabs W, Smets F, Fischer L, Offner G, et al. Patients at risk for development of posttransplant lymphoproliferative disorder: plasma versus peripheral blood mononuclear cells as material for quantification of Epstein-Barr viral load by using real-time quantitative polymerase chain reaction. Transplantation. 2001;72:1012–9.
66. Wagner H-J, Fischer L, Jabs WJ, Holbe M, Pethig K, Bucsky P. Longitudinal analysis of Epstein-Barr viral load in plasma and peripheral blood mononuclear cells of transplanted patients by real-time polymerase chain reaction. Transplantation. 2002;74:656–64.
67. Fafi-Kremer S, Brengel-Pesce K, Barguès G, Bourgeat M-J, Genoulaz O, Seigneurin J-M, et al. Assessment of automated DNA extraction coupled with real-time PCR for measuring Epstein–Barr virus load in whole blood, peripheral mononuclear cells and plasma. J Clin Virol. 2004;30:157–64.
68. Kanakry JA, Hegde AM, Durand CM, Massie AB, Greer AE, Ambinder RF, et al. The clinical significance of EBV DNA in the plasma and peripheral blood mononuclear cells of patients with or without EBV diseases. Blood. 2016;127:2007–17.
69. Tsai DE, Nearey M, Hardy CL, Tomaszewski JE, Kotloff RM, Grossman RA, et al. Use of EBV PCR for the diagnosis and monitoring of post-transplant lymphoproliferative disorder in adult solid organ transplant patients. Am J Transplant. 2002;2:946–54.
70. Fafi-Kremer S, Morand P, Barranger C, Barguès G, Magro S, Bés J, et al. Evaluation of the Epstein-Barr Virus R-gene quantification kit in whole blood with different extraction methods and PCR platforms. J Mol Diagn. 2008;10:78–84.
71. Wagner HJ, Jabs W, Smets F, Wessel M, Fischer L, Offner G, et al. Real-time polymerase chain reaction (RQ-PCR) for the monitoring of Epstein-Barr virus (EBV) load in peripheral blood mononuclear cells. Klin Padiatr. 2000;212:206–10.
72. Jabs WJ, Hennig H, Kittel M, Pethig K, Smets F, Bucsky P, et al. Normalized quantification by real-time PCR of Epstein-Barr Virus load in patients at risk for posttransplant lymphoproliferative disorders. J Clin Microbiol. 2001;39:564–9.
73. Lee T-H, Montalvo L, Chrebtow V, Busch MP. Quantitation of genomic DNA in plasma and serum samples: higher concentrations of genomic DNA found in serum than in plasma. Transfusion. 2001;41:276–82.
74. Lazzarotto T, Chiereghin A, Piralla A, Piccirilli G, Girello A, Campanini G, et al. Cytomegalovirus and Epstein-Barr Virus DNA kinetics in whole blood and plasma of allogeneic hematopoietic stem cell transplantation recipients. Biol Blood Marrow Transpl. Elsevier Inc. 2018;24:1699–706.
75. Kullberg-Lindh C, Saalman R, Olausson M, Herlenius G, Lindh M. Epstein-Barr virus DNA monitoring in serum and whole blood in pediatric liver transplant recipients who do or do not discontinue immunosuppressive therapy. Pediatr Transplant. 2017;21:e12875.
76. Morton M, Coupes B, Roberts SA, Johnson SL, Klapper PE, Vallely PJ, et al. Epstein-Barr virus infection in adult renal transplant recipients. Am J Transplant. 2014;14:1619–29.
77. Höcker B, Fickenscher H, Delecluse H-J, Böhm S, Küsters U, Schnitzler P, et al. Epidemiology and morbidity of Epstein-Barr Virus infection in pediatric renal transplant recipients: a multicenter. Prospective Study. Clin Infect Dis. 2013;56:84–92.
78. van Esser JWJ, Niesters HGM, van der Holt B, Meijer E, Osterhaus ADME, Gratama JW, et al. Prevention of Epstein-Barr virus–lymphoproliferative disease by molecular monitoring and preemptive rituximab in high-risk patients after allogeneic stem cell transplantation. Blood. 2002;99:4364–9.

79. Omar H, Hägglund H, Gustafsson-Jernberg Å, LeBlanc K, Mattsson J, Remberger M, et al. Targeted monitoring of patients at high risk of post-transplant lymphoproliferative disease by quantitative Epstein-Barr virus polymerase chain reaction. Transpl Infect Dis. 2009;11:393–9.

80. Peters AC, Akinwumi MS, Cervera C, Mabilangan C, Ghosh S, Lai R, et al. The changing epidemiology of posttransplant lymphoproliferative disorder in adult solid organ transplant recipients over 30 years. Transplantation. 2018;102:1553–62.

81. Cook L, Starr K, Boonyaratanakornkit J, Hayden R, Sam SS, Caliendo AM. Does size matter? Comparison of extraction yields for different-sized DNA fragments by seven different routine and four new circulating cell-free extraction methods. Tang Y-W, editor. J Clin Microbiol. 2018;56:1–13.

82. Niesters HGM, van Esser J, Fries E, Wolthers KC, Cornelissen J, Osterhaus ADME. Development of a real-time quantitative assay for detection of Epstein-Barr virus. J Clin Microbiol. 2000;38:712–5.

83. Kalra A, Roessner C, Jupp J, Williamson T, Tellier R, Chaudhry A, et al. Epstein-Barr virus DNAemia monitoring for the management of post-transplant lymphoproliferative disorder. Cytotherapy. Elsevier Inc. 2018;20:706–14.

84. Styczynski J, Gil L, Tridello G, Ljungman P, Donnelly JP, van der Velden W, et al. Response to rituximab-based therapy and risk factor analysis in Epstein Barr virus–related lymphoproliferative disorder after hematopoietic stem cell transplant in children and adults: a study from the infectious diseases working Party of the European Gro. Clin Infect Dis. 2013;57:794–802.

85. van Esser JWJ, Niesters HGM, Thijsen SFT, Meijer E, Osterhaus ADME, Wolthers KC, et al. Molecular quantification of viral load in plasma allows for fast and accurate prediction of response to therapy of Epstein-Barr virus-associated lymphoproliferative disease after allogeneic stem cell transplantation. Br J Haematol. 2001;113:814–21.

86. Yang J, Tao Q, Flinn IW, Murray PG, Post LE, Ma H, et al. Characterization of Epstein-Barr virus–infected B cells in patients with posttransplantation lymphoproliferative disease: disappearance after rituximab therapy does not predict clinical response. Blood. 2000;96:4055–63.

87. Oertel S, Trappe RU, Zeidler K, Babel N, Reinke P, Hummel M, et al. Epstein–Barr viral load in whole blood of adults with posttransplant lymphoproliferative disorder after solid organ transplantation does not correlate with clinical course. Ann Hematol. 2006;85:478–84.

88. Caillard S, Lamy FX, Quelen C, Dantal J, Lebranchu Y, Lang P, et al. Epidemiology of posttransplant lymphoproliferative disorders in adult kidney and kidney pancreas recipients: report of the French registry and analysis of subgroups of lymphomas. Am J Transplant. 2012;12:682–93.

89. Halliday N, Smith C, Atkinson C, O'Beirne J, Patch D, Burroughs AK, et al. Characteristics of Epstein-Barr viraemia in adult liver transplant patients: a retrospective cohort study. Transpl Int. 2014;27:838–46.

90. Schaffer K, Hassan J, Staines A, Coughlan S, Holder P, Tuite G, et al. Surveillance of Epstein-Barr virus loads in adult liver transplantation: associations with age, sex, posttransplant times, and transplant indications. Liver Transpl. 2011;17:1420–6.

91. Bamoulid J, Courivaud C, Coaquette A, Chalopin J-M, Gaiffe E, Saas P, et al. Subclinical Epstein-Barr Virus Viremia among adult renal transplant recipients: incidence and consequences. Am J Transplant. 2013;13:656–62.

92. Colombini E, Guzzo I, Morolli F, Longo G, Russo C, Lombardi A, et al. Viral load of EBV DNAemia is a predictor of EBV-related post-transplant lymphoproliferative disorders in pediatric renal transplant recipients. Pediatr Nephrol. 2017;32:1433–42.

93. L'Huillier AG, Dipchand AI, Ng VL, Hebert D, Avitzur Y, Solomon M, et al. Posttransplant lymphoproliferative disorder in pediatric patients: characteristics of disease in EBV-seropositive recipients. Transplantation. 2019;103:e369–74.

94. Gullett JC, Nolte FS. Quantitative nucleic acid amplification methods for viral infections. Clin Chem. 2015;61:72–8.

95. Preiksaitis JK, Pang XL, Fox JD, Fenton JM, Caliendo AM, Miller GG. Interlaboratory comparison of Epstein-Barr Virus viral load assays. Am J Transplant. 2009;9:269–79.

96. Perandin F, Cariani E, Pollara C, Manca N. Comparison of commercial and in-house real-time PCR assays for quantification of Epstein-Barr virus (EBV) DNA in plasma. BMC Microbiol. 2007;7:22.
97. Le QT, Zhang Q, Cao H, Cheng AJ, Pinsky BA, Hong RL, et al. An international collaboration to harmonize the quantitative plasma Epstein-Barr virus DNA assay for future biomarker-guided trials in nasopharyngeal carcinoma. Clin Cancer Res. 2013;19:2208–15.
98. Ruiz G, Pena P, de Ory F, Echevarria JE. Comparison of commercial real-time PCR assays for quantification of Epstein-Barr Virus DNA. J Clin Microbiol. 2005;43:2053–7.
99. Hayden RT, Hokanson KM, Pounds SB, Bankowski MJ, Belzer SW, Carr J, et al. Multicenter comparison of different real-time PCR assays for quantitative detection of Epstein-Barr Virus. J Clin Microbiol. 2008;46:157–63.
100. Germi R, Lupo J, Semenova T, Larrat S, Magnat N, Grossi L, et al. Comparison of commercial extraction systems and PCR assays for quantification of Epstein-Barr Virus DNA load in whole blood. J Clin Microbiol. 2012;50:1384–9.
101. Ahsanuddin AN, Standish MC, Caliendo AM, Hill CE, Nolte FS. Validation of an Epstein-Barr viral load assay using the QIAGEN Artus EBV TM PCR analyte-specific reagent. Am J Clin Pathol. 2008;130:865–9.
102. Ito Y, Takakura S, Ichiyama S, Ueda M, Ando Y, Matsuda K, et al. Multicenter evaluation of prototype real-time PCR assays for Epstein-Barr virus and cytomegalovirus DNA in whole blood samples from transplant recipients. Microbiol Immunol. 2010;54:516–22.
103. Yen-Lieberman B, Brambilla D, Jackson B, Bremer J, Coombs R, Cronin M, et al. Evaluation of a quality assurance program for quantitation of human immunodeficiency virus type 1 RNA in plasma by the AIDS Clinical Trials Group virology laboratories. J Clin Microbiol. 1996;34:2695–701.
104. Vesper HW, Miller WG, Myers GL. Reference materials and commutability. Clin Biochem Rev. 2007;28:139–47.
105. Tang L, Sun Y, Buelow D, Gu Z, Caliendo AM, Pounds S, et al. Quantitative assessment of commutability for clinical viral load testing using a digital PCR-based reference standard. McAdam AJ, editor. J Clin Microbiol. 2016;54:1616–23.
106. Tang L, Su Y, Pounds S, Hayden RT. Quantitative inference of commutability for clinical viral load testing. Tang Y-W, editor. J Clin Microbiol. 2018;56:1–3.
107. Hayden RT, Preiksaitis J, Tong Y, Pang X, Sun Y, Tang L, et al. Commutability of the first World Health Organization international standard for human cytomegalovirus. Loeffelholz MJ, editor. J Clin Microbiol. 2015;53:3325–33.
108. Preiksaitis JK, Hayden RT, Tong Y, Pang XL, Fryer JF, Heath AB, et al. Are we there yet? Impact of the first international standard for cytomegalovirus DNA on the harmonization of results reported on plasma samples. Clin Infect Dis. 2016;63:583–9.
109. Hayden RT, Sun Y, Tang L, Procop GW, Hillyard DR, Pinsky BA, et al. Progress in quantitative viral load testing: variability and impact of the WHO quantitative international standards. McAdam AJ, editor. J Clin Microbiol. 2017;55:423–30.
110. San-Juan R, Manuel O, Hirsch HH, Fernández-Ruiz M, López-Medrano F, Comoli P, et al. Current preventive strategies and management of Epstein–Barr virus-related post-transplant lymphoproliferative disease in solid organ transplantation in Europe. Results of the ESGICH questionnaire-based cross-sectional survey. Clin Microbiol Infect. Elsevier Ltd. 2015;21:604.e1–9.
111. Abbate I, Piralla A, Calvario A, Callegaro A, Giraldi C, Lunghi G, et al. Nation-wide measure of variability in HCMV, EBV and BKV DNA quantification among centers involved in monitoring transplanted patients. J Clin Virol. 2016;82:76–83.
112. Semenova T, Lupo J, Alain S, Perrin-Confort G, Grossi L, Dimier J, et al. Multicenter evaluation of whole-blood Epstein-Barr viral load standardization using the WHO international standard. Tang Y-W, editor. J Clin Microbiol. 2016;54:1746–50.
113. Rychert J, Danziger-Isakov L, Yen-Lieberman B, Storch G, Buller R, Sweet SC, et al. Multicenter comparison of laboratory performance in cytomegalovirus and Epstein-Barr virus viral load testing using international standards. Clin Transpl. 2014;28:1416–23.

114. Kuypers J, Jerome KR. Applications of digital PCR for clinical microbiology. Kraft CS, editor. J Clin Microbiol. 2017;55:1621–8.
115. Kim H, Hur M, Kim JY, Moon HW, Yun YM, Cho HC. Automated nucleic acid extraction systems for detecting Cytomegalovirus and Epstein-Barr virus using real-time PCR: a comparison study between the QIAsymphony RGQ and QIAcube systems. Ann Lab Med. 2017;37:129–36.
116. Hayden RT, Yan X, Wick MT, Rodriguez AB, Xiong X, Ginocchio CC, et al. Factors contributing to variability of quantitative viral PCR results in proficiency testing samples: a multivariate analysis. J Clin Microbiol. 2012;50:337–45.
117. Kim KY, Le QT, Yom SS, Pinsky BA, Bratman SV, Ng RHW, et al. Current state of PCR-based Epstein-Barr virus DNA testing for nasopharyngeal cancer. J Natl Cancer Inst. 2017;109:1–7.
118. Sanosyan A, Fayd'herbe de Maudave A, Bollore K, Zimmermann V, Foulongne V, Van de Perre P, et al. The impact of targeting repetitive BamHI-W sequences on the sensitivity and precision of EBV DNA quantification. Horwitz MS, editor. PLoS One. 2017;12:e0183856.
119. Le QT, Jones CD, Yau TK, Shirazi HA, Wong PH, Thomas EN, et al. A comparison study of different PCR assays in measuring circulating plasma Epstein-Barr virus DNA levels in patients with nasopharyngeal carcinoma. Clin Cancer Res. 2005;11:5700–7.
120. Baron A, Gicquel A, Plantier J-C, Gueudin M. Evaluation of four commercial extraction-quantification systems to monitor EBV or CMV viral load in whole blood. J Clin Virol. Elsevier. 2019;113:39–44.
121. Ryan JL, Fan H, Glaser SL, Schichman SA, Raab-Traub N, Gulley ML. Epstein-Barr virus quantitation by real-time PCR targeting multiple gene segments. J Mol Diagn. Association of Molecular Pathology. 2004;6:378–85.
122. Kanda T, Yajima M, Ikuta K. Epstein-Barr virus strain variation and cancer. Cancer Sci. Blackwell Publishing Ltd. 2019;110:1132–9.
123. Palser AL, Grayson NE, White RE, Corton C, Correia S, Ba Abdullah MM, et al. Genome diversity of Epstein-Barr Virus from multiple tumor types and normal infection. Longnecker RM, editor. J Virol. American Society for Microbiology. 2015;89:5222–37.
124. Neves M, Marinho-Dias J, Ribeiro J, Sousa H. Epstein-Barr virus strains and variations: geographic or disease-specific variants? J Med Virol. 2017;89:373–87.
125. Correia S, Bridges R, Wegner F, Venturini C, Palser A, Middeldorp JM, et al. Sequence variation of Epstein-Barr Virus: viral types, geography, codon usage, and diseases. Longnecker RM, editor. J Virol. American Society for Microbiology. 2018;92:e01132.
126. Santpere G, Darre F, Blanco S, Alcami A, Villoslada P, Mar Albà M, et al. Genome-wide analysis of wild-type Epstein–Barr Virus genomes derived from healthy individuals of the 1000 genomes project. Genome Biol Evol. 2014;6:846–60.
127. Navarro E, Serrano-Heras G, Castaño MJ, Solera J. Real-time PCR detection chemistry. Clin Chim Acta. Elsevier BV. 2015;439:231–50.
128. Moran J, Carr M, Waters A, Boyle S, Riordan M, Connell J, et al. Epstein-Barr Virus gene expression, human leukocyte antigen alleles and chronic high viral loads in pediatric renal transplant patients. Transplantation. 2011;92:328–33.
129. Ruf S, Behnke-Hall K, Gruhn B, Reiter A, Wagner HJ. EBV load in whole blood correlates with LMP2 gene expression after pediatric heart transplantation or allogeneic hematopoietic stem cell transplantation. Transplantation. 2014;97:958–64.
130. Kroll J, Li S, Levi M, Weinberg A. Lytic and latent EBV gene expression in transplant recipients with and without post-transplant lymphoproliferative disorder. J Clin Virol. Elsevier BV. 2011;52:231–5.
131. Qu L, Green M, Webber S, Reyes J, Ellis D, Rowe D. Epstein-Barr Virus gene expression in the peripheral blood of transplant recipients with persistent circulating virus loads. J Infect Dis. 2000;182:1013–21.
132. Hopwood PA, Brooks L, Parratt R, Hunt BJ, Maria B, Alero TJ, et al. Persistent Epstein-Barr virus infection: unrestricted latent and lytic viral gene expression in healthy immunosuppressed transplant recipients1. Transplantation. 2002;74:194–202.

133. Kasztelewicz B, Jankowska I, Pawłowska J, Teisseyre J, Dzierżanowska-Fangrat K. Epstein-Barr virus gene expression and latent membrane protein 1 gene polymorphism in pediatric liver transplant recipients. J Med Virol. 2011;83:2182–90.
134. Zawilinska B, Kosinska A, Lenart M, Kopec J, Piatkowska-Jakubas B, Skotnicki A, et al. Detection of specific lytic and latent transcripts can help to predict the status of Epstein-Barr virus infection in transplant recipients with high virus load. Acta Biochim Pol. 2008;55:693–9.
135. Münz C. Latency and lytic replication in Epstein–Barr virus-associated oncogenesis. Nat Rev Microbiol. Springer US. 2019;17:691–700.
136. Kawano Y, Iwata S, Kawada J, Gotoh K, Suzuki M, Torii Y, et al. Plasma viral MicroRNA profiles reveal potential biomarkers for chronic active Epstein–Barr Virus infection. J Infect Dis. 2013;208:771–9.
137. Kaul V, Weinberg KI, Boyd SD, Bernstein D, Esquivel CO, Martinez OM, et al. Dynamics of viral and host immune cell microRNA expression during acute infectious mononucleosis. Front Microbiol. 2018;8:1–9.
138. Bergallo M, Gambarino S, Pinon M, Barat V, Montanari P, Daprà V, et al. EBV-encoded microRNAs profile evaluation in pediatric liver transplant recipients. J Clin Virol. Elsevier. 2017;91:36–41.
139. Hassan J, Dean J, De Gascun CF, Riordan M, Sweeney C, Connell J, et al. Plasma EBV microRNAs in paediatric renal transplant recipients. J Nephrol Springer International Publishing. 2018;31:445–51.
140. Yanagisawa K, Tanuma J, Hagiwara S, Gatanaga H, Kikuchi Y, Oka S. Epstein-Barr Viral load in cerebrospinal fluid as a diagnostic marker of central nervous system involvement of AIDS-related lymphoma. Intern Med. 2013;52:955–9.
141. Ivers LC, Kim AY, Sax PE. Predictive value of polymerase chain reaction of cerebrospinal fluid for detection of Epstein-Barr Virus to establish the diagnosis of HIV-related primary central nervous system lymphoma. Clin Infect Dis. 2004;38:1629–32.
142. Corcoran C, Rebe K, van der Plas H, Myer L, Hardie DR. The predictive value of cerebrospinal fluid Epstein-Barr viral load as a marker of primary central nervous system lymphoma in HIV-infected persons. J Clin Virol. 2008;42:433–6.
143. Bossolasco S, Cinque P, Ponzoni M, Vigano MG, Lazzarin A, Linde A, et al. Epstein-Barr virus DNA load in cerebrospinal fluid and plasma of patients with AIDS-related lymphoma. J Neurovirol. 2002;8:432–8.
144. Weinberg A, Li S, Palmer M, Tyler KL. Quantitative CSF PCR in Epstein-Barr virus infections of the central nervous system. Ann Neurol. 2002;52:543–8.
145. Liu Q-F, Ling Y-W, Fan Z-P, Jiang Q-L, Sun J, Wu X-L, et al. Epstein-Barr virus (EBV) load in cerebrospinal fluid and peripheral blood of patients with EBV-associated central nervous system diseases after allogeneic hematopoietic stem cell transplantation. Transpl Infect Dis. 2013;15:379–92.
146. Michelson P, Watkins B, Webber SA, Wadowsky R, Michaels MG. Screening for PTLD in lung and heart-lung transplant recipients by measuring EBV DNA load in bronchoalveolar lavage fluid using real time PCR. Pediatr Transplant. 2008;12:464–8.
147. Parrish A, Fenchel M, Storch GA, Buller R, Mason S, Williams N, et al. Epstein-Barr viral loads do not predict post-transplant lymphoproliferative disorder in pediatric lung transplant recipients: a multicenter prospective cohort study. Pediatr Transplant. 2017;21:e13011.
148. Bauer CC, Jaksch P, Aberle SW, Haber H, Lang G, Klepetko W, et al. Relationship between cytomegalovirus DNA load in epithelial lining fluid and plasma of lung transplant recipients and analysis of coinfection with Epstein-Barr virus and human herpesvirus 6 in the lung compartment. J Clin Microbiol. 2007;45:324–8.
149. Costa C, Elia M, Astegiano S, Sidoti F, Terlizzi ME, Solidoro P, et al. Quantitative detection of Epstein-Barr Virus in Bronchoalveolar lavage from transplant and nontransplant patients. Transplantation. 2008;86:1389–94.
150. Preiksaitis JK, Diaz-Mitoma F, Mirzayans F, Roberts S, Tyrrell DLJ. Quantitative oropharyngeal Epstein-Barr Virus shedding in renal and cardiac transplant recipients: relationship to

immunosuppressive therapy, serologic responses, and the risk of posttransplant lymphoproliferative disorder. J Infect Dis. 1992;166:986–94.
151. Johnson KH, Webb C-H, Schmeling DO, Brundage RC, Balfour HH. Epstein–Barr virus
dynamics in asymptomatic immunocompetent adults: an intensive 6-month study. Clin Transl
Immunol. 2016;5:e81.
152. Balfour HH, Hokanson KM, Schacherer RM, Fietzer CM, Schmeling DO, Holman CJ,
et al. A virologic pilot study of valacyclovir in infectious mononucleosis. J Clin Virol.
2007;39:16–21.
153. Hadinoto V, Shapiro M, Sun CC, Thorley-Lawson DA. The dynamics of EBV shedding
implicate a central role for epithelial cells in amplifying viral output. Speck SH, editor. PLoS
Pathog. 2009;5:e1000496.
154. Yager JE, Magaret AS, Kuntz SR, Selke S, Huang M-L, Corey L, et al. Valganciclovir for the
suppression of Epstein-Barr virus replication. J Infect Dis. 2017;216:198–202.
155. Ling PD, Lednicky JA, Keitel WA, Poston DG, White ZS, Peng R, et al. The dynamics of
herpesvirus and polyomavirus reactivation and shedding in healthy adults: a 14-month longitudinal study. J Infect Dis. 2003;187:1571–80.
156. Haque T, Crawford DH. PCR amplification is more sensitive than tissue culture methods for
Epstein-Barr virus detection in clinical material. J Gen Virol. 1997;78:3357–60.
157. Ikuta K, Satoh Y, Hoshikawa Y, Sairenji T. Detection of Epstein-Barr virus in salivas and
throat washings in healthy adults and children. Microbes Infect. 2000;2:115–20.
158. Balfour HH, Odumade OA, Schmeling DO, Mullan BD, Ed JA, Knight JA, et al. Behavioral,
Virologic, and immunologic factors associated with acquisition and severity of primary
Epstein–Barr virus infection in university students. J Infect Dis. 2013;207:80–8.
159. Grimm JM, Schmeling DO, Dunmire SK, Knight JA, Mullan BD, Ed JA, et al. Prospective
studies of infectious mononucleosis in university students. Clin Transl Immunol. Nature
Publishing Group. 2016;5:e94.
160. Dunmire SK, Grimm JM, Schmeling DO, Balfour HH, Hogquist KA. The incubation period
of primary Epstein-Barr virus infection: viral dynamics and immunologic events. Ling PD,
editor. PLOS Pathog. Public Library of Science. 2015;11:e1005286.
161. Yao QY, Rickinson AB, Gaston JSH, Epstein MA. In vitro analysis of the Epstein-Barr virus:
host balance in long-term renal allograft recipients. Int J Cancer. 1985;35:43–9.
162. Verghese PS, Schmeling DO, Filtz EA, Grimm JM, Matas AJ, Balfour HH. Transplantation
of solid organ recipients shedding Epstein-Barr virus DNA pre-transplant: a prospective
study. Clin Transpl. 2017;31:e13116.
163. Styczynski J, Van Der Velden W, Fox CP, Engelhard D, De La Camara R, Cordonnier C, et al.
Management of Epstein-Barr virus infections and post-transplant lymphoproliferative disorders in patients after allogeneic hematopoietic stem cell transplantation: sixth European conference on infections in leukemia (ECIL-6) guidelines. Haematologica. 2016;101:803–11.
164. Hoagland CRJ. The transmission of infectious mononucleosis. Am J Med Sci. Elsevier
BV. 1955;229:262–72.
165. Svedmyr E, Ernberg I, Seeley J, Weiland O, Masucci G, Tsukuda K, et al. Virologic, immunologic, and clinical observations on a patient during the incubation, acute, and convalescent
phases of infectious mononucleosis. Clin Immunol Immunopathol. 1984;30:437–50.
166. Hadinoto V, Shapiro M, Greenough TC, Sullivan JL, Luzuriaga K, Thorley-Lawson DA. On
the dynamics of acute EBV infection and the pathogenesis of infectious mononucleosis.
Blood. 2008;111:1420–7.
167. Jayasooriya S, de Silva TI, Njie-jobe J, Sanyang C, Leese AM, Bell AI, et al. Early virological and immunological events in asymptomatic Epstein-Barr virus infection in African
children. Rochford R, editor. PLoS Pathog. 2015;11:e1004746.
168. Piriou E, Asito AS, Sumba PO, Fiore N, Middeldorp JM, Moormann AM, et al. Early age
at time of primary Epstein–Barr virus infection results in poorly controlled viral infection in
infants from Western Kenya: clues to the etiology of endemic Burkitt lymphoma. J Infect Dis.
2012;205:906–13.

169. Chan K, Tam JS, Peiris JS, Seto W, Ng M. Epstein–Barr virus (EBV) infection in infancy. J Clin Virol. 2001;21:57–62.
170. Jenson HB, Montalvo EA, McClain KL, Ench Y, Heard P, Christy BA, et al. Characterization of natural Epstein-Barr virus infection and replication in smooth muscle cells from a leiomyosarcoma. J Med Virol. 1999;57:36–46.
171. Biggar RJ, Henle G, Böcker J, Lennette ET, Fleisher G, Henle W. Primary Epstein-Barr virus infections in African infants. II. Clinical and serological observations during seroconversion. Int J Cancer. 1978;22:244–50.
172. Reynaldi A, Schlub TE, Piriou E, Ogolla S, Sumba OP, Moormann AM, et al. Modeling of EBV infection and antibody responses in Kenyan infants with different levels of malaria exposure shows maternal antibody decay is a major determinant of early EBV infection. J Infect Dis. 2016;214:1390–8.
173. Burton C, Mabilangan C, Preiksaitis J. Incidence of Epstein Barr Virus (EBV) DNAemia in EBV seronegative solid organ transplant (SOT) recipients with EBV seropositive donors. Am J Transplant. 2018;17:756.
174. Ville S, Imbert-Marcille B-M, Coste-Burel M, Garandeau C, Meurette A, Cantarovitch D, et al. Impact of antiviral prophylaxis in adults Epstein-Barr Virus-seronegative kidney recipients on early and late post-transplantation lymphoproliferative disorder onset: a retrospective cohort study. Transpl Int. 2018;31:484–94.
175. Yamada M, Nguyen C, Fadakar P, Ganoza A, Humar A, Shapiro R, et al. Epidemiology and outcome of chronic high Epstein-Barr viral load carriage in pediatric kidney transplant recipients. Pediatr Transplant. 2018;22:e13147.
176. Liu Q, Xuan L, Liu H, Huang F, Zhou H, Fan Z, et al. Molecular monitoring and stepwise preemptive therapy for Epstein-Barr virus viremia after allogeneic stem cell transplantation. Am J Hematol. 2013;88:550–5.
177. Hoshino Y, Nishikawa K, Ito Y, Kuzushima K, Kimura H. Kinetics of Epstein-Barr virus load and virus-specific CD8+ T cells in acute infectious mononucleosis. J Clin Virol. 2011;50:244–6.
178. Nakai H, Kawamura Y, Sugata K, Sugiyama H, Enomoto Y, Asano Y, et al. Host factors associated with the kinetics of Epstein-Barr virus DNA load in patients with primary Epstein-Barr virus infection. Microbiol Immunol. 2012;56:93–8.
179. Dunmire SK, Verghese PS, Balfour HH. Primary Epstein-Barr virus infection. J Clin Virol. Elsevier B.V. 2018;102:84–92.
180. Abbott RJ, Pachnio A, Pedroza-Pacheco I, Leese AM, Begum J, Long HM, et al. Asymptomatic primary infection with Epstein-Barr virus: observations on young adult cases. Longnecker RM, editor. J Virol. American Society for Microbiology. 2017;91:e00382.
181. Njie R, Bell AI, Jia H, Croom-Carter D, Chaganti S, Hislop AD, et al. The effects of acute malaria on Epstein-Barr Virus (EBV) load and EBV-specific T cell immunity in Gambian children. J Infect Dis. 2009;199:31–8.
182. Silins SL, Sherritt MA, Silleri JM, Cross SM, Elliott SL, Bharadwaj M, et al. Asymptomatic primary Epstein-Barr virus infection occurs in the absence of blood T-cell repertoire perturbations despite high levels of systemic viral load. Blood. 2001;98:3739–44.
183. Riddler S, Breinig M, McKnight J. Increased levels of circulating Epstein-Barr virus (EBV)-infected lymphocytes and decreased EBV nuclear antigen antibody responses are associated with the development of posttransplant lymphoproliferative disease in solid-organ transplant recipients. Blood. 1994;84:972–84.
184. Kenagy DN, Schlesinger Y, Weck K, Ritter JH, Gaudreault-Keener MM, Storch GA. Epstein-Barr virus DNA in peripheral blood leukocytes of patients with posttransplant lymphoproliferative disease. Transplantation. 1995;60:547–54.
185. Preiksaitis JK. Epstein—Barr viral load testing: role in the prevention, diagnosis and management of posttransplant lymphoproliferative disorders. Post-transplant lymphoproliferative disord. Berlin, Heidelberg: Springer Berlin Heidelberg; 2010. p. 45–67.

186. Cho Y-U, Chi H-S, Jang S, Park SH, Park C-J. Pattern analysis of Epstein-Barr Virus viremia and its significance in the evaluation of organ transplant patients suspected of having post-transplant lymphoproliferative disorders. Am J Clin Pathol. 2014;141:268–74.
187. Manlhiot C, Pollock-BarZiv SM, Holmes C, Weitzman S, Allen U, Clarizia NA, et al. Post-transplant lymphoproliferative disorder in pediatric heart transplant recipients. J Hear Lung Transpl. Elsevier Inc. 2010;29:648–57.
188. Fox CP, Burns D, Parker AN, Peggs KS, Harvey CM, Natarajan S, et al. EBV-associated post-transplant lymphoproliferative disorder following in vivo T-cell-depleted allogeneic transplantation: clinical features, viral load correlates and prognostic factors in the rituximab era. Bone Marrow Transpl. Nature Publishing Group. 2014;49:280–6.
189. Solano C, Mateo EM, Pérez A, Talaya A, Terol MJ, Albert E, et al. Epstein-Barr virus DNA load kinetics analysis in allogeneic hematopoietic stem cell transplant recipients: is it of any clinical usefulness? J Clin Virol. Elsevier. 2017;97:26–32.
190. Carvalho-Queiroz C, Johansson MA, Persson J-O, Jörtsö E, Kjerstadius T, Nilsson C, et al. Associations between EBV and CMV seropositivity, early exposures, and gut microbiota in a prospective birth cohort: a 10-year follow-up. Front Pediatr. 2016;4:93.
191. Balfour HH, Sifakis F, Sliman JA, Knight JA, Schmeling DO, Thomas W. Age-specific prevalence of Epstein–Barr Virus infection among individuals aged 6–19 years in the United States and factors affecting its acquisition. J Infect Dis. 2013;208:1286–93.
192. Reynaldi A, Schlub TE, Chelimo K, Sumba PO, Piriou E, Ogolla S, et al. Impact of Plasmodium falciparum coinfection on longitudinal Epstein-Barr Virus kinetics in Kenyan children. J Infect Dis. 2016;213:985–91.
193. Donati D, Espmark E, Kironde F, Mbidde EK, Kamya M, Lundkvist Å, et al. Clearance of circulating Epstein-Barr virus DNA in children with acute malaria after antimalaria treatment. J Infect Dis. 2006;193:971–7.
194. Chattopadhyay PK, Chelimo K, Embury PB, Mulama DH, Sumba PO, Gostick E, et al. Holoendemic malaria exposure is associated with altered Epstein-Barr virus-specific CD8 + T-cell differentiation. J Virol. 2013;87:1779–88.
195. Ogolla S, Daud II, Asito AS, Sumba OP, Ouma C, Vulule J, et al. Reduced transplacental transfer of a subset of Epstein-Barr virus-specific antibodies to neonates of mothers infected with Plasmodium falciparum malaria during pregnancy. Pasetti MF, editor. Clin Vaccine Immunol. 2015;22:1197–205.
196. Kumar D, Patil N, Husain S, Chaparro C, Bhat M, Kim SJ, et al. Clinical and virologic outcomes in high-risk adult Epstein-Barr virus mismatched organ transplant recipients. Clin Transpl. 2017;31(7).
197. Green M, Cacciarelli TV, Mazariegos GV, Sigurdsson L, Qu L, Rowe DT, et al. Serial measurement of Epstein-Barr viral load in peripheral blood in pediatric liver transplant recipients during treatment for posttransplant lymphoproliferative disease. Transplantation. 1998;66:1641–4.
198. Khan G, Miyashita EM, Yang B, Babcock GJ, Thorley-Lawson DA. Is EBV persistence in vivo a model for B cell homeostasis? Immunity. Cell Press. 1996;5:173–9.
199. Stowe RP, Kozlova EV, Yetman DL, Walling DM, Goodwin JS, Glaser R. Chronic herpesvirus reactivation occurs in aging. Exp Gerontol. 2007;42:563–70.
200. Smatti MK, Yassine HM, AbuOdeh R, AlMarawani A, Taleb SA, Althani AA, et al. Prevalence and molecular profiling of Epstein Barr virus (EBV) among healthy blood donors from different nationalities in Qatar. Pagano JS, editor. PLoS One. Public Library of Science. 2017;12:e0189033.
201. Vescovini R, Telera A, Fagnoni FF, Biasini C, Medici MC, Valcavi P, et al. Different contribution of EBV and CMV infections in very long-term carriers to age-related alterations of CD8+ T cells. Exp Gerontol. 2004;39:1233–43.
202. Das B, Morrow R, Huang R, Fixler D. Persistent Epstein-Barr viral load in Epstein-Barr viral naïve pediatric heart transplant recipients: risk of late-onset post-transplant lymphoproliferative disease. World J Transplant. 2016;6:729.

203. Bingler MA, Feingold B, Miller SA, Quivers E, Michaels MG, Green M, et al. Chronic high Epstein-Barr viral load state and risk for late-onset posttransplant lymphoproliferative disease/lymphoma in children. Am J Transplant. 2008;8:442–5.
204. Lau AH, Soltys K, Sindhi RK, Bond G, Mazariegos GV, Green M. Chronic high Epstein-Barr viral load carriage in pediatric small bowel transplant recipients. Pediatr Transplant. 2010;14:549–53.
205. Kamei H, Ito Y, Kawada J, Ogiso S, Onishi Y, Komagome M, et al. Risk factors and long-term outcomes of pediatric liver transplant recipients with chronic high Epstein-Barr virus loads. Transpl Infect Dis. 2018;20:e12911.
206. Green M, Soltys K, Rowe DT, Webber SA, Mazareigos G. Chronic high Epstein-Barr viral load carriage in pediatric liver transplant recipients. Pediatr Transplant. 2009;13:319–23.
207. Macedo C, Webber SA, Donnenberg AD, Popescu I, Hua Y, Green M, et al. EBV-specific CD8 + T cells from asymptomatic pediatric thoracic transplant patients carrying chronic high EBV loads display contrasting features: activated phenotype and exhausted function. J Immunol. 2011;186:5854–62.
208. Moran J, Dean J, De Oliveira A, O'Connell M, Riordan M, Connell J, et al. Increased levels of PD-1 expression on CD8 T cells in patients post-renal transplant irrespective of chronic high EBV viral load. Pediatr Transplant. 2013;17:806–14.
209. Moormann AM, Chelimo K, Sumba OP, Lutzke ML, Ploutz-Snyder R, Newton D, et al. Exposure to holoendemic malaria results in elevated Epstein-Barr virus loads in children. J Infect Dis. 2005;191:1233–8.
210. Piriou E, Dort KV, Otto S, Van Oers MHJ, Van Baarle D. Tight regulation of the Epstein-Barr Virus setpoint: interindividual differences in Epstein-Barr Virus DNA load are conserved after HIV infection. Clin Infect Dis. Oxford University Press (OUP). 2008;46:313–6.
211. Piriou E, Jansen CA, van Dort K, De Cuyper I, Nanlohy NM, Lange JMA, et al. Reconstitution of EBV latent but not lytic antigen-specific CD4 + and CD8 + T cells after HIV treatment with highly active antiretroviral therapy. J Immunol. The American Association of Immunologists. 2005;175:2010–7.
212. Piriou ER, van Dort K, Nanlohy NM, Miedema F, van Oers MH, van Baarle D. Altered EBV viral load Setpoint after HIV seroconversion is in accordance with lack of predictive value of EBV load for the occurrence of AIDS-related non-Hodgkin lymphoma. J Immunol. The American Association of Immunologists. 2004;172:6931–7.
213. Hoshino Y, Katano H, Zou P, Hohman P, Marques A, Tyring SK, et al. Long-term administration of Valacyclovir reduces the number of Epstein-Barr Virus (EBV)-infected B cells but not the number of EBV DNA copies per B cell in healthy volunteers. J Virol. 2009;83:11857–61.

Part II

Clinical Considerations in Solid Organ Transplantation (SOT)

Epidemiology of PTLD After SOT

Vikas R. Dharnidharka

Introduction

This chapter is devoted to a detailed discussion of (1) the incidence of PTLD by solid organ system and over time; (2) the time to PTLD; (3) the different risk factors involved; (4) the risk for solid organ allograft loss after PTLD; (5) mortality rates after PTLD; and (6) results of re-transplantation if PTLD occurred in a prior transplant. The equivalent epidemiologic aspects of PTLD after hematopoietic stem cell transplant (HSCT) are discussed in Chap. 12. The prognostic factors for outcomes, after PTLD has been diagnosed, are covered in Chap. 8.

Note that PTLDs after solid organ transplant include several different conditions [1, 2]. Hodgkin lymphoma (HL) and non-Hodgkin lymphoma (NHL) are considered as PTLDs by the World Health Organization (WHO) classification [3, 4], but transplant registries serve as the source of most large-scale epidemiologic information on PTLDs. Some transplant registries restrict their reporting to only lymphomas [5, 6] or only NHLs [7, 8]. Transplant registries also consider indolent lymphomas (small B cell lymphomas such as follicular lymphomas or small lymphocytic lymphomas and marginal zone lymphomas) as PTLDs, but not plasma cell neoplasms (multiple myeloma and plasmacytoma). The WHO classification does the opposite, including plasma cell neoplasms under monomorphic PTLD, but does not include indolent lymphomas [3, 4]. Also, registries can have incomplete reporting, so some groups have attempted to merge different national registries to capture more PTLD cases [9, 10].

V. R. Dharnidharka (✉)
Division of Pediatric Nephrology, Hypertension and Pheresis, Washington University School of Medicine, St. Louis, MO, USA
e-mail: vikasd@wustl.edu

Incidence of PTLD

Large registry data show that *lymphoma* (a subgroup of PTLD) incidence in transplant recipients, as compared to the general population, is several-fold elevated, as shown in Table 7.1 [7, 16]. The degree of elevation in incidence varies by recipient age. Within the Australia-New Zealand database (ANZDATA) registry of kidney transplants, recipients under 35 years old had a 23–37-fold higher incidence of lymphoma. The risk dropped with each 10-year older age group, yet the above 55-year-old recipients still experienced a sixfold increase in incidence over the general population [16]. From the Germany-based multi-national Collaborative Transplant Study (CTS) registry data across multiple different organ transplants, recipients under 10 years age experienced a 200–1200-fold increased incidence [7]; recipients above 60 years age experienced 7–16-fold increases in incidence over the general population. Compared to HIV-infected patients, the increase in lymphoma risk in transplant recipients appears to be of same magnitude [17]. Table 7.1 depicts the relative increase in standardized incidence ratios separated out for different subtypes of PTLDs, but not separated out by age groups.

Since PTLD can occur at any time post-transplant and the cumulative incidence goes up over time post-transplant [18], the appropriate unit of measurement should be incidence density, not incidence per patient. Incidence density takes into account those patients whose allografts survive longer, thus increasing their chance of developing PTLD. This is a simple concept, yet rarely followed in early PTLD publications, most of which list PTLD incidence on a per patient percentage. In the Organ Procurement and Transplantation Network database in the USA, the incidence density for PTLD ranged from 1.58 per 1000 person-years (kidney) to 2.24 (heart), 2.44

Table 7.1 Relative risk, as standardized incidence ratios (SIRs), for different types of post-transplant lymphoproliferative disorders, as compared to general population

PTLD type	Grulich et al. (2007) [5]	Engels et al. (2011) [11]	Cheung et al. (2012) [12]	Engels et al. (2013) [13]	Clarke et al. (2013) [14]	Morton et al. (2014) [15]
Non-Hodgkin lymphoma	5.5, 6.0, 9.9, 8.9	7.5	15.8		6.2	
Hodgkin lymphoma		3.58			3.6	
Plasma cell neoplasms		1.8		1.8		
Multiple myeloma	2.7, 2.7, 3.8			1.4		
Plasmacytoma				7.1		

Adapted from Ref. [1]
The Grulich et al. meta-analysis displayed SIRs from several studies. All the values shown in this table were statistically significant

Table 7.2 Reported incidence density or cumulative incidence of PTLD by organ system and recipient age

Organ	Recipient age	1 year	3 years	5 years	>5 years
Kidney[1]	Adult [25–27]	0.46%	0.87%	1.18%	2.1% (10 years)
	Pediatric [28]	1.03%	2.31%	Not stated	
Liver	Adult [29]	1.1%	3%	4%	4.7% (15 years)
	Pediatric [30]			6%	
Heart[2]	Adult (ISHLT 2015 data) [31]	0.50%	Not stated	1.1%	1.8 (10 years)
	Children (ISHLT 2008 data)	1.6%	Not stated	4.5%	9.2% (10 years)
Lung[2]	Adult (ISHLT 2008 data)	1.6%	Not stated	2.1%	5.6% (10 years)
	Children (ISHLT 2014 data) [32]	5.3%		10.7%	9.2 (at 7 years)

Footnotes:
[1]Adult kidney data are from USRDS and French PTLD registry. Pediatric kidney data are from NAPRTCS registry from 2012 to 2017 (malignancy rates, most of which are PTLD)
[2]Heart and lung data from the International Society for Heart and Lung Transplantation (ISHLT) are based on recipient survival till that time point

(liver), and 5.72 (lung) [19]. In the UK, incidence density for NHL after kidney transplant was 2.6 per 1000 person-years [20]. A very high incidence density of 1800 per 100,000 patient-years of follow-up was reported in the pediatric liver transplant population in the 1980s–1990s by McDiarmid et al. [21]. Dharnidharka et al. have shown era trends in PTLD incidence density from a multicenter pediatric kidney transplant registry [22]. In the period 1987–1992, the incidence density was 320 per 100,000 patient-years [23]; this doubled to 603 per 100,000 patient-years in the time period 1993–1998 [24]. An alternative method of displaying incidence density is rate per patient per fixed time post-transplant, e.g., rate of PTLD by 1, 3, or 5 years post-transplant, as shown in Table 7.2. In the French PTLD registry, cumulative incidence was 1% by 5 years and 2.1% by 10 years [25]. The most recent national registry data from the USA show a 5-year cumulative incidence ranging from 0.7% to 9%, based on recipient EBV serostatus and type of organ transplant [33]. Cumulative incidence implies a "fixed" cohort with no losses to follow-up, a situation that is rare in transplantation, so incidence density, where losses are acceptable, is preferable.

When analyzing PTLD incidence by the more common per patient incidence, a clear trend could be seen. Initially PTLD cases were stray and anecdotal through the 1950s–1970s. This was also a time period of two-drug immunosuppression (azathioprine and prednisone) and relatively poor graft survival. After the introduction of cyclosporine A in 1983, graft survival improved dramatically, but the frequency of PTLD reports started rising [34–37]. The pediatric kidney transplant population showed a steady increase in per patient incidence from <1% to 2.2% to 6% from the early 1990s to the early 2000s [23, 38, 39]. These rises coincided with the advent of more potent immunosuppressive agents and more intense regimens, frequently incorporating an induction antibody with three-drug maintenance immunosuppression.

In contrast, in the same time period, the pediatric liver transplant population showed reductions in per patient incidence from 10% to 5% with the use of multiple interventions [40]. It is also possible that some of the increase could be better physician awareness and recognition of PTLD and better reporting. One recent study suggested a *decrease* in PTLD incidence in patients transplanted in 2007–2009 versus 2000–2003 [41].

Time to PTLD

The time to PTLD varies greatly by series, era, and organ system. In general, time to PTLD has shortened in more recent eras with more potent immunosuppression [23, 35, 37]. Early PTLDs tend to be B cell lineage proliferations and EBV positive, while late PTLDs have higher proportions of non-B cell proliferations and EBV-negative PTLDs, albeit still a minority [29, 42]. The incidence of EBV-negative PTLD may be increasing, both as a proportion and in absolute incidence [43]. Series with predominantly adult populations [26, 44, 45] show longer median times to PTLD (25–72 months) and two spikes (early and late) of incidence (Fig. 7.1a), versus series with significant pediatric populations [27, 46–48], where the median times are shorter, ranging from 5.5 to 25 months.

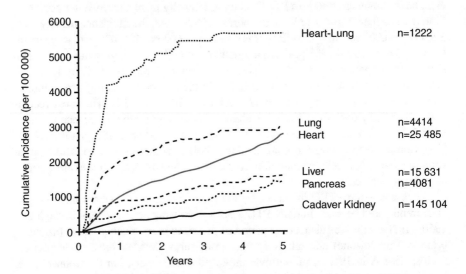

Fig. 7.1 Panel (**a**) Cumulative 5-year incidence of non-Hodgkin lymphoma by organ system, Collaborative Transplant Study [7], reproduced with permission. Panel (**b**) Incidence of PTLD by organ system, UNOS/OPTN data [38]

PTLD incidence % by organ (UNOS)

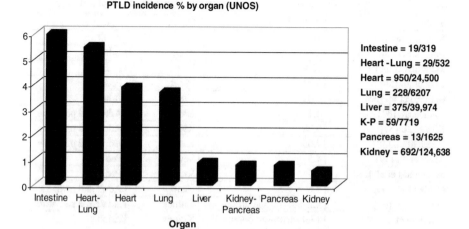

Intestine = 19/319
Heart -Lung = 29/532
Heart = 950/24,500
Lung = 228/6207
Liver = 375/39,974
K-P = 59/7719
Pancreas = 13/1625
Kidney = 692/124,638

Fig. 7.1 (continued)

Risk Factors for PTLD

There are many different risk factors for PTLD development that have been described in the medical literature. Briefly, these risk factors can be grouped under the following headings:

(a) Infectious related: Epstein-Barr virus and other infectious agents
(b) Host related
(c) Primary disease related
(d) Graft organ related
(e) Immunosuppression related

Infectious Related Risk Factors

One of the seminal events in PTLD pathogenesis was the epidemiologic linkage of PTLD risk to Epstein-Barr virus (EBV) serostatus in donor and recipient. Focus on EBV had come from the knowledge that some cases of PTLD resembled lymphomas, of which Burkitt's lymphoma was already linked to EBV. The linkage of EBV to post-transplant lymphoproliferative disease was established in the late 1970s [49, 50] and early 1980s [51, 52]. Walker et al. demonstrated that an EBV-seronegative adult recipient of a heart or lung allograft was at 24-fold higher risk for subsequent

Table 7.3 Epstein-Barr virus-associated risk ratios for PTLD or NHL development

Study	Risk ratio	Organ	Age group
Walker et al. [53]	24	Heart-lung	Adult
Cockfield et al. [54]	33	Kidney	Adult
Mendoza et al. [55]	12.84	Heart	Pediatric
Katz et al. [56]	3.94	Heart	Pediatric
Caillard et al. [26]	3.01	Kidney	Adult
Faull et al. [37]	3.1	Kidney	Adult and pediatric
Kirk et al. [57]	5.28	Kidney	Adult and pediatric
Funch et al. [58]	7.05	Kidney	Adult and pediatric
Allen et al. [59]	4.5	Several	Pediatric
McDonald et al. [39]	7.7	Kidney	Pediatric
Opelz et al. [60]	3.6	Heart	Adult and pediatric
Opelz et al. [60]	4.2–9.0 (by age group)	Kidney	Adult and pediatric
Sampaio et al. [41]	17.4 (deceased donor) 6.9 (living donor)	Kidney	Adult
Dharnidharka et al. [61]	3.58	Kidney	Adult and pediatric
Dharnidharka et al. [40]	1.48	Liver	Adult and pediatric
Dharnidharka et al. [62]	4.04	Heart	Adult and pediatric

PTLD development [53]. This finding has since been borne out by multiple other investigators in other organ type transplants and across age groups (Table 7.3). In fact, not only has this finding stood the test of time; the magnitude of risk conveyed (ranging from 3- to 33-fold in most cases) exceeds by far the magnitude of risk conveyed by any immunosuppressive agent risk factors. The reason for this strong epidemiological relationship between EBV and PTLD will become clear in Chap. 3 about the biology of EBV and pathogenesis of PTLD. EBV-positive PTLDs tend to show an early incidence spike in the first year, while EBV-negative PTLDs have a steady incidence over each year [20].

Beyond EBV, other viruses may play a role in PTLD pathogenesis. CMV co-infection or mismatch increased the risk 6–7-fold in some early studies [63, 64], but not in more recent studies [57]. A few cases of PTLD are not EBV tumor positive, and CMV co-infection cannot be documented. In these cases, it is possible that a heretofore undetected virus may play a role, though an unbiased study of PTLD tissue DNA virus genomes did not reveal any overrepresentation of other viruses [65].

With the development of peripheral blood PCR assays to measure Epstein-Barr DNAemia, the development of EB DNAemia post-transplant can also be considered a risk factor for PTLD development. This discussion is handled in great depth by Preiksaitis in Chap. 6 and hence not discussed further here.

Some PTLD types (CNS PTLD, EBV-negative PTLD, or non-B cell lineage PTLD) have different epidemiologic patterns than EBV-positive B cell PTLDs. Central nervous system localization occurs in 7–15% of PTLDs, and these have a later median time to presentation, but the majority are EBV positive [66–68].

Belatacept de novo use in EBV-seronaive transplant recipients was associated with high rates of PTLD overall, and in particular, of CNS PTLD [69].

EBV-negative PTLD comprised 33% in one series of 176 PTLDs at the University of Pennsylvania, with an increasing proportion up to 48% in more recent years [43]. The median time to presentation was later for EBV-negative PTLD and was less likely to involve the allograft and more likely monomorphic. T/NK cell PTLDs comprise 5–15% of all PTLDs, have a later median time to presentation, and are EBV positive in only 33% [70]. A meta-analysis of T cell PTLDs showed median time to presentation 72 months (versus 48 months for PTLDs in general) and median overall survival time only 6 months versus 11 months for monomorphic B cell PTLDs [71].

Host-Related Risk Factors

In data from several large registries such as the United Network for Organ Sharing/Organ Procurement and Transplantation Network (UNOS/OPTN) and North American Pediatric Renal Transplant Cooperative Studies (NAPRTCS), younger recipient age <18 years, male sex, and Caucasian race were all higher-risk factors for PTLD development individually and synergistically [38]. Hall et al. confirmed that white transplant recipients are at higher risk than black or Hispanic recipients [72]. At the other end of the age spectrum, transplant recipients above 50 or 60 years are also at higher risk for PTLD [7, 26, 47]. These host risk factors remain independently significant even after more complete reporting of donor and recipient EBV serology in the national OPTN database [57].

Caillard et al., utilizing data from the US-based United States Renal Data System (USRDS) registry, showed that pre-transplant malignancy and fewer HLA matches are also associated with higher PTLD rates [27], though one study of lung transplants showed the opposite [73]. HLA matching and specific alleles have been the subject of several studies; B mismatch, A3 allele, or Bw22 allele has all been associated with higher PTLD risk [74–76]. Most PTLDs after SOT are of recipient origin [77], but some studies have shown high proportion of donor origin also [78].

Primary Disease-Related Factors

Within the liver transplant population, some single-center series have documented certain primary liver diseases to be associated with higher risk for subsequent PTLD. These diseases include hepatitis C [79] or associated cirrhosis [47], alcoholic cirrhosis [47], autoimmune hepatitis [80], Langerhans cell histiocytosis [81], or fulminant hepatitis [29]. However, these diseases are also among the most common reasons to receive a liver transplant; hence they may have been overrepresented in individual series.

Graft Organ-Related Risk Factors

Data from the multinational CTS and the US-based OPTN/UNOS/USRDS have demonstrated differences in PTLD frequency by organ system. In general, intestinal transplants [82, 83] and thoracic organ transplants are associated with higher frequencies of PTLD, followed by liver transplants, and the lowest frequency has been in kidney transplants. From the most recent International Intestinal Transplant Registry (ITTR) report for 2003 (www.intestinaltransplant.org), the incidence of PTLD in adults was 3.3% and in children was 13.3%. Table 7.2 depicts recent incidence density or cumulative incidence data for either PTLD by organ system and recipient age at transplant. Figure 7.1 shows (A) cumulative incidence of non-Hodgkin lymphoma by organ system from the CTS or (B) incidence of PTLD by organ system from UNOS/OPTN data.

Immunosuppression-Related Risk Factors

PTLD was very rare in the era of two-drug immunosuppression with azathioprine and oral steroids. With the advent of more potent immunosuppression such as cyclosporine A, reports of PTLD started increasing [34] and then exploded in the mid-1990s with the emergence of multiple newer agents (tacrolimus, mycophenolate mofetil, OKT3, anti-thymocyte antibodies, IL-2R antibodies). Swinnen's seminal paper brought attention to the increased risk with OKT3 use [84]. Many investigators have thus focused attention on the differential risk for PTLD with individual agents. While this type of study is attractive, since immunosuppression is a modifiable risk factor, the reader should understand that cumulative totality of immunosuppression is probably the real measure of risk [18, 85]. Yet measuring totality of immunosuppression has been almost impossible so far, hence the attention to each agent.

In this regard, for most of the agents mentioned above, there are several retrospective studies that demonstrate higher PTLD risk with that agent and at least one study with each agent that does not demonstrate such increase in risk. Almost all prospective studies show no increase in PTLD risk with any agent. These prospective studies tend to have short follow-up time, patient selection biases, and more standardized follow-up than general practice. The reader is advised to look at the weight of the published literature, in both quality and quantity, as opposed to any individual study. The magnitude of risk with an immunosuppressive agent, in almost all cases, is much lower than the risk from EBV seromismatch.

Thus, some studies show higher risk of PTLD or NHL with (A) cyclosporine A [37, 86, 87] or not [88]; (B) OKT3 [7, 29, 62, 84, 89] or not [26, 56]; (C) equine anti-thymocyte polyclonal antibody [27, 89]; (D) rabbit anti-thymocyte polyclonal antibody [7, 27, 57] or not [27, 90–92]; (E) Il-2R antibodies [93] or not [7, 27, 94]; (F) tacrolimus [21, 27, 88, 95] or not [24]; and (G) alemtuzumab [61, 92] or not [57]. A meta-analysis comparison of cyclosporine to tacrolimus from prospective trials revealed no significant difference in lymphoma/PTLD rates [96]. Mycophenolate mofetil was reported to increase risk for PTLD in one study [97] but not in several other studies [58, 94, 98, 99], while high-dose steroids for acute rejection have been implicated in one study [29]. Azathioprine use was never previously considered as a risk factor for PTLD in the era of two-drug immunosuppression, but some recent studies suggest that azathioprine use (versus mycophenolate) increases PTLD risk [94], not replicated in other studies [27]. Such findings should therefore be interpreted with caution. Sirolimus is unique in that in vitro studies have suggested a protective effect from PTLD [100, 101], which seemed borne out by a clinical retrospective registry study [102]. However, more recent studies of the same database suggested the opposite [57, 61, 103]; the original registration trials showed higher PTLD rates with increasing sirolimus dose [104], and sirolimus was part of a protocol that was associated with a high PTLD frequency [39], so the issue may not be as clear-cut.

Among the newer biologic agents, alemtuzumab was not initially associated with an increased risk for PTLD, in an OPTN registry data analysis [57], but a later OPTN analysis showed higher risk [61]. As previously mentioned, belatacept showed high PTLD rates in the more and less intense arms in EBV-seronaive transplant recipients [69], leading to a black box warning to not use this drug in this specific population. Other newer biologic agents seem to share this PTLD risk. Trials of the Janus kinase inhibitor tofacitinib had to undergo a protocol modification due to high PTLD rates in the more intense arm [105]. In a small study of efalizumab, the arm receiving the highest dose of this agent and full-dose CsA experienced three PTLD cases in ten subjects, a concerning number [106].

Mortality After PTLD

In general, PTLD has been a significant cause of added mortality after transplantation [62], though at least one study suggested no increase in mortality risk [56]. The mortality rates need to be interpreted in light of the varying baseline mortality by organ system (e.g., kidney transplant recipients have lower mortality rates than heart/lung transplant recipients). Similar to incidence rates, mortality rate should ideally be expressed as a cumulative incidence over time as opposed to per PTLD percentage. The 1-year survival rates after PTLD range from 51% to 73% [7, 26, 29, 37], while 5-year survival rates are lower at 39–61% [7, 26, 29, 43, 46]. Older eras and series showed higher mortality rates [37], with improvement in each subsequent decade [10]. Children also did better than elderly adults [37]. A mid-1990s study of PTLD after pediatric kidney transplantation reported a 48% mortality [107], whereas a recent repeat study showed only 13% mortality and 5-year cumulative survival at 87.8% [108]. Higher grades of PTLD, late-onset PTLD, and central nervous system involvement are generally associated with higher mortality [26, 66, 109].

Risk for Graft Impairment and Graft Loss After PTLD

Does PTLD itself elevate the risk for earlier graft loss, independent of its effect on patient survival? Reduction of immunosuppression is typically the first strategy employed after PTLD diagnosis and can be associated with a higher risk of rejection episodes, 38% in Swinnen's prospective study of immunosuppression reduction, and sequential therapies before the advent of rituximab [110]. For thoracic organs, rejection can also be graft threatening or life-threatening. In a multicenter pediatric heart transplant study, death from graft loss was as frequent as death from PTLD. In kidney transplants, the availability of dialysis means that most clinicians might be willing to lower immunosuppression considerably and accept a risk of losing the graft. In pediatric kidney transplants, PTLD was highly significant as a predictor of worse graft survival (hazard ratio 4.3, 95% CI 3.4–4.5) after adjustment for other factors [108]. Trappe et al. have reported that patients treated with reduction of immunosuppression + chemotherapy ± rituximab had a non-inferior graft function compared with untreated controls [111]. In particular, the negative impact of reduction of immunosuppression on the renal graft function was fully compensated by the immunosuppressive effect of the CHOP regimen of chemotherapy (see Chap. 10 for more details of this regimen). The immunosuppressive effect of single-agent rituximab only partially compensated for the negative impact of reduction of immunosuppression on the graft function.

Re-transplantation After PTLD in Prior Transplant

In an UNOS/OPTN series, 69 re-transplants were recorded after PTLD [112]. Time from PTLD to re-transplant was <1 year in 24.6%, 1–3 years in 37.7%, 3–5 years in 17.4%, and 5–10 years in 20.3%. A variety of immunosuppression agents have been used in the re-transplant, and no recurrence of PTLD was reported in the re-transplants. In a more recent French series, 52 patients received 55 re-transplants after a PTLD occurrence. The time from PTLD to re-transplant was 100 months ± 44 months (range 28–224). One patient developed PTLD in a re-transplant.

Take-Home Messages

1. The incidence of PTLD varies with several host-, transplant-, and immunosuppression-related risk factors; highest risk is seen in EBV-seronegative very young or very old recipients receiving intestinal/thoracic organs and a high overall level of immunosuppression.
2. Epstein-Barr virus infection, especially primary infection acquired through the allograft, is the single most important risk factor.
3. PTLD is a significant cause of earlier graft loss and added mortality.
4. Fortunately, recurrence of PTLD in a re-transplant after prior transplant complicated by PTLD is very rare.

References

1. Dharnidharka VR. Comprehensive review of post-organ transplant hematologic cancers. Am J Transplant. 2018;18(3):537–49.
2. Dharnidharka VR, Webster AC, Martinez OM, Preiksaitis JK, Leblond V, Choquet S. Post-transplant lymphoproliferative disorders. Nat Rev Dis Primers. 2016;2:15088.
3. Campo E, Swerdlow SH, Harris NL, Pileri S, Stein H, Jaffe ES. The 2008 WHO classification of lymphoid neoplasms and beyond: evolving concepts and practical applications. Blood. 2011;117(19):5019–32.
4. Swerdlow SH, Campo E, Pileri SA, Harris NL, Stein H, Siebert R, et al. The 2016 revision of the World Health Organization classification of lymphoid neoplasms. Blood. 2016;127(20):2375–90.
5. Grulich AE, van Leeuwen MT, Falster MO, Vajdic CM. Incidence of cancers in people with HIV/AIDS compared with immunosuppressed transplant recipients: a meta-analysis. Lancet. 2007;370(9581):59–67.
6. Vajdic CM, McDonald SP, McCredie MR, van Leeuwen MT, Stewart JH, Law M, et al. Cancer incidence before and after kidney transplantation. JAMA. 2006;296(23):2823–31.
7. Opelz G, Dohler B. Lymphomas after solid organ transplantation: a collaborative transplant study report. Am J Transplant. 2004;4(2):222–30.
8. Opelz G, Henderson R. Incidence of non-Hodgkin lymphoma in kidney and heart transplant recipients. Lancet. 1993;342(8886–8887):1514–6.
9. Kasiske BL, Kukla A, Thomas D, Wood Ives J, Snyder JJ, Qiu Y, et al. Lymphoproliferative disorders after adult kidney transplant: epidemiology and comparison of registry report with claims-based diagnoses. Am J Kidney Dis. 2011;58(6):971–80.
10. Hall EC, Pfeiffer RM, Segev DL, Engels EA. Cumulative incidence of cancer after solid organ transplantation. Cancer. 2013;119(12):2300–8.
11. Engels EA, Pfeiffer RM, Fraumeni JF Jr, Kasiske BL, Israni AK, Snyder JJ, et al. Spectrum of cancer risk among US solid organ transplant recipients. JAMA. 2011;306(17):1891–901.
12. Cheung CY, Lam MF, Chu KH, Chow KM, Tsang KY, Yuen SK, et al. Malignancies after kidney transplantation: Hong Kong renal registry. Am J Transplant. 2012;12(11):3039–46.
13. Engels EA, Clarke CA, Pfeiffer RM, Lynch CF, Weisenburger DD, Gibson TM, et al. Plasma cell neoplasms in US solid organ transplant recipients. Am J Transplant. 2013;13(6):1523–32.
14. Clarke CA, Morton LM, Lynch C, Pfeiffer RM, Hall EC, Gibson TM, et al. Risk of lymphoma subtypes after solid organ transplantation in the United States. Br J Cancer. 2013;109(1):280–8.
15. Morton LM, Gibson TM, Clarke CA, Lynch CF, Anderson LA, Pfeiffer R, et al. Risk of myeloid neoplasms after solid organ transplantation. Leukemia. 2014;28(12):2317–23.
16. Webster AC, Craig JC, Simpson JM, Jones MP, Chapman JR. Identifying high risk groups and quantifying absolute risk of cancer after kidney transplantation: a cohort study of 15,183 recipients. Am J Transplant. 2007;7(9):2140–51.
17. Srisawat N, Avihingsanon A, Praditpornsilpa K, Jiamjarasrangsi W, Eiam-Ong S, Avihingsanon Y. A prevalence of posttransplantation cancers compared with cancers in people with human immunodeficiency virus/acquired immunodeficiency syndrome after highly active antiretroviral therapy. Transplant Proc. 2008;40(8):2677–9.
18. Boubenider S, Hiesse C, Goupy C, Kriaa F, Marchand S, Charpentier B. Incidence and consequences of post-transplantation lymphoproliferative disorders. J Nephrol. 1997;10(3):136–45.
19. Sampaio MS, Cho YW, Qazi Y, Bunnapradist S, Hutchinson IV, Shah T. Posttransplant malignancies in solid organ adult recipients: an analysis of the U.S. National Transplant Database. Transplantation. 2012;94(10):990–8.
20. Morton M, Coupes B, Roberts SA, Klapper PE, Byers RJ, Vallely PJ, et al. Epidemiology of posttransplantation lymphoproliferative disorder in adult renal transplant recipients. Transplantation. 2013;95(3):470–8.

21. Younes BS, McDiarmid SV, Martin MG, Vargas JH, Goss JA, Busuttil RW, et al. The effect of immunosuppression on posttransplant lymphoproliferative disease in pediatric liver transplant patients. Transplantation. 2000;70(1):94–9.
22. Dharnidharka VR, Fiorina P, Harmon WE. Kidney transplantation in children. N Engl J Med. 2014;371(6):549–58.
23. Dharnidharka VR, Sullivan EK, Stablein DM, Tejani AH, Harmon WE. Risk factors for posttransplant lymphoproliferative disorder (PTLD) in pediatric kidney transplantation: a report of the North American Pediatric Renal Transplant Cooperative Study (NAPRTCS). Transplantation. 2001;71(8):1065–8.
24. Dharnidharka VR, Ho PL, Stablein DM, Harmon WE, Tejani AH. Mycophenolate, tacrolimus and post-transplant lymphoproliferative disorder: a report of the North American Pediatric Renal Transplant Cooperative Study. Pediatr Transplant. 2002;6(5):396–9.
25. Caillard S, Lamy FX, Quelen C, Dantal J, Lebranchu Y, Lang P, et al. Epidemiology of posttransplant lymphoproliferative disorders in adult kidney and kidney pancreas recipients: report of the French registry and analysis of subgroups of lymphomas. Am J Transplant. 2012;12(3):682–93.
26. Caillard S, Lelong C, Pessione F, Moulin B. Post-transplant lymphoproliferative disorders occurring after renal transplantation in adults: report of 230 cases from the French Registry. Am J Transplant. 2006;6(11):2735–42.
27. Caillard S, Dharnidharka V, Agodoa L, Bohen E, Abbott K. Posttransplant lymphoproliferative disorders after renal transplantation in the United States in era of modern immunosuppression. Transplantation. 2005;80(9):1233–43.
28. Chua A, Cramer C, Moudgil A, Martz K, Smith J, Blydt-Hansen T, et al. Kidney transplant practice patterns and outcome benchmarks over 30 years: the 2018 report of the NAPRTCS. Pediatr Transplant. 2019;23(8):e13597.
29. Kremers WK, Devarbhavi HC, Wiesner RH, Krom RA, Macon WR, Habermann TM. Post-transplant lymphoproliferative disorders following liver transplantation: incidence, risk factors and survival. Am J Transplant. 2006;6(5 Pt 1):1017–24.
30. Ng VL, Fecteau A, Shepherd R, Magee J, Bucuvalas J, Alonso E, et al. Outcomes of 5-year survivors of pediatric liver transplantation: report on 461 children from a north American multicenter registry. Pediatrics. 2008;122(6):e1128–35.
31. Lund LH, Khush KK, Cherikh WS, Goldfarb S, Kucheryavaya AY, Levvey BJ, et al. The Registry of the International Society for Heart and Lung Transplantation: thirty-fourth adult heart transplantation report-2017; focus theme: allograft ischemic time. J Heart Lung Transplant. 2017;36(10):1037–46.
32. Benden C, Goldfarb SB, Edwards LB, Kucheryavaya AY, Christie JD, Dipchand AI, et al. The Registry of the International Society for Heart and Lung Transplantation: seventeenth official pediatric lung and heart-lung transplantation report--2014; focus theme: retransplantation. J Heart Lung Transplant. 2014;33(10):1025–33.
33. Kotton CN, Huprikar S, Kumar D. Transplant infectious diseases: a review of the scientific registry of transplant recipients published data. Am J Transplant. 2017;17(6):1439–46.
34. Harmon WE, Dharnidharka VR. Lymphoproliferative disease in children. Transplant Proc. 1999;31(2B):1268–9.
35. Alfrey EJ, Friedman AL, Grossman RA, Perloff LJ, Naji A, Barker CF, et al. A recent decrease in the time to development of monomorphous and polymorphous posttransplant lymphoproliferative disorder. Transplantation. 1992;54(2):250–3.
36. Ciancio G, Siquijor AP, Burke GW, Roth D, Cirocco R, Esquenazi V, et al. Post-transplant lymphoproliferative disease in kidney transplant patients in the new immunosuppressive era. Clin Transpl. 1997;11(3):243–9.
37. Faull RJ, Hollett P, McDonald SP. Lymphoproliferative disease after renal transplantation in Australia and New Zealand. Transplantation. 2005;80(2):193–7.

38. Dharnidharka VR, Tejani AH, Ho PL, Harmon WE. Post-transplant lymphoproliferative disorder in the United States: young Caucasian males are at highest risk. Am J Transplant. 2002;2(10):993–8.
39. McDonald RA, Smith JM, Ho M, Lindblad R, Ikle D, Grimm P, et al. Incidence of PTLD in pediatric renal transplant recipients receiving basiliximab, calcineurin inhibitor, sirolimus and steroids. Am J Transplant. 2008;8(5):984–9.
40. McDiarmid SV, Jordan S, Lee GS, Toyoda M, Goss JA, Vargas JH, et al. Prevention and preemptive therapy of posttransplant lymphoproliferative disease in pediatric liver recipients. Transplantation. 1998;66(12):1604–11.
41. Sampaio MS, Cho YW, Shah T, Bunnapradist S, Hutchinson IV. Impact of Epstein-Barr virus donor and recipient serostatus on the incidence of post-transplant lymphoproliferative disorder in kidney transplant recipients. Nephrol Dial Transplant. 2012;27(7):2971–9.
42. Leblond V, Sutton L, Dorent R, Davi F, Bitker MO, Gabarre J, et al. Lymphoproliferative disorders after organ transplantation: a report of 24 cases observed in a single center. J Clin Oncol. 1995;13(4):961–8.
43. Luskin MR, Heil DS, Tan KS, Choi S, Stadtmauer EA, Schuster SJ, et al. The impact of EBV status on characteristics and outcomes of posttransplantation lymphoproliferative disorder. Am J Transplant. 2015;15(10):2665–73.
44. Patel H, Vogl DT, Aqui N, Shaked A, Olthoff K, Markmann J, et al. Posttransplant lymphoproliferative disorder in adult liver transplant recipients: a report of seventeen cases. Leuk Lymphoma. 2007;48(5):885–91.
45. Saadat A, Einollahi B, Ahmadzad-Asl MA, Moradi M, Nafar M, Pourfarziani V, et al. Posttransplantation lymphoproliferative disorders in renal transplant recipients: report of over 20 years of experience. Transplant Proc. 2007;39(4):1071–3.
46. Cacciarelli TV, Green M, Jaffe R, Mazariegos GV, Jain A, Fung JJ, et al. Management of posttransplant lymphoproliferative disease in pediatric liver transplant recipients receiving primary tacrolimus (FK506) therapy. Transplantation. 1998;66(8):1047–52.
47. Duvoux C, Pageaux GP, Vanlemmens C, Roudot-Thoraval F, Vincens-Rolland AL, Hezode C, et al. Risk factors for lymphoproliferative disorders after liver transplantation in adults: an analysis of 480 patients. Transplantation. 2002;74(8):1103–9.
48. Fernandez MC, Bes D, De Davila M, Lopez S, Cambaceres C, Dip M, et al. Post-transplant lymphoproliferative disorder after pediatric liver transplantation: characteristics and outcome. Pediatr Transplant. 2009;13(3):307–10.
49. Chang RS, Lewis JP, Reynolds RD, Sullivan MJ, Neuman J. Oropharyngeal excretion of Epstein-Barr virus by patients with lymphoproliferative disorders and by recipients of renal homografts. Ann Intern Med. 1978;88(1):34–40.
50. Marker SC, Ascher NL, Kalis JM, Simmons RL, Najarian JS, Balfour HH Jr. Epstein-Barr virus antibody responses and clinical illness in renal transplant recipients. Surgery. 1979;85(4):433–40.
51. Hanto DW, Frizzera G, Purtilo DT, Sakamoto K, Sullivan JL, Saemundsen AK, et al. Clinical spectrum of lymphoproliferative disorders in renal transplant recipients and evidence for the role of Epstein-Barr virus. Cancer Res. 1981;41(11 Pt 1):4253–61.
52. Hanto DW, Sakamoto K, Purtilo DT, Simmons RL, Najarian JS. The Epstein-Barr virus in the pathogenesis of posttransplant lymphoproliferative disorders. Clinical, pathologic, and virologic correlation. Surgery. 1981;90(2):204–13.
53. Walker RC, Paya CV, Marshall WF, Strickler JG, Wiesner RH, Velosa JA, et al. Pretransplantation seronegative Epstein-Barr virus status is the primary risk factor for post-transplantation lymphoproliferative disorder in adult heart, lung, and other solid organ transplantations. J Heart Lung Transplant. 1995;14(2):214–21.
54. Cockfield SM, Preiksaitis JK, Jewell LD, Parfrey NA. Post-transplant lymphoproliferative disorder in renal allograft recipients. Clinical experience and risk factor analysis in a single center. Transplantation. 1993;56(1):88–96.

55. Mendoza F, Kunitake H, Laks H, Odim J. Post-transplant lymphoproliferative disorder following pediatric heart transplantation. Pediatr Transplant. 2006;10(1):60–6.
56. Katz BZ, Pahl E, Crawford SE, Kostyk MC, Rodgers S, Seshadri R, et al. Case-control study of risk factors for the development of post-transplant lymphoproliferative disease in a pediatric heart transplant cohort. Pediatr Transplant. 2007;11(1):58–65.
57. Kirk AD, Cherikh WS, Ring M, Burke G, Kaufman D, Knechtle SJ, et al. Dissociation of depletional induction and posttransplant lymphoproliferative disease in kidney recipients treated with alemtuzumab. Am J Transplant. 2007;7(11):2619–25.
58. Funch DP, Ko HH, Travasso J, Brady J, Kew CE 2nd, Nalesnik MA, et al. Posttransplant lymphoproliferative disorder among renal transplant patients in relation to the use of mycophenolate mofetil. Transplantation. 2005;80(9):1174–80.
59. Allen UD, Farkas G, Hebert D, Weitzman S, Stephens D, Petric M, et al. Risk factors for post-transplant lymphoproliferative disorder in pediatric patients: a case-control study. Pediatr Transplant. 2005;9(4):450–5.
60. Opelz G, Daniel V, Naujokat C, Dohler B. Epidemiology of pretransplant EBV and CMV serostatus in relation to posttransplant non-Hodgkin lymphoma. Transplantation. 2009;88(8):962–7.
61. Dharnidharka VR, Lamb KE, Gregg JA, Meier-Kriesche HU. Associations between EBV serostatus and organ transplant type in PTLD risk: an analysis of the SRTR National Registry Data in the United States. Am J Transplant. 2012;12(4):976–83.
62. Newell KA, Alonso EM, Whitington PF, Bruce DS, Millis JM, Piper JB, et al. Posttransplant lymphoproliferative disease in pediatric liver transplantation. Interplay between primary Epstein-Barr virus infection and immunosuppression. Transplantation. 1996;62(3):370–5.
63. Walker RC, Marshall WF, Strickler JG, Wiesner RH, Velosa JA, Habermann TM, et al. Pretransplantation assessment of the risk of lymphoproliferative disorder. Clin Infect Dis. 1995;20(5):1346–53.
64. Manez R, Breinig MC, Linden P, Wilson J, Torre-Cisneros J, Kusne S, et al. Posttransplant lymphoproliferative disease in primary Epstein-Barr virus infection after liver transplantation: the role of cytomegalovirus disease. J Infect Dis. 1997;176(6):1462–7.
65. Dharnidharka VR, Ruzinova MB, Chen CC, Parameswaran P, O'Gorman H, Goss CW, et al. Metagenomic analysis of DNA viruses from posttransplant lymphoproliferative disorders. Cancer Med. 2019;8(3):1013–23.
66. Buell JF, Gross TG, Hanaway MJ, Trofe J, Roy-Chaudhury P, First MR, et al. Posttransplant lymphoproliferative disorder: significance of central nervous system involvement. Transplant Proc. 2005;37(2):954–5.
67. Evens AM, Choquet S, Kroll-Desrosiers AR, Jagadeesh D, Smith SM, Morschhauser F, et al. Primary CNS posttransplant lymphoproliferative disease (PTLD): an international report of 84 cases in the modern era. Am J Transplant. 2013;13(6):1512–22.
68. Velvet AJJ, Bhutani S, Papachristos S, Dwivedi R, Picton M, Augustine T, et al. A single-center experience of post-transplant lymphomas involving the central nervous system with a review of current literature. Oncotarget. 2019;10(4):437–48.
69. Grinyo J, Charpentier B, Pestana JM, Vanrenterghem Y, Vincenti F, Reyes-Acevedo R, et al. An integrated safety profile analysis of belatacept in kidney transplant recipients. Transplantation. 2010;90(12):1521–7.
70. Swerdlow SH. T-cell and NK-cell posttransplantation lymphoproliferative disorders. Am J Clin Pathol. 2007;127(6):887–95.
71. Herreman A, Dierickx D, Morscio J, Camps J, Bittoun E, Verhoef G, et al. Clinicopathological characteristics of posttransplant lymphoproliferative disorders of T-cell origin: single-center series of nine cases and meta-analysis of 147 reported cases. Leuk Lymphoma. 2013;54(10):2190–9.
72. Hall EC, Segev DL, Engels EA. Racial/ethnic differences in cancer risk after kidney transplantation. Am J Transplant. 2013;13(3):714–20.

73. Sundin M, Le Blanc K, Ringden O, Barkholt L, Omazic B, Lergin C, et al. The role of HLA mismatch, splenectomy and recipient Epstein-Barr virus seronegativity as risk factors in post-transplant lymphoproliferative disorder following allogeneic hematopoietic stem cell transplantation. Haematologica. 2006;91(8):1059–67.

74. Bakker NA, van Imhoff GW, Verschuuren EA, van Son WJ, van der Heide JJ, Lems SP, et al. HLA antigens and post renal transplant lymphoproliferative disease: HLA-B matching is critical. Transplantation. 2005;80(5):595–9.

75. Pourfarziani V, Einollahi B, Taheri S, Nemati E, Nafar M, Kalantar E. Associations of Human Leukocyte Antigen (HLA) haplotypes with risk of developing lymphoproliferative disorders after renal transplantation. Ann Transplant. 2007;12(4):16–22.

76. Wheless SA, Gulley ML, Raab-Traub N, McNeillie P, Neuringer IP, Ford HJ, et al. Post-transplantation Lymphoproliferative disease: Epstein Barr virus DNA levels, HLA A3 and survival. Am J Respir Crit Care Med. 2008;178(10):1060–5.

77. Kinch A, Cavelier L, Bengtsson M, Baecklund E, Enblad G, Backlin C, et al. Donor or recipient origin of posttransplant lymphoproliferative disorders following solid organ transplantation. Am J Transplant. 2014;14(12):2838–45.

78. Olagne J, Caillard S, Gaub MP, Chenard MP, Moulin B. Post-transplant lymphoproliferative disorders: determination of donor/recipient origin in a large cohort of kidney recipients. Am J Transplant. 2011;11(6):1260–9.

79. McLaughlin K, Wajstaub S, Marotta P, Adams P, Grant DR, Wall WJ, et al. Increased risk for posttransplant lymphoproliferative disease in recipients of liver transplants with hepatitis C. Liver Transpl. 2000;6(5):570–4.

80. Shpilberg O, Wilson J, Whiteside TL, Herberman RB. Pre-transplant immunological profile and risk factor analysis of post-transplant lymphoproliferative disease development: the results of a nested matched case-control study. The University of Pittsburgh PTLD Study Group. Leuk Lymphoma. 1999;36(1–2):109–21.

81. Newell KA, Alonso EM, Kelly SM, Rubin CM, Thistlethwaite JR Jr, Whitington PF. Association between liver transplantation for Langerhans cell histiocytosis, rejection, and development of posttransplant lymphoproliferative disease in children. J Pediatr. 1997;131(1 Pt 1):98–104.

82. Quintini C, Kato T, Gaynor JJ, Ueno T, Selvaggi G, Gordon P, et al. Analysis of risk factors for the development of posttransplant lymphoproliferative disorder among 119 children who received primary intestinal transplants at a single center. Transplant Proc. 2006;38(6):1755–8.

83. Finn L, Reyes J, Bueno J, Yunis E. Epstein-Barr virus infections in children after transplantation of the small intestine. Am J Surg Pathol. 1998;22(3):299–309.

84. Swinnen LJ, Costanzo-Nordin MR, Fisher SG, O'Sullivan EJ, Johnson MR, Heroux AL, et al. Increased incidence of lymphoproliferative disorder after immunosuppression with the monoclonal antibody OKT3 in cardiac- transplant recipients. N Engl J Med. 1990;323(25):1723–8.

85. Dharnidharka VR, Harmon WE. Management of pediatric postrenal transplantation infections. Semin Nephrol. 2001;21(5):521–31.

86. Penn I. Cancers following cyclosporine therapy. Transplantation. 1987;43(1):32–5.

87. Penn I. Neoplastic complications of transplantation. Semin Respir Infect. 1993;8(3):233–9.

88. Guthery SL, Heubi JE, Bucuvalas JC, Gross TG, Ryckman FC, Alonso MH, et al. Determination of risk factors for Epstein-Barr virus-associated posttransplant lymphoproliferative disorder in pediatric liver transplant recipients using objective case ascertainment. Transplantation. 2003;75(7):987–93.

89. Opelz G, Naujokat C, Daniel V, Terness P, Dohler B. Disassociation between risk of graft loss and risk of non-Hodgkin lymphoma with induction agents in renal transplant recipients. Transplantation. 2006;81(9):1227–33.

90. Dharnidharka VR, Stevens G. Risk for post-transplant lymphoproliferative disorder after polyclonal antibody induction in kidney transplantation. Pediatr Transplant. 2005;9:622–6.

91. Hardinger KL, Rhee S, Buchanan P, Koch M, Miller B, Enkvetchakul D, et al. A prospective, randomized, double-blinded comparison of thymoglobulin versus Atgam for induction immunosuppressive therapy: 10-year results. Transplantation. 2008;86(7):947–52.

92. Hall EC, Engels EA, Pfeiffer RM, Segev DL. Association of antibody induction immunosuppression with cancer after kidney transplantation. Transplantation. 2015;99(5):1051–7.

93. Bustami RT, Ojo AO, Wolfe RA, Merion RM, Bennett WM, McDiarmid SV, et al. Immunosuppression and the risk of post-transplant malignancy among cadaveric first kidney transplant recipients. Am J Transplant. 2004;4(1):87–93.

94. Cherikh WS, Kauffman HM, McBride MA, Maghirang J, Swinnen LJ, Hanto DW. Association of the type of induction immunosuppression with posttransplant lymphoproliferative disorder, graft survival, and patient survival after primary kidney transplantation. Transplantation. 2003;76(9):1289–93.

95. Cox KL, Lawrence-Miyasaki LS, Garcia-Kennedy R, Lennette ET, Martinez OM, Krams SM, et al. An increased incidence of Epstein-Barr virus infection and lymphoproliferative disorder in young children on FK506 after liver transplantation. Transplantation. 1995;59(4):524–9.

96. Webster AC, Woodroffe RC, Taylor RS, Chapman JR, Craig JC. Tacrolimus versus ciclosporin as primary immunosuppression for kidney transplant recipients: meta-analysis and meta-regression of randomised trial data. BMJ (Clinical Research ed). 2005;331(7520):810.

97. Keay S, Meador TL, Schofield KJ, Blahut S, Anderson L, Wiland A, et al. Increased incidence of post-transplant lymphoproliferative disorder associated with mycophenolate mofetil in kidney transplant recipients. Transplantation. 1999;67(7):846A.

98. Birkeland SA, Hamilton-Dutoit S. Is posttransplant lymphoproliferative disorder (PTLD) caused by any specific immunosuppressive drug or by the transplantation per se? Transplantation. 2003;76(6):984–8.

99. Robson R, Cecka JM, Opelz G, Budde M, Sacks S. Prospective registry-based observational cohort study of the long-term risk of malignancies in renal transplant patients treated with mycophenolate mofetil. Am J Transplant. 2005;5(12):2954–60.

100. Majewski M, Korecka M, Kossev P, Li S, Goldman J, Moore J, et al. The immunosuppressive macrolide RAD inhibits growth of human Epstein-Barr virus-transformed B lymphocytes in vitro and in vivo: a potential approach to prevention and treatment of posttransplant lymphoproliferative disorders. Proc Natl Acad Sci U S A. 2000;97(8):4285–90.

101. Nepomuceno RR, Balatoni CE, Natkunam Y, Snow AL, Krams SM, Martinez OM. Rapamycin inhibits the interleukin 10 signal transduction pathway and the growth of Epstein Barr virus B-cell lymphomas. Cancer Res. 2003;63(15):4472–80.

102. Kauffman HM, Cherikh WS, Cheng Y, Hanto DW, Kahan BD. Maintenance immunosuppression with target-of-rapamycin inhibitors is associated with a reduced incidence of de novo malignancies. Transplantation. 2005;80(7):883–9.

103. Sampaio MS, Cho YW, Shah T, Bunnapradist S, Hutchinson IV. Association of immunosuppressive maintenance regimens with posttransplant lymphoproliferative disorder in kidney transplant recipients. Transplantation. 2012;93(1):73–81.

104. Mathew T, Kreis H, Friend P. Two-year incidence of malignancy in sirolimus-treated renal transplant recipients: results from five multicenter studies. Clin Transpl. 2004;18(4):446–9.

105. Busque S, Vincenti FG, Tedesco Silva H, O'Connell PJ, Yoshida A, Friedewald JJ, et al. Efficacy and safety of a tofacitinib-based immunosuppressive regimen after kidney transplantation: results from a long-term extension trial. Transplant Direct. 2018;4(9):e380.

106. Vincenti F, Mendez R, Pescovitz M, Rajagopalan PR, Wilkinson AH, Butt K, et al. A phase I/II randomized open-label multicenter trial of efalizumab, a humanized anti-CD11a, anti-LFA-1 in renal transplantation. Am J Transplant. 2007;7(7):1770–7.

107. Hebert D, Sullivan EK. Malignancy and post transplant lymphoproliferative disorder (PTLD) in pediatric renal transplant recipients: a report of the North American Pediatric Renal Transplant Cooperative Study (NAPRTCS). Pediatr Transplant. 1998;2(S1):107:57A.

108. Dharnidharka VR, Martz KL, Stablein DM, Benfield MR. Improved survival with recent Post-Transplant Lymphoproliferative Disorder (PTLD) in children with kidney transplants. Am J Transplant. 2011;11(4):751–8.

109. Hayashi RJ, Kraus MD, Patel AL, Canter C, Cohen AH, Hmiel P, et al. Posttransplant lymphoproliferative disease in children: correlation of histology to clinical behavior. J Pediatr Hematol Oncol. 2001;23(1):14–8.
110. Swinnen LJ, Leblanc M, Grogan TM, Gordon LI, Stiff PJ, Miller AM, et al. Prospective study of sequential reduction in immunosuppression, interferon alpha-2B, and chemotherapy for posttransplantation lymphoproliferative disorder. Transplantation. 2008;86(2):215–22.
111. Trappe R, Hinrichs C, Appel U, Babel N, Reinke P, Neumayer HH, et al. Treatment of PTLD with rituximab and CHOP reduces the risk of renal graft impairment after reduction of immunosuppression. Am J Transplant. 2009;9(10):2331–7.
112. Johnson SR, Cherikh WS, Kauffman HM, Pavlakis M, Hanto DW. Retransplantation after post-transplant lymphoproliferative disorders: an OPTN/UNOS database analysis. Am J Transplant. 2006;6(11):2743–9.

Clinical Features and Diagnostic Considerations

8

Upton D. Allen and Daan Dierickx

Introduction

The Epstein-Barr virus (EBV) is associated with the majority of cases of post-transplant lymphoproliferative disorder (PTLD). This condition encompasses a spectrum of clinical entities in the post-transplant period. These syndromes range from the manifestations of non-destructive lesions, including infectious mononucleosis-like pathologies, to true malignancies [1]. While these manifestations of PTLD are often conveniently classified into discreet entities, in reality they often represent a spectrum of illnesses where more benign entities may be followed by more serious syndromes. The heterogeneous nature of PTLD makes generalization problematic. This notwithstanding, one can recognize two primary modes of presentation of PTLD in the solid organ transplant recipient, namely, early-onset PTLD and later-onset PTLD. Although the time demarcation between these entities is somewhat arbitrary, the former occurs within the first 1–2 years, while the latter occurs after the first 1–2 years [2].

U. D. Allen (✉)
Department of Paediatrics, Division of Infectious Diseases, The Hospital for Sick Children, University of Toronto, Toronto, ON, Canada
e-mail: upton.allen@sickkids.ca

D. Dierickx
Department of Hematology, University Hospitals Leuven, Leuven, Belgium
e-mail: daan.dierickx@uzleuven.be

© Springer Nature Switzerland AG 2021
V. R. Dharnidharka et al. (eds.), *Post-Transplant Lymphoproliferative Disorders*,
https://doi.org/10.1007/978-3-030-65403-0_8

Severe Infectious Mononucleosis, Clinical Categories, and Sites of PTLD

Severe Infectious Mononucleosis Infectious mononucleosis is the prototype of primary EBV infection [3, 4]. The clinical spectrum of infection ranges from asymptomatic infection to severe, sometimes fatal disease in immunocompromised patients. Infectious mononucleosis is typically characterized by fever, exudative pharyngitis, lymphadenopathy, hepatosplenomegaly, and atypical lymphocytosis. In symptomatic individuals, adenotonsillar disease is often a prominent feature (Fig. 8.1). The features of severe infectious mononucleosis may be seen in some cases of acutely symptomatic PTLD. In complicated cases or the more severe cases in the immunocompromised host, patients may develop hepatitis, upper airway obstruction due to enlarged adenotonsillar tissue, pneumonitis, encephalitis, aseptic meningitis, splenic rupture, decreased blood cellular elements, disseminated intravascular coagulation and hemophagocytic syndrome, bacterial superinfection, and renal, cardiac, and other complications [3, 4]. In the transplant setting, certain features (e.g., hepatitis) may be accentuated or represent diagnostic dilemmas as this relates to the role that the virus is having versus non-EBV-related complications of transplantation.

PTLD Presenting Early After Organ Transplantation PTLD presenting within the first 1–2 years after transplantation may be characterized by marked constitutional symptoms and rapid enlargement of lymphoreticular tissue. The vast majority of these lesions during this time are EBV-positive. Although less commonly seen in recent years, this entity is characterized by rapidly progressive disease of a disseminated nature and a systemic sepsis-like syndrome as a result of a cytokine storm. The clinical picture includes some features that are consistent with severe EBV disease [5], as outlined above (e.g., hemophagocytosis and disseminated intravascular coagulation). In some patients, the diagnosis of PTLD is unfortunately

Fig. 8.1 Exudative tonsillopharyngitis in infectious mononucleosis. (Footnote: Reproduced with permission, Slide Library, Hospital for Sick Children, Toronto)

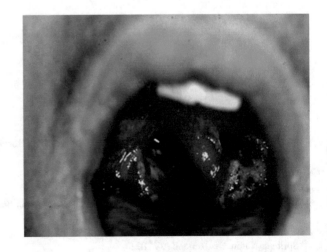

made at autopsy due to difficulty in diagnosis [6, 7]. Mass lesions may not be present; pyrexia is present and the disease may be extranodal. It can be difficult to separate this entity from patients who have overwhelming sepsis and multiorgan failure. The above notwithstanding, some cases of early PTLD may present in less aggressive forms with nodal involvement and less constitutional symptomatology. In the adult patient, this presentation is the most frequent presentation of the early-onset PTLD.

PTLD Presenting Late After Organ Transplantation PTLD that presents after the first 1–2 years after transplantation is likely to be more anatomically defined, has few systemic symptoms, and is less rapidly progressive. This form of PTLD is now the form that is frequently seen in most centers, as the early-onset, rapidly progressive form is less frequently seen in recent years [8, 9]. Proportionately more cases of EBV-negative PTLD occur in the late-onset category in contrast to the early-onset category. One possible explanation is that in recent years, the enhanced surveillance for EBV after transplantation has enabled the early recognition of upregulation of EBV activity prior to the development of PTLD, allowing for early intervention, including reduction in immunosuppression.

PTLD Occurring After Hematopoietic Stem Cell Transplantation This is addressed elsewhere in this book and will only be briefly mentioned here for context and contrast. In the HSCT patients, PTLD usually affects recipients of allogeneic grafts. Among affected patients, very few cases of PTLD occur after the first year in the absence of chronic graft versus host disease. This is due to the fact that immune restoration occurs as engraftment takes place with advancing time after HSCT. This is in contrast to solid organ transplant recipients who require varying degrees of ongoing immunosuppression to prevent organ rejection. The occurrence of PTLD at a relatively early stage after HSCT poses a challenge with a tendency for fulminant multi-system disease in some patients. While HSCT patients may experience the full spectrum of PTLD seen in solid organ transplantations, it occurs significantly less frequently after hematopoietic stem cell transplantation (HSCT) compared with solid organ transplantation. Among HSCT recipients, PTLD lesions are usually of donor origin in contrast to recipient origin in the majority of solid organ transplant recipients [10–12].

Sites of PTLD Lesions The dominant presenting signs and symptoms of PTLD are related to the organs affected and the sites of PTLD lesions. In contrast to lymphomas in immunocompetent patients, PTLD is associated with a very high incidence of extranodal involvement, with published rates of 60–90%. Virtually no site is exempt from PTLD involvement, and a high index of suspicion is required when assessing lesions in any location in the body of patients after transplantation. In this regard, PTLD has been documented at the following sites: bone, bone marrow, small bowel, large bowel, stomach, central nervous system, diaphragm, kidneys, liver, lung, lymph nodes, orbits, ovary, paraspinal tissues, salivary glands, paranasal sinuses, skin, soft palate, spleen, stomach, testes, tonsils, and uterus. In addition,

EBV-positive (+) mucocutaneous ulcers involving the oropharyngeal mucosa, skin, or gastrointestinal tract may occur and have been added to the WHO classification system [1, 13].

The vast majority of cases involve the organs of the reticuloendothelial systems and the transplanted organs. With respect to the transplanted organs, the heart is the only organ that is not usually the primary site of PTLD. Data from a recent review of PTLD cases in children over a 15-year period at The Hospital for Sick Children in Toronto revealed that the sites most frequently affected at the diagnosis of PTLD were tonsillar/adenoidal (34%), gastrointestinal (GI) tract (32%), lymph node (LN) 11%), and multisite (11%) [14]. Among adult patients, Caillard et al. described a temporal sequence of sites of PTLD among renal transplant recipients, with disease localized to the graft occurring within the first 2 years, primary CNS lymphoma (PCNSL) occurring between years 2 and 7, and gastrointestinal disease occurring between years 6 and 10 and being the predominant site of late disease [15], the latter supporting the observation of the relatively high frequency of involvement of the GI tract in cases of PTLD [16–18].

With respect to GI tract disease, the nature of organ involvement may include isolated solitary or multisite lesions or disease that is part of a more disseminated process. Easily resectable intestinal lesions that are solitary are associated with better outcomes compared with disease that is either multisite or part of a more generalized PTLD process. Patients with GI PTLD may present with a variety of gastrointestinal manifestations, including vomiting, diarrhea, evidence of protein-losing enteropathy, intussusception, bleeding, and in some cases evidence of bowel perforation. The latter is also a known complication during the treatment phase of intestinal PTLD during which necrosis of transmural lesions can occur.

Patients with head and neck PTLD disease may present with a spectrum of findings including asymptomatic adenotonsillar hypertrophy, tonsillitis, palatal ulcerative lesions, cervical lymphadenopathy, and disease of the paranasal sinuses [19–24]. The latter has been documented to be one of the manifestations of PTLD in patients who have undergone lung transplantation [24]. Among these findings, enlarged adenoids and tonsils represent the most frequent presentation of head and neck PTLD (Fig. 8.2). In one series, adenotonsillar biopsies yielded PTLD in approximately 40% of children who were referred to the otolaryngology service for assessment to rule out PTLD following initial screening by clinicians [19].

Pulmonary involvement is most frequently seen in heart and lung transplant patients. In most cases it is characterized by solitary or multiple pulmonary nodules or an infiltrative process [7, 15, 25, 26]. In addition, there may be pulmonary dysfunction in the lung allograft. In the latter situation, clearly discernible lesions might not be apparent in the setting of diffuse consolidation on chest X-rays.

Liver involvement usually occurs in liver transplant recipients where there may be evidence of diffuse hepatitis or nodular disease. Non-liver transplant recipients may also have liver involvement as a component of multi-system disease.

Among renal transplant recipients, PTLD may involve the allograft or distant sites. This influences the nature of the presenting signs and symptoms. When PTLD

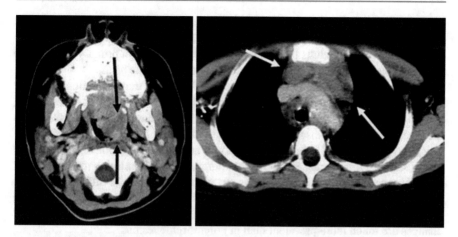

Fig. 8.2 Older child after liver transplantation. CT reveals left tonsillar nodal mass and mediastinal adenopathy. (Courtesy of Dr. David Manson, Hospital for Sick Children, Toronto)

affects the renal graft, a significant proportion of patients may present with renal dysfunction [15]. However, when alterations in renal function occur presumably due to PTLD affecting the kidneys, other cause of renal dysfunction after transplant should be considered in the differential diagnosis. These conditions include rejection and BK polyoma virus nephropathy.

Patients may also present with skin nodules. These should be differentiated from non-PTLD malignancies, including donor-derived malignancies in adult patients. Rarely, EBV-associated smooth muscle tumors have been described [27].

Central nervous system (CNS) disease is usually seen in the setting of extensive multi-system disease. However, solitary CNS disease may occur, which is an important consideration in the diagnostic evaluation of transplant patients with sustained elevations of EBV loads. In this regard, patients with CNS lesions might not have symptoms or signs referable to the CNS during the early stages of disease. The time to primary CNS PTLD may be less than 2 years and exceed 10 years post-transplant [15, 28, 29]. When symptomatic, patients may present with evidence of intracranial pathology with headaches, seizures, and focal neurologic deficits. Generally, patients presenting with CNS PTLD tend to have poorer prognoses [8, 15, 25].

As indicated above, several other sites may be affected by PTLD. Their clinical importance may relate to the fact that their involvement may be indicative of disseminated disease and/or may be suggestive of poorer outcomes. For example, as is the case with CNS PTLD, bone marrow involvement is regarded as a poor prognostic indicator.

Histopathologic Correlates

The histopathologic examination of suspected PTLD lesions is crucial for the diagnosis of PTLD [1, 30, 31]. A detailed description is provided in Chap. 2; PTLD lesions presenting early after transplantation are generally EBV-associated.

Non-destructive lesions of the plasmacytic and infectious mononucleosis types tend to occur at a younger age than other forms of PTLD and are thus more likely to be seen in children than adults [1]. These lesions tend to occur in primary EBV where infection occurs in the setting of no previous exposure to the virus.

The histology of PTLD lesions presenting late after transplantation is highly variable. In children and adults experiencing late-onset primary EBV infection, "non-destructive PTLD" and/or other forms of PTLD may still be observed. With increasing time from transplantation, a greater proportion of lesions are monomorphic, and many are EBV-negative, notably in adults. These lesions may resemble non-Hodgkin lymphomas, Hodgkin lymphoma, or malignancies with plasma cell predominance. Their clinical behaviors are variable and may be different from the histologically equivalent lesions in non-transplant recipients. Monomorphic lesions are clonal proliferations, and genetic abnormalities and structural chromosomal changes are much more prevalent than in polymorphic lesions.

Diagnostic Evaluation

Early diagnosis of PTLD is essential in order to maximize favorable outcomes. The initial diagnostic evaluation of patients with suspected PTLD is influenced by the appropriate historical information, as this relates to symptoms as well as background patient information and the physical examination findings. The diagnostic workup is guided by the presenting symptoms and signs as outlined above and in Table 8.1, taking into account the differential diagnosis. Therefore, clinicians need to be aware of the conditions that must be differentiated from PTLD in order that these alternative diagnoses are not missed and are managed appropriately.

Table 8.1 Presenting symptoms and signs in patients with lymphoproliferative disorder

Symptoms/complaints	Signs
Swollen lymph glands	Lymphadenopathy
Weight loss	Hepatosplenomegaly
Fever or night sweats	Subcutaneous nodules
Sore throat	Tonsillar enlargement
Malaise and lethargy	Tonsillar inflammation
Chronic sinus congestion and discomfort	Signs of bowel perforation
Anorexia, nausea, and vomiting	Focal neurologic signs
Abdominal pain	
Gastrointestinal bleeding	
Symptoms of bowel perforation	
Cough and shortness of breath	
Headache	
Focal neurologic deficits	

Background Information on Patients

Clinical information that should be recorded includes the patient's age, the underlying disease resulting in transplantation, the date(s) and type(s) of transplant received, and the date of onset of symptoms. It is also necessary to obtain other information that will assist in determining the risk of PTLD or guide the subsequent management of the patient [32, 33]. This is covered in detail in Chap. 10. The donor and recipient EBV serostatus is important given the fact that the primary risk factor for PTLD in the SOT patient is primary EBV infection [32, 33]. Pediatric patients are more likely to have primary EBV infection after transplantation, due to the fact the majority are EBV-seronegative at transplantation compared with their adult counterparts. Additional data include the types of organ transplanted and the dose and types of immunosuppression used. In this regard, the risk of PTLD depends on the types of organ transplanted. Patients who have received specific anti-T cell therapies may be at an increased risk of PTLD [33], although in recent years, clinical experiences are less convincing. The types and doses of antiviral agents used and the CMV donor and recipient serostatus are relevant, given the possibility that CMV infection/disease may be a risk factor 32–33],

Initial Clinical Examination

In keeping with regular clinical practice, a thorough physical examination is required to detect the manifestations of PTLD, which may be quite nonspecific (Table 8.1). The general physical examination might elicit evidence of pallor or signs referable to the site(s) of organs affected by PTLD. Given the predilection for the reticuloendothelial system to be involved, the clinical examination should include a meticulous assessment for lymphadenopathy. In selected cases, clinicians may choose to supplement clinical examinations with chest radiographs and abdominal ultrasounds as they screen for lymphadenopathy. The clinical examination should include periodic assessments by an otolaryngologist in high-risk cases, given the frequency with which the adenotonsillar tissues are involved, notably in the setting of primacy EBV infection.

Diagnostic and Screening Tests

The diagnostic tests that are performed for PTLD can be group into four main categories (Table 8.2). These are (1) general tests; (2) non-EBV-specific tests; (3) EBV-specific tests; and (4) histopathology. Given the importance of early diagnosis, the development of screening tests has been the subject of research for many years. Such screening is aimed at detecting subclinical PTLD or more overt PTLD in its earliest stages. There are data to suggest that in some patients, a definite subclinical phase of PTLD exists [34]. This is based on examination of liver biopsy samples

Table 8.2 Diagnostic evaluation of patients with symptoms or signs consistent with PTLD

General tests	Selective diagnostic tests	EBV-specific
CBC, WBC differential	Evaluation for specific infectious agents based on clinical presentation	EBV serologies (anti-EA, EBNA, and VCA)
Liver function tests	Lumbar puncture	EBV viral load in peripheral blood/blood compartments
Renal function tests	Bone scan	EBV status of lesions (PCR, in situ hybridization)
Serum electrolytes, calcium	Bone marrow biopsy	Excision or core needle biopsy of lesions for histopathology
Lactate dehydrogenase	Brain CT/MRI	
Uric acid	Gastrointestinal endoscopy	
Serum immunoglobulins	PET scan	
Stools for occult blood		
Chest radiographs		
CT scan of chest/abdomen/pelvis		

obtained prior to the diagnosis of PTLD. Examination of such samples have indicated the presence of EBV by PCR or EBER staining in 70% of patients who went on to develop PTLD compared with 10% of those who did not develop PTLD [34]. In addition, the histopathological examination of enlarged adenoidal tissue may indicate evidence of occult PTLD in asymptomatic individuals. In order to assist in the early diagnosis of PTLD, viral load surveillance is employed in most centers. This utility of viral load testing is discussed below and further elucidated in Chap. 6.

Tests are performed to rule out other diagnoses, as appropriate. This takes into account the likely differential diagnosis (see section "Differential Diagnoses"). Specific tests are performed to establish the histologic diagnosis of PTLD and to characterize PTLD lesions, including the presence or absence of EBV in biopsy tissue. General tests are performed to determine the presence or absence of complications of PTLD or related conditions. Depending on the nature of the tests, these are performed concurrently or sequentially.

General Tests and Non-EBV-Specific Tests

Blood Tests Initial tests include a complete blood count with white blood cell differential. In some patients with PTLD, there may be evidence of anemia which is usually normochromic, normocytic. In patients with gastrointestinal tract PTLD and occult bleeding over a prolonged period of time, there may be evidence of iron deficiency anemia with hypochromia and microcytosis. The source of bleeding can be determined by performing additional testing, namely, examination of the stools for occult blood. The blood elements may be depressed with evidence of leucopenia, atypical lymphocytosis, and thrombocytopenia. Thrombocytopenia and neutropenia have been shown to be associated with poorer outcomes, although the precise mechanism underlying this association is unclear [8, 9].

Depending on the location of PTLD lesions, there may be evidence of disturbance in serum electrolytes, liver, and renal function tests. Elevations in serum uric acid and lactate dehydrogenase may occur. Serum immunoglobulin levels may be elevated as part of an acute phase reaction. However, serum IgE levels have been observed to be elevated in some cases of PTLD [35]. Serum IgE levels may be elevated in the setting of a TH2 response profile which is thought be seen in patients with PTLD. The presence of elevated serum IgE may function as a proxy assay for TH2 activity. However, the relationship between PTLD and serum IgE levels has been found to be inconsistent. The presence of monoclonal or oligoclonal gammopathy has been shown to precede the detection of overt PTLD, but the specificity of this maker is poor [36].

Adjunctive tests that might predict PTLD risk or indicate the presence of PTLD have been investigated. Potential biomarkers studied include serum IL-6 [37], serum/plasma free light chains [38, 39], serum sCD30 [40], serum CXCL13 [41], and host genetic factors including HLA type [42] and polymorphisms in cytokine genes [43] but require further validation. How these markers relate to each other and to EBV viral load in predicting PTLD risk is the subject of current and future research. To date none of these markers should be definitively used for detection and follow-up.

Evaluation for the presence of cytomegalovirus is usually performed in patients with suspected PTLD. Diagnostic tests would include CMV quantitative PCR on blood as well as the examination of biopsy tissue for viral inclusions, PCR testing and immunohistochemistry for CMV. Cytomegalovirus may contribute to the net state of immunosuppression and is regarded by some experts to be a risk factor for PTLD. However, analyses of the impact of CMV disease or CMV mismatch have yielded conflicting results [44, 45]. HHV6 may also be an indirect co-factor for PTLD due to the potential for interaction with CMV [46].

Radiographic Imaging Imaging is essential in the evaluation of PTLD. Most centers employ a total body CT scan (head to pelvis) as part of the initial assessment. Beyond this, the choice of tests depends largely on the location of suspected lesions and the historical sequence of prior recent radiographic testing. Many experts recommend that a head CT or MRI be included as part of the initial workup. This is due to the fact that the presence of central nervous system lesions will influence treatment and such lesions may be solitary and may not be associated with disease in extracranial locations. CNS lesions often tend to fail therapy and are associated with high relapse rates, based on the fact that the CNS is a site that is relatively immunologically privileged.

Given the frequency of adenotonsillar involvement in PTLD, CT scanning of the neck may help to define the extent of involvement or detect subtle early changes that necessitate biopsy to rule out PTLD. Figure 8.2 shows the CT findings in a patient who was subsequently shown to have PTLD involving the adenoids. In some patients, adenotonsillar involvement is the only site of PTLD. It is likely that at least a proportion of these asymptomatic cases with adenotonsillar involvement resolve spontaneously as immunosuppression is minimized and stabilized beyond the early months after organ transplantation.

Pulmonary lesions that are visible on chest radiographs may require high-resolution CT scanning for better delineation prior to biopsy (Fig. 8.3). Furthermore, CT of the chest may reveal mediastinal adenopathy and small pulmonary nodules that are not visible on the plain chest radiograph. Suspected intra-abdominal lesions may be evaluated with ultrasonography and CT scanning. This is in addition to other modalities of assessment, including GI endoscopy in the case of intestinal hemorrhage. Figure 8.4 shows peripancreatic and retroperitoneal node involvement in a patient with PTLD. Such findings are not specific for PTLD, and other causes of lymphadenopathy should be considered in the differential diagnosis.

PET-CT (positron emission tomography-computerized tomography) has emerged to be a useful test in the evaluation of PTLD [47, 48]. PET is a diagnostic scanning method that directly measures metabolic, physiological, and biochemical functions

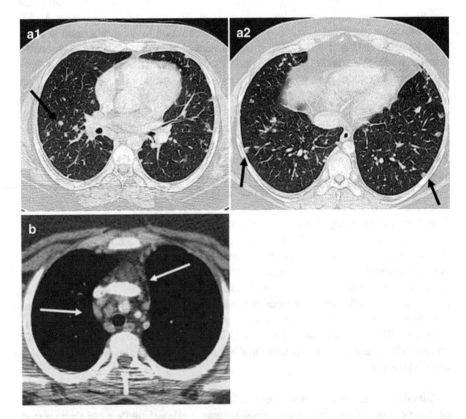

Fig. 8.3 CT (**a**) reveals multiple pulmonary parenchymal nodules and small mediastinal lymph nodes. (**b**) Biopsy of the parenchymal nodules confirmed PTLD. (Courtesy of Dr. David Manson, Hospital for Sick Children, Toronto)

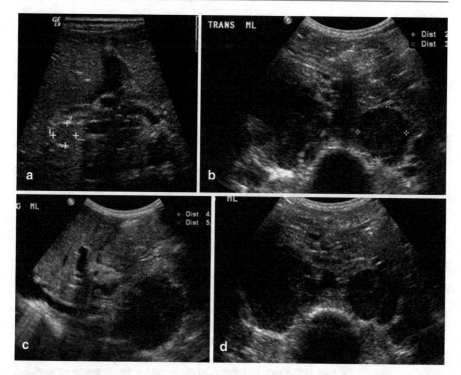

Fig. 8.4 Abdominal US of PTLD lesions: older child after HSCT and liver transplantation with elevated EBV titers. Multiple images show peri-pancreatic and retroperitoneal lymphadenopathy. (Courtesy of Dr. David Manson, Hospital for Sick Children, Toronto)

of the human body. A PET scan uses a small dose of a radionuclide combined with glucose (fluoro-2-deoxy-D-glucose, FDG) [47, 48]. The radionucleotide enables glucose metabolism to be traced, and it emits positrons, which are then detected by a scanner. Since certain tumors or lesions are known to grow at a fast rate compared to healthy tissue, the former cells will use up more of the glucose that is coupled with the radionuclide attached. The PET scan computer uses the measurements of glucose consumed to produce a color-coded picture. PET-CT utilizes a PET scanner with a computed tomography scanner in an integrated system, such that the CT provides accurate localization of lesions and the PET scan assists in interpretation of the suspected PTLD lesions. It has also proved to be of value in assessing the extent of remission after treatment (Fig. 8.5a, b). In the case of FDG-avid lymphomas, 18F-FDG-PET-CT has become the standard to assess treatment response [18, 49, 50]. Data in PTLD patients are limited and are largely confined to reports from single centers, where PET-CT has been used in diagnosis and more selectively in the follow-up of PTLD. However, a report from a registry of adult PTLD cases reported that end of treatment PET-CT had a 92% negative predictive value for disease relapse [51]. A major disadvantage is the amount of radiation delivered by PET-CT, which makes it difficult to make all-encompassing recommendations for all patients.

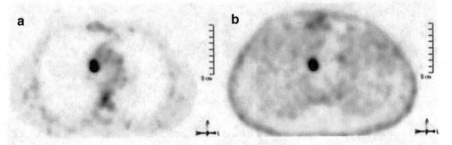

Fig. 8.5 Pretreatment PET-CT (**a**) reveals FDG-avid right paratracheal lymph node in a teenager after lung transplantation. Posttreatment study (**b**) reveals resolution of the FDG avidity and diminution of the node. (Courtesy of Dr. David Manson, Hospital for Sick Children, Toronto)

Once the diagnosis of PTLD has been determined, or is highly suspected, additional diagnostic tests may be performed to assist in defining the extent of disease. These investigations may include but are not limited to a bone scan, a bone marrow biopsy, and a lumbar puncture to assist in ruling out bone, bone marrow, and CNS disease, respectively.

EBV-Specific Tests

EBV Serology In immunocompetent patients, primary EBV infection can be determined by measuring EBV antiviral capsid antigen IgM and IgG antibodies, anti-early antigen (EA), and anti-Epstein-Barr nuclear antigen. Persistence of anti-EA antibodies has been previously shown to be more likely in PTLD patients [52], and patients who are known to be seropositive before transplantation may have falling anti-EBNA-1 titers in the setting of elevated EBV loads and the presence of PTLD [53]. However, experience has shown that serology is unreliable as a diagnostic tool for either PTLD or primary EBV infection in immunocompromised patients. These patients show a marked delay in their humoral response to EBV antigens, and many fail to develop immunoglobulin (Ig) M antibodies altogether. Another important drawback is that these patients may have received blood or blood products with the passive transfer of antibodies that render EBV IgG antibody assays difficult to interpret. In the above context, the most important role of EBV serology in the setting of transplantation is the categorization of serostatus of donors and recipients in order to determine the likely risk of PTLD.

Detection of EBV Nucleic Acids or Protein in Tissue It has been determined that 85–90% of PTLD lesions are EBV-positive. In situ analysis of biopsy specimens by polymerase chain reaction, viral antigen [54], and EBV-encoded small nuclear RNA (EBER) [54, 55] are of value in the diagnosis of EBV-associated PTLD. These modalities establish the presence or absence of EBV in the PTLD lesions. Polymerase chain reaction detection of EBV DNA in tissue is more useful in ruling out the presence of EBV in lesions than in indicating its presence as it is difficult to determine if the DNA is originating in the specific tissue as opposed to being deposited in the tissue by passenger lymphocytes. Immunohistochemistry staining may indicate the presence of viral genes, such as LMP-1. In situ hybridization for EBER labels EBV-encoded early RNA transcripts in infected cells. This is a rapid and reliable approach that is performed in most transplant centers.

Viral Load Determination in the Peripheral Blood   Technical aspects of the measurement of Epstein-Barr virus load are addressed in detail in Chap. 6. This test was first shown to be of value in the surveillance for PTLD as a result of work by Rocchi et al. [56], who indicated a relationship between PTLD and the number of EBV-infected cells in the peripheral blood. In 1994, Riddler et al. [57] and Savoie et al. [58] independently reported that an abnormally elevated EBV DNAemia correlated with PTLD development. Data from the Riddler et al. study indicated that using semi-quantitative polymerase chain reaction (PCR), patients with PTLD had a viral load greater than 5000 EBV genome copies/10^6 PBMC [57]. Other studies confirmed this relationship between viral loads and PTLD [59–64]. An association between PTLD and EBV detection in plasma has also been reported along with an increased specificity of plasma viral load in the diagnosis of EBV-positive PTLD [65]. These studies have advocated for the establishment of a threshold value for EBV DNAemia to distinguish patients at high risk for PTLD from those at low risk. The characteristics of this test as a diagnostic indicator of the presence of PTLD indicate that it is more useful in ruling out PTLD than in indicating its presence, in keeping with a low positive predictive value and a high negative predictive value.

Serial measurements of EBV load are more useful than single values. The addition of complimentary tests might increase the overall utility of viral load in the diagnostic evaluation of PTLD. In the future, these tests might include EBV-specific cytotoxic T lymphocyte measurements with or without the integration of cytokine/chemokine or viral gene expression profiling, using quantitative real-time reverse transcription-PCR and/or microarray technology.

Patients with asymptomatic sustained high loads (chronic high load carriers) require monitoring, as a proportion of these patients' clinical course evolves into PTLD. In this situation, the risk is represented by the sustained load as opposed to a specific quantifiable viral load threshold. Pediatric heart transplant recipients followed by intestinal recipients are more likely than their liver and kidney counterparts to develop PTLD in the setting of chronic high viral load carriage [66–68]. Data from prospective studies are needed to confirm these observations. In HSCT patients chronic high viral load carriage is not a frequent occurrence in the absence of chronic graft versus host disease with the resulting need for ongoing immunosuppression.

Histopathology

The pathologic examination of biopsy material is the gold standard for the diagnosis of PTLD. This is discussed in detail in Chap. 2. The presence of certain features in the lesions might assist in indicating malignant transformation and prognosis. Such criteria include monoclonality, oncogene rearrangements, and presence of specific mutations. Depending on the location of lesions, particular procedures may be needed to obtain tissue for histopathologic examination to rule out non-PTLD diagnoses, establish the diagnosis of PTLD, and characterize PTLD lesions. These procedures may include transbronchial biopsies; surgical biopsies of internal organs, skin lesions, tissues, or lymph nodes; CT-guided needle biopsies; and endoscopic gastrointestinal biopsies, as indicated.

Clinical Staging of PTLD

No staging system currently exists for PTLD, and no single system total captures the full spectrum of what is classified as PTLD. Most centers use systems that have been developed for lymphoma staging in immunocompetent hosts, the Lugano classification system in adults [69] and the International Pediatric Non-Hodgkin Lymphoma Staging System (IPNHLSS) in children [70]. The need for routine bone marrow biopsy and lumbar puncture for staging, particularly in the absence of symptoms or signs of involvement at these sites is uncertain; routine bone marrow biopsies are not recommended in immunocompetent hosts with DLBCL if PET-CT is performed [18].

At the very minimum, staging should document the presence or absence of symptoms, the precise location of lesions, the involvement of the allograft, and the presence or absence of CNS involvement. A simple clinical categorization of lesions based on location has been proposed [14]. In EBV-positive PTLD, the virologic status should be categorized as reflected by the level of viral load. While, conceptually, an increase in load from "remission levels" after therapy may be an indicator of relapse following successful initial treatment of PTLD, this may not be consistently accurate and notably so after rituximab-based treatment [71].

Differential Diagnoses

Some conditions may mimic PTLD depending on the nature of the presenting symptoms and the location of lesions. Rejection may be confused with PTLD affecting the transplanted organs [43]. This is an important consideration, given that the former requires augmentation of immunosuppression, while reduction in immunosuppression is required in the management of PTLD.

The presence of nonspecific constitutional symptoms might suggest the presence of an infectious etiology. Critically ill patients with an acute fulminant presentation may be confused with those with sepsis. Such patients may need to be empirically treated for infections other than EBV, while the diagnosis of PTLD is being established.

Patients presenting with pulmonary nodules might have a variety of conditions that can cause these lesions, including infections due to *Mycobacteria tuberculosis*, atypical mycobacteria, *Nocardia*, *Actinomyces*, and fungal species, among other pathogens. In lung transplant patients in particular, the differential diagnosis of pulmonary lesions includes *Aspergillus*. This deserves special mention, as in cases of pulmonary aspergillosis, careful consideration has to be given to the safety of using CT-guided needle biopsies to obtain tissue. These procedures are generally safe to do if the lesions are PTLD but may result in life-threatening pulmonary hemorrhage, if the lesions are due to *Aspergillus* [72]. In hematopoietic stem cell transplant recipients, the differential diagnosis includes graft versus host disease, particularly when the lesions are less well circumscribed with more diffuse involvement of lung parenchyma.

The differential diagnosis of lymphadenopathy includes the above entities as well as other condition causing localized or generalized lymphadenopathy. Examples include, but are not limited to, infections caused by *Bartonella* species and *Toxoplasma gondii* [73–75].

Patients with gastrointestinal symptomatology, such as diarrhea, may have a variety of other diagnoses other than PTLD. This can be particularly problematic when these symptoms occur in the setting of elevated EBV viral loads. In some patients with EBV enteritis, the boundaries of separation of this entity from PTLD can be blurred. Conditions to rule out besides PTLD or EBV disease include de novo bowel lymphomas, adenoviral disease, rejection in intestinal transplant patients, graft versus host disease in HSCT patients, cytomegalovirus disease, *Clostridium difficile* infection, intestinal mycobacterial infection and other infectious etiologies, and medication-induced diarrhea (in particular mycophenolate mofetil).

Clinicians should always be reminded that non-EBV-related malignancies may arise in the post-transplant period and enter into the differential diagnosis of PTLD [73–77]. These malignancies may be classified into three categories: preexisting recipient malignancies, de novo malignancies originating in the recipient, and donor-transmitted malignancies. These entities are generally more frequently seen in adult patients compared with children. The skin represents the most frequently documented site of involvement by these non-PTLD malignancies. A detailed discussion of these is beyond the scope of this chapter.

In disseminated PTLD, the extent of hemophagocytosis can be significant enough to create a syndrome that mimics hemophagocytic lymphohistiocytosis (HLH) [78, 79]. The latter is characterized by fever, splenomegaly, jaundice, and the pathologic finding of hemophagocytosis (phagocytosis by macrophages of erythrocytes, leukocytes, platelets, and their precursors) in the bone marrow and other tissues. Epstein-Barr virus infection is one of the etiologic agents that have been linked with HLH, even if the patient does not have PTLD. This gives rise to diagnostic confusion between PTLD with some elements of hemophagocytosis and HLH that is driven by Epstein-Barr virus in the absence of PTLD. Treatment of the latter includes, but is not limited to, chemotherapy with etoposide and dexamethasone, while the former requires reduction in immunosuppression as discussed elsewhere in this publication.

Ten Take-Home Pearls

- Early detection of PTLD is important in maximizing the chances for a successful outcome.
- Epstein-Barr virus load is more useful in ruling out PTLD than in indicating its presence.
- Epstein-Barr virus serology is unreliable as a diagnostic tool for PTLD and primary EBV infection in immunocompromised patients.
- Clinicians should have a high index of suspicion for PTLD in at-risk patients, including but not limited to those who have no pre-transplant EBV immunity.
- PTLD often affects the transplanted organ with the exception of the heart.
- Lymphoid tissues, including nodes, adenoids, and tonsils, are frequently the primary sites affected by PTLD.
- PTLD affecting the central nervous system may present as a solitary lesion.
- Knowledge of the differential diagnosis is important in preventing missed diagnoses of non-PTLD diseases.
- *Positron emission tomography-computerized tomography* has emerged to be a useful test in the evaluation of PTLD.
- Histopathologic examination is the gold standard for the diagnosis of PTLD.

References

1. Swerdlow SH, Campo E, et al. The 2016 revision of the World Health Organization classification of lymphoid neoplasms. Blood. 2016;127:2375–90.
2. Dierickx D, Habermann TM. Post-transplant lymphoproliferative disorder in adults. N Engl J Med. 2018;378(6):549–62.
3. Grotto I, Mimouni D, Huerta M, et al. Clinical and laboratory presentation of EBV positive infectious mononucleosis in young adults. Epidemiol Infect. 2003;131:683–9.
4. Tattevin P, Le Tulzo Y, Minjolle S, et al. Increasing incidence of severe Epstein-Barr virus-related infectious mononucleosis: surveillance study. J Clin Microbiol. 2006;44:1873–4.
5. Imashuku S. Systemic type Epstein–Barr virus-related lymphoproliferative diseases in children and young adults: challenges for pediatric hemato-oncologists and infectious disease specialists. Pediatr Hematol Oncol. 2007;24:563–8.
6. Nalesnik MA, Makowa L, Starzl TE. The diagnosis and treatment of posttransplant lymphoproliferative disorders. Curr Probl Surg. 1988;25:367–472.
7. Swinnen LJ, Mullen GM, Carr TJ, et al. Aggressive treatment for postcardiac transplant lymphoproliferation. Blood. 1995;86:3333–40.
8. Dror Y, Greenberg M, Taylor G, et al. Lymphoproliferative disorders after organ transplantation in children. Transplantation. 1999;67:990–8.
9. Green M, Webber S. Posttransplantation lymphoproliferative disorders. Pediatr Clin N Am. 2003;50:1471–91.
10. Cen H, Breinig MC, Atchison RW, et al. Epstein-Barr virus transmission via donor organ in solid organ transplantation: polymerase chain reaction and restriction fragment length polymorphism analysis of IR2, IR3 and IR4. J Virol. 1991;65:976–80.
11. Larson RS, Scott MA, McCurley TL, et al. Microsatellite analysis of posttransplant lymphoproliferative disorders: determination of donor/recipient origin and identification of putative lympho-magnetic mechanism. Cancer Res. 1996;56:4378–81.

12. Shapiro RS, McClain K, Frizzera G, et al. Epstein-Barr virus associated B-cell lymphoprolif-
    erative disorders following bone marrow transplantation. Blood. 1988;71:1234–43.
13. Dojcinov SD, Venkataraman G, Raffeld M, Pittaluga S, Jaffe ES. EBV positive mucocutane-
    ous ulcer–a study of 26 cases associated with various sources of immunosuppression. Am J
    Surg Pathol. 2010;34(3):405–17. https://doi.org/10.1097/PAS.0b013e3181cf8622.
14. L'Huillier AG, Dipchand AI, Ng VL, et al. Posttransplant lymphoproliferative disorder in pedi-
    atric patients: survival rates according to primary sites of occurrence and a proposed clini-
    cal categorization. Am J Transplant. 2019;19(10):2764–74. https://doi.org/10.1111/ajt.15358.
    Epub 2019 Apr 22
15. Caillard S, Lamy FX, Quelen C, et al. Epidemiology of post-transplant lymphoproliferative
    disorders in adult kidney and kidney pancreas recipients: report of the French registry and
    analysis of subgroups of lymphomas. Am J Transplant. 2012;12:682–93.
16. Bishnoi R, Bajwa R, Franke AJ, et al. Post-transplant lymphoproliferative disorder (PTLD):
    single institutional experience of 141 patients. Exp Hematol Oncol. 2017;6:26. https://doi.
    org/10.1186/s40164-017-0087-0. eCollection 2017
17. Caillard S, Porcher R, Provot F, et al. Post-transplantation lymphoproliferative disorder after
    kidney transplantation: report of a Nationwide French registry and the development of a new
    prognostic score. JCO. 2013;31:1302–9.
18. Dierickx D, Tousseyn T, Sagaert X, et al. Single-center analysis of biopsy-confirmed posttrans-
    plant lymphoproliferative disorder: incidence, clinicopathological characteristics and prognos-
    tic factors. Leuk Lymphoma. 2013;54(11):2433–40.
19. Campisi P, Allen UD, Ngan BY, et al. Utility of head and neck biopsies in the evaluation of post-
    transplant lymphoproliferative disorder. Otolaryngol Head Neck Surg. 2007;137:296–300.
20. Herrmann BW, Sweet SC, Hayashi RJ, et al. Otolaryngological manifestations of posttrans-
    plant lymphoproliferative disorder in pediatric thoracic transplant patients. Int J Pediatr
    Otorhinolaryngol. 2006;70:303–10.
21. Herrmann BW, Sweet SC, Molter DW. Sinonasal posttransplant lymphoproliferative disorder
    in pediatric lung transplant patients. Otolaryngol Head Neck Surg. 2005;133:38–41.
22. Roy S, Vivero RJ, Smith LP. Adenotonsillar pathology in post-transplant patients. Int J Pediatr
    Otorhinolaryngol. 2008;72:865–8.
23. Shapiro NL, Strocker AM. Adenotonsillar hypertrophy and Epstein-Barr virus in pediatric
    organ transplant recipients. Laryngoscope. 2001;111:997–1001.
24. Williamson RA, Huang RY, Shapiro NL. Adenotonsillar histopathology after organ transplan-
    tation. Otolaryngol Head Neck Surg. 2001;125:231–40.
25. Leblond V, Sutton L, Dorent R, et al. Lymphoproliferative disorders after organ transplanta-
    tion: a report of 24 cases observed in a single institution. J Clin Oncol. 1995;13:961.
26. Starzl TE, Nalesnik MA, Porter KA, et al. Reversibility of lymphomas and lymphoprolifera-
    tive lesions developing under cyclosporin-steroid therapy. Lancet. 1984;1:583–7.
27. Lee ES, Locker J, Naslesnik M, et al. The association of Epstein–Barr virus with smooth
    muscle tumors occurring after organ transplantation. N Engl J Med. 1995;332:19–25.
28. Evens A, Choquet S, Kroll-Desrosiers A, et al. Primary CNS posttransplant lymphoprolifera-
    tive disease (PTLD): an international report of 84 cases in the modern era. Am J Transplant.
    2013;13:1512–22.
29. Mahale P, Shiels M, Lynch C, Engels E. Incidence and outcomes of primary central nervous
    system lymphoma in solid organ transplant recipients. Am J Transplant. 2018;18:453–61.
30. Knowles DM, Cesarman E, Chadburn A, et al. Correlative morphologic and molecular genetic
    analysis demonstrates three distinct categories of posttransplant lymphoproliferative disorders.
    Blood. 1995;85:552–65.
31. Ranganathan S, Webber SA, Ahuja S, et al. Hodgkin's-like posttransplant lymphoproliferative
    disorder in children: does it differ from posttransplant Hodgkin's lymphoma? Pediatr Dev
    Pathol. 2004;7:348–60.
32. Allen UD, Farkas G, Hébert D, et al. Risk factors for post-transplant lymphoproliferative dis-
    order in pediatric patients: a case-control study. Pediatr Transplant. 2005;9:450–5.

33. Walker RC, Marshall WF, Strickler JG, et al. Pretransplantation assessment of the risk of lymphoproliferative disorder. Clin Infect Dis. 1995;20:1346–53.
34. Randhawa PS, Jaffe R, Demetris AJ, et al. Expression of Epstein–Barr virus-encoded small RNA (by the EBER-1 gene) in liver specimens from transplant recipients with post- transplantation lymphoproliferative disease. N Engl J Med. 1992;327:1710–4.
35. Mathur A, Kamat DM, Filipovich AH, et al. Immunoregulatory abnormalities in patients with Epstein-Barr virus-associated B cell lymphoproliferative disorders. Transplantation. 1994;57:1042–5.
36. Badley AD, Portela DF, Patel R, et al. Development of monoclonal gammopathy precedes the development of Epstein–Barr virus-induced posttransplant lymphoproliferative disorder. Liver Transpl Surg. 1996;2(5):375–82.
37. Barton M, Wasfy S, Hébert D, and the EBV and Associated Viruses Collaborative Research Group, et al. Exploring beyond viral load testing for EBV lymphoproliferation: role of serum IL6 and IgE assays as adjunctive tests. Pediatr Transplant. 2009;13:990–8.
38. Engels EA, Preiksaitis JK, Zingone A, Landgren O. Circulating antibody free light chains and risk of posttransplant lymphoproliferative disorder. Am J Transplant. 2012;12:1268–74.
39. Borrows R, Scheer A, Cockwell P, et al. Serum-free light chains adjusted for renal function are a potential biomarker for post-transplant lymphoproliferative disorders. Ann Hematol. https://doi.org/10.1007/s00277-018-03591-w.
40. Haque T, Chaggar T, Schafers J, Atkinson C, McAulay K, Crawford D. Soluble CD30: a serum marker for Epstein-Barr virus- associated lymphoproliferative diseases. J Med Virol. 2011;83:311–6.
41. Schiffer L, Henke-Gendo C, Wilsdorf N, et al. CXCL13 as a novel marker for diagnosis and disease monitoring in pediatric PTLD. Am J Transplant. 2012;12:1610–7.
42. Kinch A, Sundstrom C, Tufveson G, Glimelius I. Association between HLA-A1 and A2 types and Epstein-Barr virus status of post-transplant lymphoproliferative disorder. Leuk Lymphoma. 2016;57(10):2351–8.
43. Howard TK, Klintmalm GB, Stone MJ. Lymphoproliferative disorder masquerading as rejection in liver transplant recipients – an early aggressive tumor with atypical presentation. Transplantation. 1992;53:1145–7.
44. Courtwright AM, Burkett P, Divo M, et al. Posttransplant lymphoproliferative disorders in Epstein-Barr virus donor positive/recipient negative lung transplant recipients. Ann Thorac Surg. 2018;105:441–7.
45. Huang JG, Tan MYQ, Quak SH, Aw MM. Risk factors and clinical outcomes of pediatric liver transplant recipients with post-transplant lymphoproliferative disease in a multi-ethnic Asian cohort. Transpl Infect Dis. 2018;20(1) https://doi.org/10.1111/tid.12798. Epub 2017, Nov 28
46. Humar A, Malkan G, Moussa G, et al. Human herpesvirus-6 is associated with cytomegalovirus reactivation in liver transplant recipients. J Infect Dis. 2000;181:1450–3.
47. Bianchi E, Pascual M, Nicod M, et al. Clinical usefulness of FDG-PET/CT scan imaging in the management of posttransplant lymphoproliferative disease. Transplantation. 2008;85:707–12.
48. McCormack L, Hany TI, Hübner M, et al. How useful is PET/CT imaging in the management of post-transplant lymphoproliferative disease after liver transplantation? Am J Transplant. 2006;6:1731–6.
49. von Falck C, Maecker B, Schirg E, et al. Post-transplant lymphoproliferative disease in pediatric solid organ transplant patients: a possible role for [18F]-FDG-PET(/CT) in initial staging and therapy monitoring. Eur J Radiol. 2007;63(3):427–35.
50. Vali R, Punnett A, Bajno L, Moineddin R, Shammas A. The value of 18F-FDG PET in pediatric patients with post-transplant lymphoproliferative disorder at initial diagnosis. Pediatr Transplant. 2015;19(8):932–9. https://doi.org/10.1111/petr.12611. Epub 2015 Oct 30
51. Zimmermann H, Denecke T, Dreyling MH, et al. End-of-treatment positron emission tomography after uniform first-line therapy of B cell posttransplant lymphoproliferative disorder identifies patients at low risk of relapse in the prospective German PTLD registry. Transplantation. 2018;102(5):868–75.

52. Carpentier L, Tapiero B, Alvarez F, et al. Epstein–Barr virus (EBV) early-antigen serologic testing in conjunction with peripheral blood EBV DNA load as a marker for risk of posttransplantation lymphoproliferative disease. J Infect Dis. 2003;188:1853–64.
53. Preiksaitis JK, Diaz-Mitoma F, Mirzayans F, et al. Quantitative oropharyngeal Epstein–Barr virus shedding in renal and cardiac transplant recipients: relationship to immunosuppressive therapy, serologic responses, and the risk of posttransplant lymphoproliferative disorder. J Infect Dis. 1992;166:986–94.
54. Young L, Alfieri C, Hennessy K, et al. Expression of Epstein–Barr virus transformation-associated genes in tissues of patients with EBV lymphoproliferative disease. N Engl J Med. 1989;321:1080–5.
55. Fanaian N, Cohen C, Waldrop S, EBER, et al. Automated in situ hybridization (ISH) vs. manual ISH and immunohistochemistry (IHC) for detection of EBV in pediatric lymphoproliferative disorders. Pediatr Dev Pathol. 2008;1:195–9. [Epub ahead of print]
56. Rocchi G, de Felici A, Ragona G, et al. Quantitative evaluation of Epstein–Barr virus- infected mononuclear peripheral blood leukocytes in infectious mononucleosis. N Engl J Med. 1977;296:132–4.
57. Riddler SA, Breinig MC, McKnight JLC. Increased levels of circulating Epstein–Barr virus (EBV)-infected lymphocytes and decreased EBV nuclear antigen antibody responses are associated with the development of posttransplant lymphoproliferative disease in solid-organ transplant recipients. Blood. 1994;84:974–84.
58. Savoie A, Perpête C, Carpentier L, et al. Direct correlation between the load of Epstein–Barr virus-infected lymphocytes in the peripheral blood of pediatric transplant patients and risk of lymphoproliferative disease. Blood. 1994;83:2715–22.
59. Allen UD, Hébert D, Tran D, et al. Utility of semiquantitative polymerase chain reaction for Epstein–Barr virus among pediatric solid organ transplant recipients with and without transplant lymphoproliferative disease. Clin Infect. 2001;33:145–50.
60. Bai X, Hosler G, Rogers BB, et al. Quantitative polymerase chain reaction for human herpesvirus diagnosis and measurement of Epstein-Barr virus burden in posttransplant lymphoproliferative disorder. Clin Chem. 1997;43:1843–9.
61. Kenagy DN, Schlesinger Y, Wesk K, et al. Epstein-Barr virus DNA in peripheral blood leukocytes of patients with posttransplant lymphoproliferative disease. Transplantation. 1995;60:547–54.
62. Lucas KG, Burton RL, Zimmerman SE, et al. Semiquantitative, Epstein-Barr virus (EBV) polymerase chain reaction for the determination of patients at risk for EBV-induced lymphoproliferative disease after stem cell transplantation. Blood. 1998;91:3654–61.
63. Nakazawa Y, Chisuwa H, Ikegami T, et al. Efficacy of quantitative analysis of Epstein-Barr virus-infected peripheral blood lymphocytes by in situ hybridization of EBER-1 after living-related liver transplantation: a case report. Transplantation. 1997;63:1363–6.
64. Rowe DT, Qu L, Reyes J. Use of quantitative competitive PCR to measure Epstein-Barr virus genome load in the peripheral blood of pediatric transplant patients with lymphoproliferative disorders. J Clin Microbiol. 1997;35:1612–5.
65. Allen UD, Preiksaitis JK, AST Infectious Diseases Community of Practice. Post-transplant lymphoproliferative disorders, Epstein-Barr virus infection, and disease in solid organ transplantation: guidelines from the American Society of Transplantation Infectious Diseases Community of Practice. Clin Transpl. 2019:e13652. https://doi.org/10.1111/ctr.13652.
66. Green M, Soltys K, Rowe DT, et al. Chronic high Epstein-Barr viral load carriage in pediatric liver transplant recipients. Pediatr Transplant. 2008;13:319–23.
67. Bingler MA, Feingold B, Miller SA, et al. Chronic high Epstein-Barr viral load state and risk for late-onset posttransplant lymphoproliferative disease/lymphoma in children. Am J Transplant. 2008;8:442–5.
68. Yamada M, Nguyen C, Fadakar P, et al. Epidemiology and outcome of chronic high Epstein-Barr viral load carriage in pediatric kidney transplant recipients. Pediatr Transplant. 2018;22(3):e13147. https://doi.org/10.1111/petr.13147. Epub 2018 Feb 6

69. Cheson BD, Fisher RI, Barrington SF, et al. Recommendations for initial evaluation, staging, and response assessment of Hodgkin and non-non-Hodgkin lymphoma: the Lugano classification. J Clin Oncol. 2014;32(27):3059–68.
70. Rosolen A, Perkins SL, Pinkerton CR, et al. Revised international pediatric Non-Hodgkin lymphoma staging system. J Clin Oncol. 2015;33(18):2112–8.
71. Oertel S, Trappe RU, Zeidler K, et al. Epstein–Barr viral load in whole blood of adults with posttransplant lymphoproliferative disorder after solid organ transplantation does not correlate with clinical course. Ann Hematol. 2006;85:478–84. https://doi.org/10.1007/s00277-006-0109-1.
72. Slatore CG, Yank V, Jewell KD, et al. Bronchial-pulmonary artery fistula with fatal massive hemoptysis caused by anastomotic bronchial *Aspergillus* infection in a lung transplant recipient. Respir Care. 2007;52:1542–5.
73. American Academy of Pediatrics. *Toxoplasma gondii* infections. In: Kimberlin W, Brady MT, Jackson MA, Long SL, editors. Red book: 2018 report of the committee on infectious diseases. 27th ed. Elk Grove Village: American Academy Pediatrics; 2018. p. 809–19.
74. Dharnidharka VR, Richard GA, Neiberger RE, et al. Cat scratch disease and acute rejection after pediatric renal transplantation. Pediatr Transplant. 2002;6:327–31.
75. Friedman AM. Evaluation and management of lymphadenopathy in children. Pediatr Rev. 2008;29:53–60.
76. Penn I. De novo malignancies in pediatric organ transplant recipients. Pediatr Transplant. 1998;2:56–63.
77. Penn I. Neoplastic complications of organ transplantation. In: Ginns LC, Cosimi AB, Morris PJ, editors. Transplantation. Malden: Blackwell Science; 1999. p. 770–86.
78. Fisman DN. Hemophagocytic syndromes and infection. Emerg Infect Dis. 2000;6:601–8.
79. Imashuku S. Clinical features and treatment strategies of Epstein-Barr virus-associated hemophagocytic lymphohistiocytosis. Crit Rev Oncol Hematol. 2002;44:259–72.

Prognostic Factors of PTLD after SOT

9

Donald E. Tsai and Mitchell E. Hughes

Historical Background

Prognosis of post-transplant lymphoproliferative disorders (PTLD) follows the principles of other B-cell lymphomas. The prognosis of Hodgkin lymphoma patients has been established using the Ann Arbor staging system (Table 9.1) [1]. Originating in 1971, the Ann Arbor system classifies patients into risk categories based on anatomic stage. The Ann Arbor system was further validated in 1977 for non-Hodgkin lymphoma (NHL) and is currently the primary prognostic tool for both Hodgkin lymphoma and NHL [2]. However, anatomic staging alone is inadequate for estimating prognosis in NHL due to the hematogenous spread of disease characteristic of these lymphomas, a nonspecific clinical presentation, advanced Ann Arbor stage often present upon initial diagnosis, and outcomes better correlated with histopathology. Given the aforementioned challenges with prognostication of lymphomas, in 1993, the International Prognostic Index (IPI) was published. The IPI was the culmination of international level data to help develop a better prognostic-factor model for NHL [3]. NHL continues to follow IPI, or a modification of IPI, for assessment of prognosis (Tables 9.2 and 9.3).

Prognostic Factors for PTLD

Identification of prognostic factors for PTLD is complicated and tortuous due to the rapid changes in the understanding and management of this heterogeneous group of disorders. Similar to the treatment paradigm shift in NHL, the introduction of the anti-CD20 monoclonal antibody, rituximab, has drastically changed the treatment

D. E. Tsai (✉) · M. E. Hughes
Abramson Cancer Center, University of Pennsylvania, Philadelphia, PA, USA
e-mail: dtsai@loxooncology.com; mitchell.hughes@pennmedicine.upenn.edu

© Springer Nature Switzerland AG 2021
V. R. Dharnidharka et al. (eds.), *Post-Transplant Lymphoproliferative Disorders*,
https://doi.org/10.1007/978-3-030-65403-0_9

Table 9.1 Ann Arbor staging classification for Hodgkin and non-Hodgkin lymphomas

Stage	Description
Stage I	Involvement of a single lymph node region (I) or of a single extralymphatic organ or site (IE)
Stage II	Involvement of two or more lymph node regions or lymphatic structures on the same side of the diaphragm alone (II) or with involvement of limited, contiguous extralymphatic organ or tissue (IIE)
Stage III	Involvement of lymph node regions on both sides of the diaphragm (III) which may include the spleen (IIIS) or limited, contiguous extralymphatic organ or site (IIIE) or both (IIIES)
Stage IV	Diffuse or disseminated foci of involvement of one or more extralymphatic organs or tissues, with or without associated lymphatic involvement
A	No symptoms
B	Fever (temperature > 38.0 °C), drenching night sweats, unexplained loss of >10% of body weight in the past 6 months
E	Refers to extranodal contiguous extension
S	Splenic involvement

Adapted from Refs. [1, 4]

Table 9.2 The International Prognostic Index (IPI) historic survival data [3]

One point for each risk factor present	Prognosis
Age greater than 60 years Stage III or IV disease	Low risk (0–1 points) – 5-year survival of 73%
Elevated serum lactate dehydrogenase (LDH) ECOG performance status of 2, 3, 4 (see Table 9.3)	Low-intermediate risk (2 points) – 5-year survival of 51%
More than one extranodal site	High-intermediate risk (3 points) – 5-year survival of 43% High risk (4–5 points) – 5-year survival of 26%

Table 9.3 ECOG performance status [5]

Grade	ECOG
0	Fully active, able to carry on all pre-disease performance without restrictions
1	Restricted in physically strenuous activity, but ambulatory and able to carry out work of a light or sedentary nature, e.g., lighthouse work and office work
2	Ambulatory and capable of all self-care, but unable to carry out any work activities. Up and about more than 50% of waking hours
3	Capable of only limited self-care, confined to bed or chair more than 50% of waking hours
4	Completely disabled. Cannot carry on any self-care. Totally confined to bed or chair
5	Dead

approach of PTLD. Thus, the assembly for prognostic outcomes in patient with PTLD has shifted.

In the current era, there continues to be modest, often conflicting, and outdated or non-generalizable data regarding prognostic factors for PTLD. The large majority of the data include retrospective literature from the pre-rituximab era, heavily weighted in renal transplant patients. Despite this heterogeneity and lack of robust consistency in the literature, we attempt to assemble a clinically meaningful overview of the information published to date (Table 9.4).

Table 9.4 Summary of recent studies on PTLD prognostic factors [6]

Study	Design	Size (N)	Population	Significant prognostic factors for poorer survival	Prognostic index development
Leblond et al. [7]	Retrospective analysis	61	Solid organ txp[a]	High PS, multifocal dz	Yes
Tsai et al. [8]	Retrospective analysis	42	Solid organ txp	Elevated LDH, organ dysfunction, multiorgan dz, B sx, increased age	Yes
Muti et al. [9]	Retrospective and prospective analysis	40	Solid organ txp	High PS, multifocal dz, elevated LDH, high Ann Arbor stage	No
Ghobrial et al. [10]	Retrospective analysis	30	Solid organ txp in rituximab era	High PS, CD-20 negative	No
Bakker et al. [11]	Retrospective analysis	40	Lung and kidney txp	High PS	No
Ghobrial et al. [12]	Retrospective analysis	107	Solid organ txp	PS 3 or 4, graft organ involvement, monomorphic dz[b]	Yes
Trofe et al. [13]	Retrospective registry analysis	402	Kidney	PTLD within 6 months of txp, multifocal dz, increased age	No
Caillard et al. [14]	Prospective registry analysis	230	Kidney	Multifocal dz, azathioprine	No
Maecker et al. [15]	Retrospective registry analysis	55	Kidney, liver, heart/lung	Stage IV disease, BM involvement, CNS involvement	No
Hourigan et al. [16]	Retrospective analysis	42	Kidney	Elevated LDH, PS >1, B sx	No
Oton et al. [17]	Retrospective analysis	84	Solid organ txp	Increased age, multiorgan transplant, ECOG >2, grafted organ involvement, extranodal disease, early (< 1 year) PTLD, stage IV, EBV+, BCL2+, elevated WBC	No

(continued)

Table 9.4 (continued)

Study	Design	Size (N)	Population	Significant prognostic factors for poorer survival	Prognostic index development
Knight et al. [18]	Retrospective registry analysis	78	Solid organ txp	CNS involvement, IPI 3–5	No
Evens et al. [19]	Retrospective analysis	80	Solid organ txp	CNS involvement, BM involvement	No
Yoon et al. [20]	Retrospective analysis	43	Heart, kidney, liver	Early onset (<1 year) PTLD, monomorphic dx	No
Trappe et al. [21]	Prospective clinical trial analysis	70	Solid organ txp	Age, ECOG, type of transplant, response to rituximab	Yes
Bishnoi et al. [22]	Retrospective analysis	141	Solid organ txp	Male gender, PMH of malignancy, increased age, lung allograft, BMT, EBV+, monomorphic dz, pts experiencing multiple rejections	Yes
Trappe et al. [23]	Prospective clinical trial	152	Solid organ txp	Response to rituximab, type of transplant, IPI <3 vs. ≥3	Yes

dz disease. *sx* symptoms, *txp* transplantation
See Table 9.5 for a summary of prognostic indices
[a]Implies at least heart, lung, liver, and kidney and can include pancreatic and dual organ
[b]Monomorphic disease was not significant by univariate analysis, but was useful as part of multivariable model using all three prognostic factors

Of all prognostic factors, performance status has the most supporting evidence in the body of PTLD literature [7, 9–12, 15]. As ECOG PS increases, prognosis worsens, with poorer survival appearing to be most pronounced in PS greater than 1. PS may not be the most intuitive prognostic factor for PTLD, as compared to NHL, because PS is, in part, a marker of tolerance to chemotherapy regimens, whereas PTLD treatment in the current era involves reduced immunosuppression and rituximab, which are well-tolerated therapies. PTLD itself may resonate the toll the disease has on patients and is therefore a marker of tumor biology and behavior. PS is likely a reflection of a patient's overall stamina and capacity to endure the disease process itself.

Patient age at diagnosis of PTLD is the next prognostic factor with the most supporting studies [8, 12, 24]. The International Prognostic Index defines age greater than 60 as the benchmark definition; in contrast, PTLD prognosis worsens in a relatively linear fashion as age advances beyond 55–60 [12]. Advanced age in patients with NHL is a poor prognostic factor due to comorbidities and is associated with a reduced capacity to tolerate chemotherapy. Patients with PTLD of advanced age, similar to PS, may be a surrogate marker for overall health and stamina to fight or endure PTLD. It is also postulated that a younger patient with PTLD may have different disease biology than PTLD in patients with advanced age. EBV status is by and large less likely to be negative in younger patients. Younger patients also have different exposures and different immune systems as compared to older patients. Finally, the biology of EBV-driven PTLD in younger patients, particularly children, arising from primary infection, is likely different from older patients who develop PTLD through viral re-activation [25, 26].

The presence of multifocal disease is an additional well-supported poor prognostic factor in PTLD [7–9, 12, 13, 24]. This is akin to the IPI in NHL, where both extranodal disease and advanced Ann Arbor stage confer poorer prognosis. In contrast to NHL, PTLD often present with allograft involvement. Even though allograft involvement qualifies as organ involvement by strict definition, it does not appear to confer as much risk of a poorer outcome as involvement of a non-allograft organ, and clearly is not as strong a risk factor alone as the presence of multifocal or multiorgan involvement. In renal transplant, isolated allograft involvement alone can be managed with surgical resection and therefore may improve prognosis [12].

Another poor prognostic factor is CD-20-negative status, mainly because this debars the use of rituximab therapy [12]. The lack of CD-20 suggests a divergent underlying cell of origin that leads to a different disease behavior, whether it be immature B cells who have yet to acquire CD-20 or a mature plasmacytic B cell that has shed CD-20. Rituximab will likely continue to be the predominant agent used in CD-20-positive PTLD, and therefore, it will be difficult to parse out the prognostic significance of CD-20 status outside the context of the effect of rituximab.

The introduction of rituximab in the current era and its relationship to prognostic factors are weighed in an article published in 2005 by Ghobrial and colleagues [10]. The study retrospectively evaluated 30 consecutive patients at a single center diagnosed with PTLD between 1999 and 2002. Rituximab was administered to 15 patients who were CD-20 positive and EBV positive and did not respond to front-line treatment with reduction in immunosuppression. There were 15 patients who did not meet the aforementioned criteria and had received alternative therapy, including observation, surgery, radiation, chemotherapy, or a combination of these therapies. There were differences observed in a number of characteristics between the rituximab group and the other treatment group. The average age was younger in the rituximab group (average age 37 vs. 50) and they developed disease sooner after transplant (average 8 months vs. >5 years out). Multivariate analysis for all 30 patients identified important prognostic factors. Overall survival in patients with CD-20-positive PTLD, low IPI ($P = 0.004$), and rituximab therapy ($P = 0.03$) was significant on multivariate analysis.

Prognostic factors for response to rituximab have been evaluated in two prospective clinical trials. Choquet and colleagues conducted a phase 2 multicenter trial of 46 solid organ transplant recipients with B-cell PTLD. The only factor predictor of response at 80 days in patients receiving rituximab was a normal LDH level (odds ratio = 6.9; $P = 0.007$) [27]. Lack of CNS disease is hypothesized to be a positive predictive marker for response to rituximab; however, clinical trials exclude patients with CNS disease and thus have not been evaluated prospectively. Furthermore, Oertel and colleagues conducted a prospective multicenter trial of 17 PTLD patients administered with rituximab therapy. The two factors predictive of response were

EBV positivity ($P < 0.0001$) and a shorter time from transplantation to diagnosis ($P = 0.036$) [28]. These predictive markers to rituximab are logical given elevated LDH and EBV-negative PTLD are known poor prognostic features in PTLD. Response to rituximab can also be used as a prognostic feature to predict which patients will require subsequent therapy with chemotherapy. Trappe and colleagues suggest that PTLD patients treated sequentially with 4 infusions of rituximab followed by chemotherapy is preferable to rituximab monotherapy plus chemotherapy at disease progression [21, 23, 29]. If a patient is noted to respond well to rituximab, then chemotherapy is not necessary, and consolidation of a CR with four applications of rituximab with four additional courses of rituximab is even superior to chemotherapy consolidation.

The presence of CNS involvement signifies poorer outcomes [30]. One study, published by Trofe and colleagues, reviewed the Israel Penn registry specifically identifying cases of PTLD with CNS involvement [13]. Out of 910 cases, 15% had CNS involvement. Patients with CNS disease had a 3-year survival of 9.4% compared to those without CNS disease which was 49.4%. Isolated CNS disease conferred a 3-year overall survival of 29%. Patients with both CNS and non-CNS involvement of PTLD had a 3-year overall survival of 0. Another multicenter study of 80 solid organ transplant recipients removed treatment on Cox regression multivariate analysis and identified CNS disease, in addition to hypoalbuminemia, and bone marrow involvement as the most significant prognostic markers [19]. Hypoalbuminemia was later found to be non-significant in a subsequent single-center analysis [22].

The majority of PTLD cases are of B-cell origin; however, there are many case reports and small case series of T-cell PTLD. Classic PTLD arise from suppressed T-cell activity leading to EBV, which reside in B cells, ultimately inducing B-cell proliferation and transformation. In contrast, T-cell PTLD, in most cases, are not EBV positive and follow a distinct biologic mechanism, conceivably through altered T-cell proliferation related to T-cell-suppressive therapies. The onset of T-cell PTLD usually presents later and more commonly is associated with a primary extranodal site [31]. There remains a lack of large analyses of this rare subgroup; however, based on case reports and clinical experience, T-cell PTLD have been observed to have a poorer prognosis compared to classic B-cell PTLD [31, 32].

The type of organ transplanted noticeably has an impact on the incidence of PTLD. From highest to lowest, the incidence of PTLD occurs in the following order among solid organ transplants: intestinal, lung, heart, liver, and kidney. The intensity and duration of immunosuppression required for organ transplantation is related to incidence, as well as the mass of lymphoid tissue associated with a particular organ, which is why intestinal transplantation has the highest incidence of PTLD. Kidney and liver recipients who have PTLD appear to have better outcomes as compared to lung and heart recipients, which is related to the ease and safety of immunosuppression reduction [20, 33]. Kidney and liver rejection is reasonably easy to monitor with laboratory observation, and both organs are relatively tolerant of rejection allowing for more aggressive reduction in immunosuppression. In contrast, cardiac and lung transplant rejection is more likely to manifest as sudden death or rapid and frequently irreversible decompensation. The risks in rejection in these organs temper the extent to which immunosuppression is reduced. The opportunity of initiating a patient on dialysis makes kidney rejection manageable compared to other organ decompensation from rejection. In addition to the difficulty of immune suppression reduction, heart and lung transplant recipients treated for PTLD have a more aggressive disease course. A lack of response to rituximab monotherapy in the heart and lung transplant population predicts a lack of response to CHOP and early relapse as compared to liver or kidney transplant patients refractory to rituximab monotherapy [21, 23].

It was once thought that EBV-positive PTLD carried a more favorable prognosis compared to EBV-negative PTLD. Several biologic inferences with similar favorable prognosis supported this assumption. EBV-driven PTLD are primarily B cell in origin, conferring favorable prognosis compared to T-cell PTLD. EBV-positive PTLD are more likely to be CD-20 positive, which can be treated with rituximab, and therefore more favorable. Additionally, EBV-positive PTLD biology is more often polymorphic, which is observed to have more favorable outcomes compared to monomorphic disease. Finally, children have better outcomes compared to adults and are more likely to have EBV-positive disease. Despite these strong correlative observations, studies discussed elsewhere in this chapter have not found EBV status to be a reliable prognostic factor [7–9, 12, 13, 16]. By the same token, a 2006 study by Kremers and colleagues investigated 35 adult liver transplant patients and the prognostic significance of EBV status. Their study found the outcomes among 22 EBV-positive patients and 13 EBV-negative patients were nearly identical at both 1- and 5-year follow-up [34]. Ultimately, the data does not support EBV as a marker useful for prognostication. While EBV positivity may not be a useful prognosticator, patients who are EBV-naïve receiving an EBV-infected organ seem to be at the highest risk for PTLD development [18].

Another potential prognostic factor without robust evidence is the presence of monomorphic disease. Monomorphic disease suggests a clonal process resisted the natural checks on cell growth and survival. PTLD with monomorphic disease resemble traditional NHL in immunocompetent patients. A multi-institutional retrospective analysis of 56 pediatric heart transplant patients with PTLD identified 35 polymorphic cases and 19 monomorphic cases. Early onset PTLD were observed to be more commonly polymorphic. Nonetheless, there was no survival difference identified between these two histologic categories [26]. Curiously, one study of 107 PTLD patients identified monomorphic disease was not a significant prognostic factor by univariate analysis; however, upon multivariable analysis, it was identified as a poor prognostic factor in the author's proposed PTLD prognostic index [35] (Table 9.5).

There are many other prognostic factors hypothesized to confer a negative prognostic value in PTLD; however, there remains scant or contradictory evidence supporting them. One of these factors is early vs. late onset of PTLD after transplantation. Some clinicians posit early onset PTLD indicate worse outcomes under the assumption early disease designates aggressive disease. In 2005, a large retrospective analysis of the Israel Penn registry between 1968 and 2004 was conducted, identifying

Table 9.5 Prognostic indices in PTLD [6]

Index name	Population	Risk factors	Prognosis
Leblond index [7]	31 patients, two institutions, solid organ transplants	PS >1 dz sites >1	0 RFs = median survival >100 months 1 RF = 1 month 2 RF = 1 month
Ghobrial et al. [35]	107 patients, single institution, solid organ transplants	Monomorphic disease Graft organ involvement	Pts with 2–3 RFs had 5.31 RR of death compared with 0–1 RFs
Choquet et al. [24]	60 patients, solid organ transplants receiving rituximab	Age > 60 PS >1 Elevated LDH Time from transplant[a]	2-year survival 0 RFs = 88% 1 = 50% 2–3 RFs = 0%
Oton et al. [17]	84 patients, single institution, solid organ transplant	ECOG >2 Elevated WBC 1 month prior to diagnosis BCL-2 overexpression	Three risk factors = median survival 10 days (95% CI:0–41) No RFs = median survival of 1414 days
Hourigan et al. [16]	42 patients, single institution, kidney transplants	B-symptoms Elevated LDH	Reduced survival with the presence of each RF – see Fig. 9.1
Caillard et al. [36]	500 patients, multicenter, solid organ transplant	Age > 55 Serum creatinine >1.5 mg/dL Elevated LDH PTLD localization Monomorphic disease T-cell PTLD[b]	Mortality using a 5-point scale: 0 (3.3%; CI, 0.4%–9.5%) 1 (18.7%; CI, 10.7%–28.4%) 2–3 (35.8%; CI, 29%–42.6%) 4–5 (60.8%; CI, 40.5%–76.1%)
Trappe et al. [21]	70 patients, multicenter, solid organ transplant	Age ECOG Type of transplant Response to rituximab	Age > 60 ($p = 0.001$, HR 4.423) Thoracic organ txp ($p < 0.001$, HR 7.827) Overall response to rituximab at interim staging ($P = 0.017$, HR 0.322) IPI ≥3 ($p = 0.032$, CI 1.052–4.981, HR 2.289)
Trappe et al. [23]	152 patients, multicenter, solid organ transplant	Response to rituximab Type of transplant IPI <3 vs. ≥3	IPI ≥3 overall survival ($p = 0.001$, CI 1.461–4.418, HR 2.540) Response to rituximab overall survival ($p < 0.001$, CI 0.180–0.571, HR 0.320)
Bishnoi et al. [21]	141 patients, single institution, solid organ transplant	Age at diagnosis Recipient EBV status Bone marrow involvement Initial best response	Female gender HR 0.553 (p: 0.0427, CI 0.311–0.981) Elderly patient HR 3.543 ($p < 0.0001$, CI 1.894–6.628)

[a]Time from transplant not included in prognostic index
[b]Excluded from five-point Caillard prognostic index

402 kidney transplant patients diagnosed with PTLD [12]. Survival was identified to be poorer in those patients diagnosed within 6 months of transplant (64%) compared to diagnosis beyond 6 months (54%, $P = 0.04$), as well as those diagnosed within 1 year compared to after 1 year from transplantation (60% vs. 55%, $p < 0.04$). A dissimilar report was published in 2001, reporting a single institution retrospective study of 30 lung transplant patients diagnosed with PTLD observed no survival difference between patients diagnosed before or after 1 year from transplant [37]. Another negative retrospective single-center analysis of 107 solid organ transplant patients found early onset PTLD, defined as within 1 year of transplant, commonly were EBV-positive, were CD-20-positive, and involved grafted organs. In spite of these biological markers, there were no differences observed in survival [35]. Given the conglomerate of literature, it is fair to presume both early and late PTLD can either behave as indolent in nature or behave aggressively, often leading to rapid decline.

Similar to adults, PTLD in children are a heterogeneous group of diseases. PTLD in children often have better outcomes compared to adults. The timing of PTLD in children is generally earlier after transplantation, is commonly EBV positive, and associated with primary EBV infection. There remains little data on prognostic factors in children with PTLD, although there remain some analyses [38].

A retrospective analysis of 55 pediatric patients with PTLD after solid organ transplant, by Maecker and colleagues, suggested prognostic factors in children largely mirror those in adults [15]. The authors identified stage IV disease, bone marrow involvement, CNS disease, and poor response to initial therapy were significantly associated with poor outcomes. EBV negativity and early onset of PTLD after transplantation were not significantly associated with poor outcomes. These findings are consistent with those identified in adult patients with PTLD. Additionally, as similar to adult NHL patients, children with c-*myc* translocation had worse outcomes. The presence of c-*myc* translocation may poorly predict event-free survival; therefore, as more robust data presents itself, it is not uncommon to recommend a cytogenetic analysis of patients. While monomorphic disease was not associated with prognostic value in this study, another single-center retrospective analysis of 32 patients showed conflicting results [39].

A recent publication studied the efficacy of low-dose chemotherapy in 36 children diagnosed with PTLD after failing first-line therapy. Patients in this study responded well to chemotherapy; however, patients who presented with fulminant disseminated disease ($N = 4$) did poorly [40].

As previously mentioned, one retrospective, multi-institutional analysis of 56 pediatric heart transplant patients with PTLD observed no survival difference between monomorphic and polymorphic diseases [26].

Compared to adult patients, there is less data on prognostic factors for PTLD in children, leading clinicians to extrapolate based on adult literature. The retrospective questionnaire study of centers who participate in the NAPRTS database investigated the pediatric kidney transplant population. There were 92 survey questionnaires evaluated from 35 different centers. Pediatric patients with PTLD within 1 year post-transplant were associated with better survival outcomes compared to PTLD after 1 year of transplantation ($p = 0.032$). The presence of EBV, CD20 positivity, and clonality were not found to be negative prognostic factors; however, several confounders in this study leave room for further investigation of these factors [41]. Additional research in the pediatric population is required to shed additional light on prognostic factors given the pitfalls of extrapolating data from adults, especially given the biologic and phenotypic differences recognized in each population.

Prognostic Indices

There have been several authors who attempted to develop a PTLD-specific prognostic index to replace the International Prognostic Index, which was developed for aggressive NHL who are otherwise immunocompetent. Unfortunately, these indices are restricted by the nature of their small sample sizes and generalizability of the patient populations being studied. However, clinicians still may find these other indices useful as long as they match their patient population where applicable. We summarize several of these articles in Table 9.5 to provide a comparison.

In 2001, Leblond and colleagues published a retrospective analysis from two institutions examining 61 patients diagnosed with PTLD between 1980 and 1999. There were 34 patients who had kidney transplants, 19 cardiac transplants, and all other patients had a lung or liver transplant [7]. The authors acknowledged two of the risk factors identified, PS and number of involved sites, could define a risk index by sorting patients into three groups: low-risk patients (PS <2 and <2 sites) whose median survival time had not yet been reached at well over 100 months of follow-up, intermediate-risk patients (PS ≥2 or ≥2 sites involved) with a median survival time of 34 months, and high-risk patients (PS ≥2 and ≥2 sites involved) with a median survival time of 1 month. The authors concluded this PTLD-specific index had a slight advantage when predicting survival as compared to the International Prognostic Index.

Another study in 2001, by Tsai and colleagues, examined prognostic factors in 42 patients who were treated with reduction in immunosuppression as initial therapy for PTLD [8]. Multivariable analysis identified that an elevated lactate dehydrogenase (LDH) ratio, organ dysfunction, and multiorgan involvement by PTLD were independent prognostic factors for lack of response to reduction of immunosuppression. Of the 18 patients lacking these poor prognostic factors, 89% responded to reduction in immunosuppression as opposed to three of five (60%) in patients with one risk factor and zero out of seven patients who had two to three risk factors. The notable overlap of the prognostic factors discovered in this study with the IPI suggests that PTLD behave much like lymphomas in immunocompetent hosts, despite a stark difference in management.

In 2005, Ghobrial and colleagues published a prognostic study including 107 patients diagnosed with PTLD at the Mayo Clinic between 1970 and 2003 [35]. The median survival for the entire cohort was 31.5 months (95% CI, 10.7–72.5 months). The median follow-up of living patients was 51.8 months (range, 5.6–202.6 months).

An easy-to-use multivariable model for survival was created, which included poor performance status (3–4), monomorphic disease, and graft organ involvement. Patients who were identified with two or three of these factors had a 5.31 relative risk of death during follow-up compared with patients with zero or one factor present. As previously mentioned, monomorphic disease was useful in the multivariable model; however, it was not a prognostic factor in univariate analysis. When compared to the IPI, the authors concluded their three-variable model was superior ($P = 0.006$).

A 2007 study by Choquet and colleagues investigated the long-term efficacy of single-agent rituximab in PTLD patients [24]. Predictors of survival in patients treated with rituximab were age at diagnosis, performance status, LDH, and time from transplantation. The authors developed a PTLD-specific prognostic index in the setting of rituximab treatment, using LDH, age > 60, PS >1, and time from transplant as risk factors. Patients with no risk factors had an 88% 2-year survival. Patients with one risk factor had a 50% 2-year survival and no patients with two risk factors survived to 2 years. Compared to the IPI, the author's PTLD prognostic index appeared to predict survival better.

A 2008 paper published by Oton and colleagues studied 84 solid organ transplant patients at a single center diagnosed with PTLD. The authors identified patients who had overexpression of BCL-2 (>50% staining), ECOG >2, and elevated white blood cell count had a median survival of 10 days. Patients with none of the aforementioned risk factors had a median survival of 1414 days [17]. Strong expression of the proto-oncogene, BCL-2, seemed to correlate with inferior outcomes, as similar to NHL. BCL-2 overexpression is proposed to provide prognostic significance and requires confirmatory studies to validate.

In 2008, Hourigan and colleagues published correspondence describing their retrospective study of 42 patients with PTLD after renal transplant [16]. The authors identified elevated LDH, PS >1, and presence of B symptoms were significantly associated with decreased survival. An analysis of this index was compared to the IPI, the Leblond (2001) PTLD prognostic index, the Choquet (2007) index, and the Ghobrial (2005) index. The authors found all indices, except the Ghobrial index, could separate patients into clinically meaningful survival groups (Fig. 9.1). It is important to note that the correspondence described an analysis of only renal transplant patients, while the other indices, including the Ghobrial index, identified a more diverse group of transplant recipients.

The French registry investigation by Caillard and colleagues in 2013 identified age > 55 years, serum creatinine >133 μmol/L (1.5 mg/dL), elevated LDH, disseminated lymphoma, brain localization, invasion of serous membranes, monomorphic PTLD, and T-cell PTLD as independent poor prognostic indicators of survival. The investigators incorporated age, serum creatinine, LDH, PTLD localization, and histology as a five-point prognostic score. PTLD mortality was low in patients with a score of 0 (3.3%; 95% CI, 0.4–9.5%), intermediate in a score of 1 (18.7%; 95% CI, 29–42.6%), high in a score of 2 or 3 (35.8%; 95% CI, 29–42.6%), and very high in patients with a score of 4 or 5 (60%; 95% CI, 40.5–76.1%). Patients with a score of 0 have a 5-year survival rate of 92%, whereas patients with a score of 4 to 5 have a

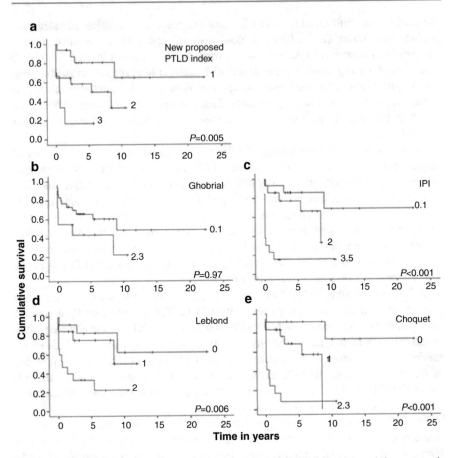

Fig. 9.1 Overall survival according to the proposed renal (PTLD) index (**a**), and the prognostic groupings according to Ghobrial and colleagues [33] (**b**), the international prognostic index (IPI) (**c**), Leblond and colleagues [7] (**d**), and Choquet and colleagues [22] (**e**). + refers to censored points

5-year survival rate of 35% [36]. This study was missing performance status, so it was unable to assess IPI and thus unable to compare this prognostic system against the IPI to see whether it is a suitable alternative. The scale was able to correctly prognosticate survival in this patient population and requires independent validation.

In 2015, Trappe and colleagues analyzed a cohort of 70 patients treated in the international multicenter phase II PTLD-1 trial in order to identify the risk factors for PTLD. The analysis confirmed the prognostic role of IPI, Ghobrial score, and PTLD prognostic index in relation to the overall survival. A high IPI and high PTLD prognostic index were associated with higher treatment-related mortality, primarily driven by age and ECOG performance status. It was identified that thoracic organ transplantation and response to rituximab were prognostic indicators for both time to progression and overall survival. IPI was broken down into low (<3) and high (≥3) [21].

With low sample size as a limitation, Trappe and colleagues followed up their survey in 2016 with a prospective, international, multicenter phase II trial. Response to weekly doses of rituximab (375 mg/m² IV) for 4 weeks was a significant predictor of time to progression and overall survival ($P < 0.001$). IPI <3 or ≥3 was confirmed in this trial to be a significant prognostic factor for overall survival. An IPI ≥3 conferred a negative prognostic value for overall survival ($p = 0.001$; 95% HR 2.540; CI, 1.461–4.418) and time to progression ($p = 0.001$; HR 3.338; 95% CI, 1.624–6.862). Overall survival and time to progression were further broken down according to IPI <3 or ≥3 (Fig. 9.2). Response to rituximab conferred a positive prognostic value for overall survival ($p < 0.001$; HR 0.320; 95% CI, 0.180–0.571) and time to progression ($p < 0.001$; HR 0.256; 95% CI, 0.119–0.549) [23]. Patients who did not respond to rituximab tended to have more aggressive disease when treated with CHOP and were more likely to have refractory disease and early treatment relapse [23].

A 2017 single institution study by Bishnoi and colleagues identified older age at PTLD diagnosis, recipient EBV status, bone marrow involvement, and initial best response were statistically significant prognostic factors ($p < 0.05$) [19]. Female gender was found to have a statistically significant better prognosis compared to males [Female gender HR 0.553 (p: 0.0427, CI 0.311–0.981)]. Similar to other studies, monomorphic PTLD performed poorly; however, it was not significant. EBV was not supported for predicting survival, yet it is still important for predicting pathogenesis. Interestingly, rituximab as upfront therapy did not impact overall

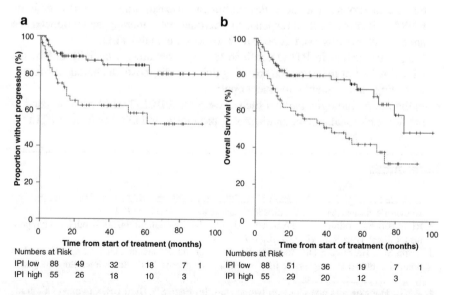

Fig. 9.2 IPI index <3 and ≥3 by Trappe and colleagues. 143 patients included in analysis; solid line: $n = 88$; dashed line: $n = 55$. **Panel a** time to progression ($p = 0.001$). **Panel b** overall survival ($p = 0.001$)

survival and had a poor hazard ratio [0.589 (95% CI: 0.289–1.201)]. This single institution study confirmed previous risk factors associated with predicting PTLD.

As research will illuminate further dichotomy, PTLD will undoubtedly separate into various histologic, molecular, and clinical diagnoses, as similar to NHL. The perpetual forward momentum of our understanding of these disease processes, in addition to the foreseeable arrival of new treatment options, will make prognosis an ever-evolving issue for clinicians and patients. Biologic markers, such as BCL-2 and c-*myc*, will be more closely scrutinized to help refine diagnosis, prognosis, and management of PTLD. When considering the various prognostic factors identified in the heterogeneous body of PTLD literature, age, PS, sites of disease/extranodal disease, and LDH remain consistent. The IPI has helped predict response in the prior era of chemotherapy-based treatment, and newer PTLD indices now account for rituximab-based therapies and reduction of immunosuppression. In the face of evolving therapies in PTLD with newer options in the clinical setting, the prognostic factors have by and large remained the same. Regardless of the therapy used, in the end, the biology of PTLD has endured to follow similar principles as lymphoma.

Take-Home Pearls

- The identification of prognostic factors for PTLD is complicated by the rapid changes in the understanding and management of what is a heterogeneous group of disorders.
- Several factors such as poor PS, multifocal disease, tumor CD-20 negativity, CNS involvement, lack of response to rituximab monotherapy, and advanced age are consistently observed as poor prognostic features in PTLD.
- Prognostic factors in PTLD continue to vary over time, especially due to the wide timeline of investigation spanning different diagnostic techniques, molecular testing, and available treatment options.
- In the future, biologic markers such as c-*myc* and BCL-2 will be investigated to provide additional insight on diagnosis, prognosis, and management of PTLD.

References

1. Carbone PP, Kaplan HS, Musshoff K, Smithers DW, Tubiana M. Report of the committee on Hodgkin's disease staging classification. Cancer Res. 1971;31:1860–1.
2. Rosenberg SA. Validity of the Ann Arbor staging classification for the non-Hodgkin's lymphomas. Cancer Treat Rep. 1977;61:1023–7.
3. Shipp MA, Harrington DP, Anderson JR, Armitage JO, Bonadonna G, Brittinger G, et al. A predictive model for aggressive non-Hodgkin's lymphoma. The international non-Hodgkin's lymphoma prognostic factors project. N Engl J Med. 1993;329(14):987–94.
4. AJCC: Hodgkin and non-Hodgkin lymphomas. In: Edge SB, Byrd DR, Compton CC, et al., editors. AJCC cancer staging manual. 7th ed. New York: Springer; 2010.p. 607–11.
5. Oken MM, Creech RH, Tormey DC, Horton J, Davis TE, McFadden ET, Carbone PP. Toxicity and response criteria of the Eastern Cooperative Oncology Group. Am J Clin Oncol. 1982;5:649–55.

6. Maniar T, Tsai D. Prognostic Factors for PTLD. Post-Transplant Lymphoproliferative Disorders [Internet]. Springer Berlin Heidelberg; 2010;105–16. Available from: http://dx.doi.org/10.1007/978-3-642-01653-0_8.

7. Leblond V, Dhedin N, Brunee MF, Choquet S, Hermine O, Porcher R, et al. Identification of prognostic factors in 61 patients with post-transplantation lymphoproliferative disorders. J Clin Oncol. 2001;19(3):772–8.

8. Tsai DE, Hardy CL, Tomasezewski JE, Kotloff RM, Oltoff KM, Somer BG, et al. Reduction in immunosuppression as initial therapy for posttransplant lymphoproliferative disorder: analysis of prognostic variables and long-term follow-up of 42 adult patients. Transplantation. 2001;71(8):1076–88.

9. Muti G, Cantoni S, Oreste P, Klersy C, Gini G, Rossi V, et al. Post-transplant lymphoproliferative disorders: improved outcome after clinic-pathologically tailored treatment. Haematologica. 2002;87(1):67–77.

10. Ghobrial IM, Habermann TM, Ristow KM, Ansell SM, Macon W, Geyer SM, et al. Prognostic factors in patients with post-transplant lymphoproliferative disorders (PTLD) in the rituximab era. Leuk Lymphoma. 2005;46:191–6.

11. Bakker NA, van Imhoff GW, Verschuuren EAM, van Son WJ, Homan van der Heide JJ, Veeger NJGM, et al. Early onset post-transplant lymphoproliferative disease is associated with allograft localization. Clin Transpl. 2005;19(3):327–34.

12. Ghobrial IM, Haberman TM, Macon WR, Ristow KM, Larson TS, Walker RC, et al. Differences between early and late posttransplant lymphoproliferative disorders in solid organ transplant patients: are they two different diseases? Transplantation. 2005;79(2):244–7.

13. Trofe JT, Buell JF, Beebe TM, Hanaway MJ, First MR, Alloway RR, et al. Analysis of factors that influence survival with post-transplant lymphoproliferative disorder in renal transplant recipients: the Israel Penn international transplant tumor registry experience. Am J Transplant. 2005;5(4):775–80.

14. Caillard S, Lelong C, Pessione F, Moulin B. Post-transplant lymphoproliferative disorders occurring after renal transplantation in adults: report of 230 cases from the French registry. Am J Transplant. 2006;6:2735–42.

15. Maecker B, Jack T, Zimmerman M, Abdul-Khalig H, Burdelski M, Fuchs A, et al. CNS or bone marrow involvement as risk factors for poor survival in post-transplantation lymphoproliferative disorders in children after solid organ transplantation. J Clin Oncol. 2007;31:4902–8.

16. Hourigan MJ, Doecke J, Mollee PN, Gill DS, Norris D, Johnson DW, et al. A new prognosticator for post-transplant lymphoproliferative disorders after renal transplantation. Br J Haematol. 2008;141(6):904–7.

17. Oton AB, Wang H, Leleu X, Melhem MF, George D, Lacasce A, et al. Clinical and pathological prognostic markers for survival in adult patients with post-transplant lymphoproliferative disorders in solid transplant. Leuk Lymphoma. 2008;49:1738–44.

18. Knight JS, Tsodikov A, Cibrik DM, Ross CW, Kaminski MS, Blayney DW. Lymphoma after solid organ transplantation: risk, response to therapy, and survival at a transplantation center. J Clin Oncol. 2009;27:3354–62.

19. Evens AM, David KA, Helenaowski I, Nelson B, Kaufman D, Kircher SM, et al. Multicenter analysis of 80 solid organ transplantation recipients with post-transplantation lymphoproliferative disease: outcomes and prognostic factors in the modern era. J Clin Oncol. 2010;28(6):1038–46.

20. Yoon SO, Cho YE, Suh C, Kim KM, Han DJ, Lee SG, et al. Post-transplant lymphoproliferative disorders: clinicopathological analysis of 43 cases in a single center, 1990–2009. Clin Transpl. 2012;26:67–73.

21. Trappe RU, Choquet S, Dierickx D, Mollee P, Zaucha JM, Dreyling MH, et al. International prognostic index, type of transplant and response to rituximab are key parameters to tailor treatment in adults with CD20-positive B cell PTLD: clues from the PTLD-1 trial. Am J Transplant. 2015;15:1091–100.

22. Bishnoi R, Bajwa R, Franke AJ, Skelton WP, Wang Y, Patel N, et al. Post-transplant lympho-proliferative disorder (PTLD): single institutional experience of 141 patients. Exp Hematol Oncol. 2017;6:1–14.
23. Trappe RU, Dierickx D, Zimmermann H, Morschhauser F, Mollee P, Zaucha JM, et al. Response to rituximab induction is a predictive marker in B-cell post-transplant lymphoprolif-erative disorder and allows successful stratification into rituximab or R-CHOP consolidation in an international, prospective, multicenter phase II trial. J Clin Oncol. 2017;35:536–43.
24. Choquet S, Oertel S, Leblond V, Riess H, Varoqueaux N, Dörken B, et al. Rituximab in the management of post-transplant lymphoproliferative disorder after solid organ transplantation: proceed with caution. Ann Hematol. 2007;86(8):599–607.
25. Lucas KG, Burton RL, Zimmerman SE, Wang J, Cornetta KG, Robertson KA, et al. Semiquantitative Epstein-Barr virus polymerase chain reaction for the determination of patients at risk for EBV-induced lymphoproliferative disease after stem cell transplantation. Blood. 1998;92(10):3977–8.
26. Webber SA, Naftel DC, Fricker FJ, Olesnevich P, Blume ED, Addonizio L, et al. Lymphoproliferative disorders after paediatric heart transplantation: a multi-institutional study. Lancet. 2006;367:233–9.
27. Choquet S, Leblond V, Herbrecht R, Socié G, Stoppa AM, Vandenberghe P, et al. Efficacy and safety of rituximab in B-cell post-transplantation lymphoproliferative disorders: results of a prospective multicenter phase 2 study. Blood. 2006;107:3503–7.
28. Oertel SH, Vershuuren E, Reinke P, Zeidler K, Papp-Váry M, Babel N, et al. Effect of anti-CD 20 antibody rituximab in patients with post-transplant lymphoproliferative disorder (PTLD). Am J Transplant. 2005;5:2901–6.
29. Trappe R, Oertel S, Leblond V, Mollee P, Sender M, Reinke P, et al. Sequential treatment with rituximab followed by CHOP chemotherapy in adult B-cell post-transplant lymphoprolifera-tive disorder (PTLD): the prospective international multicentre phase 2 PTLD-1 trial. Lancet Oncol. 2012;13:196–206.
30. Buell JF, Gross TG, Hanaway MJ, Trofe J, Roy-Chaudhury P, First MR, et al. Posttransplant lymphoproliferative disorder: significance of central nervous system involvement. Transplant Proc. 2005;37(2):954–5.
31. Haldas J, Wang W, Lazarchick J. Post-transplant lymphoproliferative disorders: T-cell lym-phoma following cardiac transplant. Leuk Lymphoma. 2002;43(2):447–50.
32. Lundell R, Elenitoba-Johnson KSJ, Lim MS. T-cell posttransplant lymphoproliferative disorder occurring in a pediatric solid-organ transplant patient. Am J Surg Pathol. 2004;28(7):967–73.
33. Benkerrou M, Jais J-P, Leblond V, Durandy A, Sutton L, Bordigoni P, et al. Anti-B-cell mono-clonal antibody treatment of severe posttransplant B-lymphoproliferative disorder: prognostic factors and long-term outcome. Blood. 1998;92(9):3137–47.
34. Kremers WK, Devarbhavi HC, Wiesner RH, Krom RAF, Macon WR, Habermann TM. Post-transplant lymphoproliferative disorders following liver transplantation: incidence, risk factors and survival. Am J Transplant. 2006;6:1017–24.
35. Ghobrial IM, Habermann TM, Maurer MJ, Geyer SM, Ristow KM, Larson TS, et al. Prognostic analysis for survival in adult solid organ transplant recipients with post-transplantation lym-phoproliferative disorders. J Clin Oncol. 2005;23:7574–82.
36. Caillard S, Porcher R, Provot F, Dantal J, Choquet S, Durrbach A, et al. Post-transplantation lymphoproliferative disorder after kidney transplantation: report of a nationwide French regis-try and the development of a new prognostic score. J Clin Oncol. 2013;31:1302–9.
37. Paranjothi S, Yusen RD, Kraus MD, Lynch JP, Patterson GA, Trulock EP. Lymphoproliferative disease after lung transplantation: comparison of presentation and outcome of early and late cases. J Heart Lung Transplant. 2001;20:1054–63.

38. Gross TG, Bucuvalas JC, Park JR, Greiner TC, Hinrich SH, Kaufman SS, et al. Low-dose chemotherapy for Epstein-Barr virus-positive post-transplantation lymphoproliferative disease in children after solid organ transplantation. J Clin Oncol. 2005;23:6481–8.
39. Hayashi RJ, Kraus MD, Patel AL, Canter C, Cohen AH, Hmiel P, et al. Posttransplant lymphoproliferative disease in children: correlation of histology to clinical behavior. J Pediatr Hematol Oncol. 2001;23:14–8.
40. Fohrer C, Caillard S, Koumarianou A, Ellero B, Woehl-Jaeglé M-L, Meyer C, et al. Long-term survival in post-transplant lymphoproliferative disorders with a dose-adjusted ACVBP regimen. Brit J Haem. 2006;134:602–12.
41. Dharnidharka VR, Martz KL, Stablein DM, Benfield MR. Improved survival with recent post-transplant lymphoproliferative disorder (PTLD) in children with kidney transplants. Am J Transplant. 2011;11:751–8.

Management of PTLD after SOT

10

Ralf Ulrich Trappe and Steven A. Webber

Introduction

Despite a growing understanding of the pathophysiology of PTLD, its optimal management remains controversial. There is an increasing armamentarium of treatments available to the clinician, but the evidence to define how and when to use these treatments, or how best to combine therapies, is restricted to discrete patient populations and cannot be generalized. Of note, no randomized trials of any form of therapy for PTLD have been performed. In the first part of this review, we summarize the rationale and evidence to support individual treatments. Following this, we discuss combinations of therapies and how they might be best applied as first- or second-line therapies. It should be noted that the choice of therapy is often arbitrary (e.g., institutional preference) but may also be driven by predictive factors (real or perceived) such as pathological findings, age at onset, organ transplanted, disease stage, presence or absence of EBV, comorbid conditions, and prior rejection history. This chapter focuses on treatment of PTLD after solid organ transplantation. Management of PTLD within the context of hematopoietic stem cell transplantation is dealt with in detail in Chap. 14.

R. U. Trappe (✉)
Department of Hematology and Oncology, Christian-Albrechts-University Kiel, Kiel, Germany

Division of Hematology and Oncology, Department of Medicine, DIAKO Ev. Diakonie-Krankenhaus Bremen, Bremen, Germany
e-mail: rtrappe@gwdg.de

S. A. Webber
Department of Pediatrics, Vanderbilt University School of Medicine, Monroe Carell Jr. Children's Hospital at Vanderbilt, Nashville, TN, USA
e-mail: steve.a.webber@vumc.org

© Springer Nature Switzerland AG 2021
V. R. Dharnidharka et al. (eds.), *Post-Transplant Lymphoproliferative Disorders*,
https://doi.org/10.1007/978-3-030-65403-0_10

167

Optimal Therapy for PTLD

The optimal treatment regimen for PTLD is one that rapidly eradicates the disease, does not increase the risk of allograft rejection (acute or chronic), and is simple to give, cost-effective, and is associated with minimal adverse events. It is apparent that no single treatment fulfills all these criteria. Furthermore, the treatment must be geared to the individual patient, since the appropriate treatment, for example, for severe PTLD in a lung recipient early after transplant with adverse rejection profile, is likely to be very different from that of a renal recipient with benign rejection history late out from transplant. Moreover, organ involvement has a considerable impact on the choice of treatment including occasional need for surgery in patients with gastrointestinal involvement (e.g., with perforation or uncontrolled bleeding) or specific CNS-directed therapies in patients with CNS involvement. These considerations underscore the enormous challenges involved in designing clinical trials for a rare disease with such clinical heterogeneity. Clinical response is also likely to depend on intrinsic characteristics of the tumor such as rate of mitosis, presence or absence of EBV, and the ability to be controlled by reconstitution of T-cell immune surveillance. Unfortunately, it is currently very hard to predict tumor behavior, even after extensive pathological evaluation is completed. Even the presence of cytogenetic alterations, for example, the t(8;14)-translocation in Burkitt PTLD, does not necessarily predict an aggressive clinical course [92]. However, response to rituximab monotherapy and a baseline international prognostic index (IPI) score of three or higher (risk factors are age > 60 years, Ann Arbor stage ≥ III, ECOG performance status ≥2, elevated LDH, and more than one extranodal disease manifestation) have been identified as prognostic markers in prospective clinical trials in adult PTLD, and response to rituximab monotherapy already has been validated prospectively [76, 79].

Reduction of Immunosuppression

In 1984, Starzl and colleagues reported the reversibility of PTLD by reduction in immunosuppression in cyclosporine-treated patients [66]. This strategy remains the initial mainstay of therapy for most patients with non-destructive lesion and polymorphic PTLDs across all age groups. It is also used as initial therapy in monomorphic disease, though most patients require subsequent treatment. The goal of reduction (or cessation) of immunosuppression is to allow the host to recover natural immune surveillance and subsequently gain control over the proliferation of EBV-infected B cells. Restitution of immune surveillance may also be associated with resolution of EBV-negative PTLD, though this seems to occur with lower frequency [20]. The majority of PTLD in children (especially non-destructive and polymorphic lesions) will respond to reduction in immunosuppression, though with significant rates of rebound acute cellular rejection that may vary by organ [34, 86]. The reported response rates of PTLD to reduction of immunosuppression among adults are highly variable, with excellent results reported by some groups [81] and very poor results by others [1] including a 6% overall response rate in the only clinical trial evaluating reduction of immunosuppression prospectively [68]. The diverse outcomes may reflect differing referral patterns and patient characteristics, differences in range of pathology, and perhaps differences in use of adjunctive therapies that are not always well described. As for children, rebound rejection rates in adults are significant and are an important cause of death after treatment of PTLD by reduced immunosuppression, especially after heart transplantation [1].

In general, patients show evidence of clinical response within 2–4 weeks of reduction of immune suppression, though a delayed response has been observed as long as several months in some patients. Significant responses to immunosuppression reduction alone are unlikely in Burkitt, DLBCL, Hodgkin, and T-cell PTLD [20, 68], and although there is no evidence to guide the decision when to initiate further treatment, there is increased reluctance to wait especially in Burkitt PTLD, due to very fast cell replication times [93].

The approach to reduction in immunosuppression varies widely. Most authorities initially reduce or hold calcineurin inhibitors (CNIs) and adjunctive antiproliferative agents and maintain any corticosteroids that the patient might be receiving. Tacrolimus and cyclosporine levels may initially be high due to impaired hepatic metabolism. Subsequent practice varies widely. Among liver transplant programs, there is a tendency to withhold CNIs long term or even indefinitely [34]. This is unlikely to be possible in thoracic and intestinal transplantation. There has been considerable interest in replacing CNIs with inhibitors of the mammalian target of rapamycin (mTOR) once immunosuppression is reintroduced. Sirolimus has frequently been used in this setting. Interest in the use of this group of agents in PTLD, in part, reflects the anti-neoplastic properties of this class of agents, including inhibition of EBV-driven B-cell lymphomas [45, 84]. However, mTOR inhibitors are also potent T-cell inhibitors, and patients managed with CNI-free immunosuppression, using mTOR inhibitors, may still develop PTLD [80]. Recent data suggest that while mTOR-associated PTLD more frequently is of early onset and less frequently shows nodal involvement, it is important to notice that the clinical course of PTLD treated with anti-CD20-directed therapy (+/− chemotherapy) does not differ significantly with respect to the class of immunosuppression under which it develops [76].

The effect of reduced immunosuppression on the risk of relapse after successful treatment has been analyzed in depth in a prospective, international, multicenter trial in 159 adults with B-cell PTLD after solid organ transplantation treated with rituximab ± CHOP after an initial attempt of immunosuppression reduction [89]. The most common immunosuppressive drug regimens before diagnosis were the triple combination of CNI, antimetabolite, and corticosteroid and the doublet of CNI and antimetabolite. The focus of the analysis was the use of different classes of maintenance immunosuppression and late relapse risk after successful PTLD therapy. Although antimetabolites have been singled out for discontinuation in guidelines [19, 49, 51, 57, 68], patients on immunosuppression containing an antimetabolite after diagnosis had a very similar relapse risk, and there was no difference in the risk of relapse between patients who had stopped the antimetabolite and those who had not. In contrast, patients on immunosuppression containing a corticosteroid after diagnosis of PTLD had a higher relapse risk compared to those on steroid-free immunosuppression, and corticosteroid-containing maintenance immunosuppression after diagnosis of PTLD was identified as an independent risk factor for PTLD relapse. In addition, the corticosteroid dose as a percent of the dose pre-PTLD correlated with a patient's absolute risk of relapse. Patients on tacrolimus after diagnosis of PTLD had a significantly lower relapse risk than patients on cyclosporine, and tacrolimus-containing immunosuppression after diagnosis of PTLD was a protective risk factor. Thus, data from a large prospective clinical trial now suggest that maintaining corticosteroid-containing immunosuppression after diagnosis might be a risk factor for PTLD relapse and should be avoided, if not indicated, from a transplant perspective. In contrast, stopping antimetabolites appears to not be essential for long-term PTLD outcome [89].

Surgery and Radiation Therapy

Excisional biopsy, generally performed for diagnostic purposes, may be curative for solitary PTLD lesions but is usually combined with some reduction in immunosuppression. Thus, almost all patients do receive a systemic approach to treatment and PTLD is probably best thought of as a systemic process. In certain histologies solitary lesions are common. For example, in adults with plasmacytoma-like PTLD, resection combined with irradiation is the mainstay of treatment and is usually followed by an excellent long-term outcome [75]. In children with disease isolated to the tonsils, resection and transient reduction of immunosuppression usually suffice to achieve long-term disease-free state. These lesions are typically of the non-destructive and polymorphic types. In most other settings surgery may be indicated for management of local complications such as gastrointestinal hemorrhage, obstruction, or perforation. Radiation therapy has a limited role in the management of systemic PTLD, although many lesions will be responsive. It has been used when rapid local responses are required, for example, when there is acute airway compression from tumor mass or compression of other critical structures. It has also been shown to be effective in combination with anti-CD20-directed strategies as radioimmunotherapy (^{90}Y-ibritumomab tiuxetan) in patients with prior exposure to rituximab [62]. In combination with systemic rituximab, it can be an effective strategy for the treatment of central nervous system (CNS) PTLD (see below).

Antiviral Therapy

Initial interest in the role of antiviral chemotherapy for treatment of PTLD arose in 1982 when Hanto described a patient whose EBV-associated PTLD lesion appeared to wax and wane in association with starting and stopping acyclovir [31]. Both acyclovir and ganciclovir inhibit lytic EBV DNA replication in vitro and may be of value in treating the lytic phase of EBV infection. Cidofovir and foscarnet may also be active in the latent phase of EBV infection but are much more toxic. Ganciclovir is approximately 6–10-fold more potent than acyclovir at inhibiting lytic EBV replication in vitro and has the additional advantage of inhibiting CMV that may be present at the same time in some patients with PTLD. Use of acyclovir, ganciclovir, or valganciclovir for the treatment of PTLD has become routine in many centers. However, their efficacy has not been established in prospective clinical trials, and many investigators have questioned their role in the treatment of PTLD. This may reflect the fact that the vast majority of EBV-infected cells within PTLD lesions are believed to be transformed B cells that are not undergoing lytic infection, although more recently, quantitative RT-PCR analyses of EBV gene expression profiles in primary CNS and systemic EBV-associated PTLD have shown that EBER-positive PTLD samples frequently express at least one of the latent transcripts EBNA2, EBNA3A, or LMP1 and one of the early lytic transcripts BZLF1, BRLF, or BLLF1 [22]. However the expression pattern is highly variable in the majority of EBV-associated PTLDs, and transcript expression alone does not infer that antiviral agents will be effective in eradicating PTLD. This must be confirmed, or refuted, in appropriately designed clinical trials.

There also has been progress in the development of other types of antiviral agents for the treatment of severe human herpes virus infections, including those due to EBV [55, 87]. Drugs that act independently of the viral enzyme target, thymidine kinase, may be particularly suitable candidates for investigation for the treatment of PTLD [73]. Cidofovir has potential in this regard, and recent work suggests that lipid ester analogues of cidofovir and cyclic cidofovir may have much greater activity against EBV than the parent drug and may be suitable drugs for phase I clinical studies [87].

The strategy to induce EBV thymidine kinase in EBV-infected tumors, thus making the tumors sensitive to nucleoside-type antiviral agents such as ganciclovir, has become outdated because the agent that may achieve this goal (arginine butyrate) has not become licensed [25, 54].

In primary CNS PTLD that is closely EBV-associated, and where rituximab monotherapy and systemic chemotherapy have limited efficacy and high toxicity, antiviral therapy with zidovudine (AZT), ganciclovir, dexamethasone, and rituximab has demonstrated high efficacy [18]. In a clinical phase II trial, 13 SOT recipients initially underwent reduction or withdrawal of immunosuppression followed by twice-daily, intravenous AZT (1500 mg), ganciclovir (5 mg/kg), and dexamethasone (10 mg given for 14 days). Weekly rituximab (375 mg/m^2) was delivered for the first 4 weeks. Twice-daily valganciclovir (450 mg) and AZT (300 mg) started day 15. The overall response rate in this trial was 92% (95% CI, 64–100). The median time to response was 2 months. Median therapy duration was 26.5 months. With a median follow-up of 52 months, the estimated 2-year overall survival was 76.9% (95% CI, 44–92).

Interferon and Other Cytokines

The use of interferon has been described in anecdotal reports as a therapeutic option in the management of PTLD [15, 65]. Interferon is both a pro-inflammatory cytokine and a natural antiviral agent and appears capable of controlling proliferation of

EBV-infected B cells. Since it is a non-specific immune stimulant, anti-donor responses are often seen and severe rejection can develop during therapy. In a series of adult PTLD patients unresponsive to reduction in immunosuppression, only 1 of 13 (7%) achieved durable complete remission with interferon-alpha 2b [68]. At the present time, almost no center is using interferon in the management of PTLD.

Interleukin 6 (IL6) has been described as a growth factor for EBV-infected B cells. For this reason, an anti-IL6 monoclonal antibody has been tested in a phase I/II clinical trial [14]. This was well tolerated and complete response was observed in approximately 40% of patients that had not responded to a brief period of reduction in immunosuppression. It is not currently used in routine clinical care of patients with PTLD [30] although it has become commercially available for the treatment of rheumatoid arthritis in 2005. As the biology of PTLD is further unraveled (see Chaps. 3 and 4), more targets for biologic intervention are likely to be identified.

Intravenous Immune Globulin

A potential role for the use of intravenous immune globulin (IVIG) for the treatment of PTLD has also been suggested. Several reports have documented an association between loss and absence of antibody against at least one of the Epstein-Barr nuclear antigens (EBNA) in EBV-infected organ recipients and the subsequent development of PTLD [58]. In addition, a correlation between an increasing level of anti-EBNA antibodies (including those introduced through transfusions) with a decrease in EBV viral load has been demonstrated. Taken together, these reports may provide a rationale for considering the use of antibodies in the prevention and/or treatment of EBV disease and EBV-associated PTLD even though the primary mechanism for controlling EBV infection appears to be cytotoxic T-cell-mediated immunity. IVIG has been used alone and in combination with interferon-alpha as treatment for PTLD [65]. Both IVIG and CMV-IVIG have been used in the treatment of some patients with PTLD, and IVIG may be effective even in patients not responding to anti-CD20 strategies or even chemotherapy [73]. But there are no clinical trials that have evaluated the role of IVIG in general, or CMV-IVIG in particular, in the treatment of PTLD.

Anti-B-Cell Antibodies

Most PTLDs are of B-cell origin, and the use of anti-CD21 and anti-CD24 monoclonal antibodies has been reported for the treatment of B-cell PTLD in recipients of solid organ and bone marrow transplantation in early clinical trials [23]. Neither products were commercialized; however, an anti-CD20 human/mouse chimeric monoclonal antibody (rituximab) has become the mainstay of treatment in CD20-positive B-cell PTLD in the last decade, either alone or in combination with subsequent chemotherapy (see below) [16]. In 2000, clinical investigators in France published the first retrospective analysis of the use of rituximab in 32 patients with

PTLD [43]. The overall response rate was 65% in solid organ transplant recipients, most of whom experienced long-term remission. Relapse of PTLD developed in approximately 20% of responders a median of 7 months after completing their therapeutic course of rituximab. Several subsequent reports have emerged from single centers [3, 20, 35, 37] and from prospective multicenter phase II trials [10, 26, 48] using a treatment schedule of 375 mg/m^2 IV once a week for 4 consecutive weeks after an initial attempt of reduction of immunosuppression. Overall response rates for adults varied, with complete response rates ranging from 28% to 59% [3, 10, 48], while a realistic approximation of the complete response rate is 25% based on clinical trials with substantial numbers of patients [72, 79]. Late follow-up of one series to date (60 patients) revealed that 57% had progressive disease 1 year after completing treatment with a median progression-free survival of only 6 months [11]. However, response to rituximab was validated as a predictor of time to progression and overall survival, and rituximab monotherapy resulted in excellent long-term outcome in patients with complete response after 4 weekly doses of rituximab that had subsequent rituximab consolidation with four additional doses in 3-week intervals [79]. This data from a prospective multicenter clinical phase II trial that enrolled 152 adult patients strongly suggests that eight, not four, doses of rituximab are the best available therapy for patients in complete response after 4 weekly doses of rituximab induction. Freedom from disease progression in the patient cohort receiving rituximab consolidation was 89% at 3 years (95% CI 76–100) and overall survival was 91% at 3 years (95% CI 82–100) [79]. With a significant amount of data from clinical trials, it has been pointed out that the drug is well tolerated and those that do demonstrate progressive disease or relapse can still undergo chemotherapy [20, 79]. Rituximab seems to be equally effective in patients who relapsed after chemotherapy [77].

The results of rituximab monotherapy in PTLD may be superior in children, though less data are available. Two pediatric, prospective studies evaluated the efficacy of single agent rituximab in solid organ transplant patients with PTLD that failed reduction in immunosuppression. 49 and 12 patients, respectively, received 3–4 weekly doses of rituximab, and if complete or partial response was achieved, patients received an additional 0–4 doses. Complete response was achieved in 60–75% and 53–67% remained alive and in complete response after a median follow-up of 4.9 and 1.5 years, respectively [40, 85]. Based on these data, an expert consensus meeting (International Pediatric Transplant Association) of hematologists, oncologists, pathologists, infectious disease specialists, and transplant physicians and surgeons recommended in 2019 that children with CD20-positive B-cell PTLD who do not respond to reduction of immunosuppression should receive 3–4 weekly doses of rituximab (375 mg/m^2), and if partial response or better is achieved, additional rituximab (3–4 doses) should be considered. If no partial response is achieved, other treatment modalities should be evaluated. There is no data available on maintenance rituximab therapy after the initial course(s), so recommendations on "rituximab consolidation" in children are not possible.

There still remain several questions regarding the use of rituximab in the transplant setting. Will the prolonged elimination of B cells and immunodeficiencies result in additional opportunistic infections or other sequelae? Should rituximab be used in all patients at diagnosis, or only those who fail an initial period of reduced immunosuppression? Are clinicians less aggressive in immunosuppression reduction when they use rituximab from the time of diagnosis? Might there be a role for next-generation monoclonal anti-B-cell antibodies like the anti-CD79a antibody drug conjugate polatuzumab vedotin?

Supportive and prophylactic management of patients receiving rituximab seems necessary, and clinicians should be aware of the indications for these treatments and the potential for specific clinical adverse events, which include PJP prophylaxis, prolonged hypogammaglobulinemia, and possible need for replacement therapy, an effect of rituximab-induced B-cell depletion on vaccine responses, and potential for cellular lysis and sepsis-like picture following rituximab.

Chemotherapy

First-line chemotherapy is used for T-cell PTLD [70], for advanced Hodgkin PTLD [60], for Burkitt PTLD [40, 92], for stage III/IV plasma cell myeloma [61, 75], and for plasmablastic lymphoma [91]. Over the last 20 years, first-line treatment with single agent rituximab for all other types of B-cell PTLD has evolved as the standard of care in most adult transplant programs. However, CHOP (cyclophosphamide, vincristine, doxorubicin, prednisone) still is used after upfront rituximab monotherapy for consolidation (sequential treatment [72]) and treatment intensification (risk-stratified sequential treatment [79]). While mortality of first-line chemotherapy is high [12, 20, 24, 68, 69, 74], it was considerably lower after (successful) debulking with upfront rituximab [72], and sequential treatment with rituximab and CHOP became a treatment standard in adult PTLD in 2012 based on the results of the European PTLD-1 trial.

The European PTLD-1 trial employed frontline weekly rituximab treatment for 4 weeks followed by four courses of CHOP in adult solid organ transplant recipients with CD20-positive PTLD [72]. Seventy-four patients were enrolled, median overall survival was 6.6 years, and 11% of patients experienced treatment-related mortality. The overall response rate to 4 doses of rituximab followed by 4 courses of CHOP was 90% with 68% of patients achieving a complete response. A subsequent trial (Fig. 10.1) established that patients with complete response to frontline rituximab had a favorable survival if consolidated with rituximab alone (Fig. 10.2), leading to a recommendation to avoid chemotherapy in this specific patient subgroup [79]. One hundred fifty-two treatment-naïve adult solid organ transplant recipients with CD20-positive PTLD unresponsive to immunosuppression reduction were included in this prospective, international, multicenter phase II trial and treated with 4 weekly doses of rituximab as induction. After restaging, complete responders continued with four single doses of rituximab every 3 weeks; all others received four 3-weekly courses of combined rituximab and CHOP chemotherapy. The primary endpoint was treatment efficacy measured as response rate in patients who completed therapy and response duration in those who completed therapy and responded. One hundred eleven of 126 patients had a complete or partial response (88%, 95%

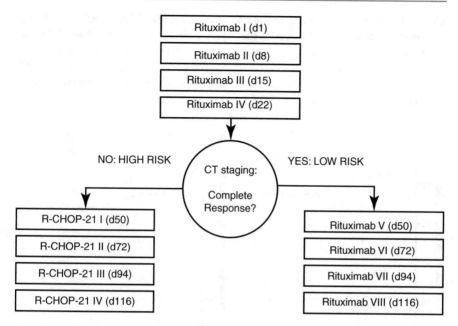

Fig. 10.1 Risk-stratified sequential treatment (RSST) schedule for adults with PTLD [79]. Rituximab signifies rituximab 375 mg/m² IV, R-CHOP21 signifies rituximab 375 mg/m² IV day (d) 1, cyclophosphamide 750 mg/m² IV d1, doxorubicin 50 mg/m² IV d1, vincristine 1·4 mg/m² (max. 2 mg) IV d1, and prednisone 50 mg/m² PO d1–5. In case of progressive disease from d1 to d50, patients proceeded to R-CHOP21 immediately

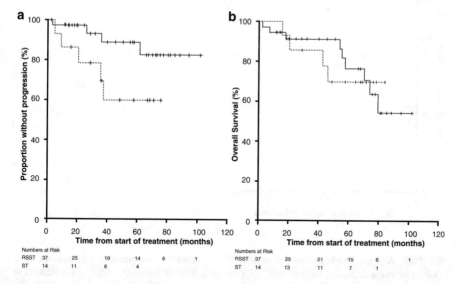

Fig. 10.2 Sequential treatment (ST) [72] and risk-stratified sequential treatment among adult PTLD patients (RSST) [79]: patients in complete response after rituximab induction (low-risk group). Time to progression and overall survival in the RSST cohort (n = 37, solid line) and the ST cohort (n = 14, dashed line). Numbers at risk for both populations (RSST and ST) are indicated at the bottom of each graph. (**a**) Time to progression. (**b**) Overall survival

CI 81–93), of which 88 were complete responses (70%, 95% CI 61–77). Median response duration was not reached; the 3-year estimate was 82% (95% CI 74–90). Median time to progression also was not reached; the 3-year estimate was 75% (95% CI 67–82). Median overall survival was 6.6 years (95% CI 5·5–7·6), Fig. 10.3. The frequencies of grade 3/4 infections and of treatment-related mortality were 34% (95% CI 27–42) and 8% (95% CI 5–14), respectively.

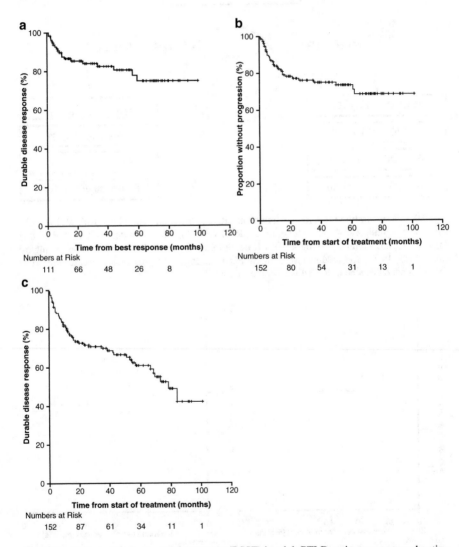

Fig. 10.3 Risk-stratified sequential treatment (RSST) in adult PTLD patients: response duration, time to progression, and overall survival [79]. Median time of follow-up: 4.5 years. Numbers at risk are indicated at the bottom of each graph. (**a**) Response duration (patients in CR or PR). (**b**) Time to progression (all patients). (**c**) Overall survival (all patients)

Chemotherapy for pediatric PTLD can be divided into different intensity levels. Highly intense regimens used for lymphoma in immunocompetent children (NHL-BFM regimen, FAB-/LMB-type regimen) are often not tolerated in PTLD and lead to high morbidity and mortality [39]. Therefore, chemotherapy regimens with low to moderate intensity have been developed for pediatric PTLD patients. A first multicenter phase II study tested prednisone plus cyclophosphamide in 36 children with an overall response rate of 83% and a 2-year overall and failure-free survival of 73% and 67%, respectively [27]. Treatment was well tolerated with acceptable treatment-related mortality (5.5%) and graft loss rates (8.3%). In a subsequent phase II trial, six doses of rituximab were added to this chemotherapy [28]. Fifty-five patients were enrolled, 2-year overall survival was improved to 83%, and 2-year event-free survival was 71%. A German trial in 49 children with B-cell PTLD that used sequential rituximab followed by mCOMP (cyclophosphamide, vincristine, prednisone, low-dose MTX) in patients not responding to rituximab achieved similar survival rates [40]. In this trial patients with Burkitt PTLD were subjected to primary immunochemotherapy due to rapid progression with rituximab alone in three patients. In the European PTLD-1 ST [72] and RSST [79] trials, adult patients with Burkitt PTLD were included, and although all patients received chemotherapy, sequential treatment was safe and effective [79]. It is important to note that none of the chemotherapy trials in pediatric PTLD have directly compared rituximab to cyclophosphamide plus prednisone with or without rituximab (so-called CHOP lite) in patients failing to respond to reduced immunosuppression alone. Thus, it is unclear which strategy is the optimal treatment in this setting. The addition of chemotherapy may help protect the allograft during reduced immunosuppression, but at the cost of additional treatments, greater expense, and potentially more adverse events. A direct comparison of the two strategies is warranted.

T-cell PTLDs comprise a heterogeneous group of EBV-positive (30%) and EBV-negative lymphomas occurring late after transplantation [70]. While ALK+ anaplastic large cell lymphoma has a reasonable prognosis, other entities like peripheral T-cell lymphoma not otherwise specified (PTCL/NOS) or hepatosplenic lymphoma have an extremely bad prognosis [33]. No prospective trials are available for T-cell PTLD patients. Most patients (adults and children) that survived T-cell PTLD received intensive chemotherapy of various kinds and/or radiation therapy [70]. However, both treatment-related mortality and mortality due to PTLD are high in this patient cohort. Occasionally, targeted therapies (ALK inhibitors, CD30-directed therapies) have been added to, or were substituted for, intensive chemotherapy in selected cases [9, 52].

In a phase I/II trial of the anti-CD30 antibody drug conjugate brentuximab vedotin plus rituximab as frontline therapy for immunosuppression-associated CD30-positive and/or EBV-positive lymphomas, 12 patients with PTLD following solid organ transplantation were included and evaluable (most of them had CD20-positive B-cell PTLD). Treatment consisted of two 28-day cycles of brentuximab vedotin (1.2 mg/kg on days 1, 8, and 15) combined with 8 applications of weekly rituximab (375 mg/m^2) followed by brentuximab vedotin and rituximab maintenance (1.8 mg/kg every 3 weeks and 375 mg/m² every 6 weeks, respectively) for 1 year. The overall response rate was 70% (14/20: 95% CI 48–86), which is similar to overall response with rituximab monotherapy in the PTLD-1 trials (129/218: 59%, 95% CI 52–65) [78]. 60% reached complete response. With limited follow-up, survival data are not yet mature. Treatment-related mortality was 10% and thus similar to CHOP in the PTLD-1 trials. One transplant recipient developed graft rejection (7%). Many patients deviated from the treatment schedule due to toxicity with 35% deviating from induction therapy and 45% discontinuing maintenance [52]. In summary, this treatment approach has limited additional effect compared to rituximab monotherapy, is associated with significant treatment-related mortality, and results in the overtreatment of those patients (approximately 25%) who can safely be treated with rituximab alone. The data therefore do not support the frontline treatment with brentuximab vedotin in addition to rituximab in EBV-associated B-cell PTLD.

Classical Hodgkin lymphoma PTLD is usually a late event (>5 years) after solid organ transplantation. It is commonly EBV-positive. Published data on treatment outcomes is scarce and limited to case reports and small retrospective series. The picture is further complicated by the different management of limited vs. disseminated disease in immunocompetent patients. Reduction of immunosuppression followed by radiotherapy in stage I disease and systemic chemotherapy (ABVD: adriamycin, bleomycin, vinblastine, and dacarbazine) as tolerated in stage II to IV is the common treatment option. However, it should be noted that ABVD in PTLD is associated with significant (infectious) mortality. In a series of adult Hodgkin PTLD, patients receiving ABVD had an improved probability of survival compared to no chemotherapy or other chemotherapy [60]. Similar results were seen in a case series of 17 pediatric patients with classical Hodgkin PTLD that reports an excellent outcome with a 5-year overall survival of 86% and a 5-year event-free survival of 81% using chemotherapy regimens similar to non-immunocompromised patients [36].

PTLD with plasmacellular differentiation has been reported as a rare subtype of monomorphic B-cell PTLD with histological and immunophenotypical features of plasmacytoma in the non-transplant population. In adults with plasmacytoma-like PTLD, extranodal manifestations are common, while osteolytic lesions are rare and patients usually do not show bone marrow involvement. Immunohistochemistry shows light chain restriction and expression of CD138 without CD20 expression. An association with EBV is found in about half of the patients. Patients generally respond well to treatment including reduction of immunosuppression and surgery and irradiation in localized disease and to conventional chemotherapy similar to myeloma regimens in the non-transplant population [75].

Chemotherapy in PTLD will generally protect the graft against rejection [71], but is associated with a much higher infectious morbidity and mortality than comparable regimes used in the non-transplant setting [12, 20, 24, 42, 46]. Nonetheless, ongoing careful surveillance of the graft is imperative as rejection events can occur during chemotherapy, especially with less intense regimens such as those used in pediatric settings.

Cellular Immunotherapy

Inadequate EBV-specific T-cell responses are an important, if not critical, pathologic step in the development of EBV-driven PTLD, though other mechanisms may contribute. Infusion of EBV-specific CTLs has been employed both as treatment and prophylaxis against PTLD in bone marrow/stem cell transplantation [59]. In this setting, the PTLDs are generally of donor origin, and the donor is usually available to provide a source of CTL for the recipient. The success of this adoptive immunotherapy in stem cell recipients has stimulated investigation into applying this approach as a therapy for PTLD in solid organ transplant recipients [67]. This is a logical therapy, as it is directed against the PTLD, and should (in theory) cause little anti-donor response (i.e., rejection). However, the use of CTL infusions in solid organ recipients is made more difficult by the fact that the EBV-infected cells within PTLD lesions are typically of recipient origin. For this reason, autologous CTLs are the obvious source for development of EBV-specific CTL infusions for solid organ transplant recipients. However, the development of EBV-specific CTLs from organ recipients is challenging since patients at risk for EBV-associated PTLD may be EBV-naïve at transplant, CTL generation is impaired by the presence of immunosuppression, and T-cell responses are further severely suppressed at the time of development of PTLD. Accordingly, techniques for adoptive immunotherapy of EBV-associated PTLD in solid organ transplant recipients have focused on developing strategies to immunize and stimulate the organ recipient's own T cells against EBV ex vivo and then subsequently infusing these EBV-specific CTLs back into the recipient at a time when the patient develops refractory EBV infection/EBV-associated PTLD [13, 63, 67]. Such an approach could also be used for prevention, with infusion performed when EBV viral loads start to climb after primary post-transplant EBV infection [63]. Ideally, the cells for culture should be obtained prior to transplantation and the initiation of immunosuppression in high-risk recipients, i.e., those that are EBV seronegative at the time of transplantation. Such an approach is expensive and labor intensive as most candidates will never require CTL therapy. Furthermore, at this time, the success of adoptive immunotherapy using autologous CTLs after solid organ transplantation has not paralleled that seen after bone marrow/stem cell transplantation.

An alternate approach is the use of allogeneic T-cell infusions from EBV-positive blood donors that are as closely matched as possible to the recipient's HLA type. The first and still largest multicenter clinical trial of third-party EBV-CTLs in SOT patients with PTLD was reported by Haque and colleagues in 33 patients with EBV-positive PTLD. 31/33 patients had PTLD following SOT. Nearly 50% had early lesion or polymorphic B-cell histology. One third of patients were children. The group reported an overall response rate of 53% at 6 months, with 14 CRs, following 4 weekly infusions of the EBV-CTLs [32]. In a retrospective review of ten pediatric SOT patients who received third-party EBV-CTLs for PTLD in the UK from 1999 to 2018, seven had monomorphic, two had polymorphic, and one had Hodgkin-type PTLD. Third-party EBV-CTLs achieved an overall response rate of 80%. Transient adverse effects included fever, tachycardia, and vomiting. None developed graft-versus-host disease or opportunistic infections [8].

Feasibility, response rates, and safety profile of third-party EBV-CTL banks have led to partnerships with industry and attempts to integrate third-party EBV-CTLs earlier in treatment. In June 2015, Atara Biotherapeutics, Inc. licensed allogeneic EBV-CTL technology from Memorial Sloan Kettering Cancer Center and designated the EBV-CTL cell product as tabelecleucel. Currently tabelecleucel has orphan status in the USA and EU and is in phase III clinical development for the treatment of EBV-positive PTLD following allogeneic stem cell transplantation (HCT) or solid organ transplantation (SOT). Tabelecleucel has been evaluated in phase I/II and II studies in allogeneic HCT and SOT subjects with EBV-positive PTLD, for whom treatment with rituximab or rituximab plus chemotherapy had failed and currently is being evaluated for the treatment of EBV-associated PTLD failing rituximab in phase III. Between 2005 and 2015, a total of 46 patients with EBV-associated B-cell PTLD that either progressed during rituximab treatment, failed to fully respond to, or had relapsed after rituximab were treated in a single center cohort at the Memorial Sloan Kettering Cancer Center with banked third-party EBV-CTL lines, including 13 patients with PTLD following SOT (median age 19 years). Prior therapy had included chemotherapy in 12/13 SOT patients. 8/13 SOT patients had been diagnosed with DLBLC-type PTLD. EBV-CTL lines were matched with the patient for $\geq$2/10 HLA alleles and restricted by $\geq$1 HLA allele shared by the lymphoma. EBV-CTL lines were given at 1×10^6 cells/kg/dose (protocol 1) or 2×10^6 cells/kg/dose (protocol 2) on days 1, 8, and 15 followed by a 3-week observational period. Patients failing to achieve complete response who had no therapy-related toxicity could receive additional cycles. Only 1/13 SOT patients achieved a CR after the first cycle of EBV-CTLs. Two additional patients achieved a partial response. However, response rates increased with additional cycles, with maximal response achieved after a median of 2 cycles. Ultimately, 2/13 SOT patients achieved a CR and 5/13 a durable PR. Thus, the final ORR was 54%. With a median follow-up of 2 years, 2-year OS was 54% as well. There were no immediate adverse reactions and only one de novo grade I acute GVHD of the skin, which resolved with topical steroids. No patient experienced CTL-related de novo suppression of neutrophils, red cells, or platelet counts and no SOT patient experienced graft rejection [56].

Role of Combination Therapies

Since no therapies have been tested in randomized controlled trials, it is evident that the use of combination therapies is also not evidence based. Nonetheless, as with other diseases, there may be logic in combining therapies that work by different mechanisms of action. However, multi-modality therapies might lead to a belief that individual therapies can be given at lower doses or for reduced lengths of time. This could lead to reduced efficacy. For example, if rituximab is used without significant reduction in immunosuppression, then there may be little or no recovery in CTL responses. Such responses might be critical for long-term disease control and relapse may be common without them. The use of combination therapies also makes it very challenging to identify the efficacious components of a treatment regimen. For example, autologous EBV-specific CTLs have been used immediately following polychemotherapy combined with rituximab with success of the combined regimen. Combination therapies are likely to remain largely empiric given the enormous challenges of performing randomized controlled trials in this disease.

Central Nervous System Disease

CNS disease may be primary [4, 6] or may be an additional site of disease in patients with extracranial disease [4] and is EBV-associated in more than 90% of cases [22]. In both situations, the prognosis has generally been considered to be very poor with a survival ranging from 9% to 43% [5, 7, 21, 53]. The CNS is generally considered a protected site in which it is harder for normal immune surveillance to gain control of disease. Nonetheless, reestablished immune surveillance may be sufficient to control disease. Unfortunately, this occurs with insufficient frequency to justify reduction in immunosuppression as the only therapy.

Therapies cover a broad scope of interventions including reduction of immunosuppression [83]; administration of antiviral agents [18]; administration of rituximab, both intravenously and intrathecally [14, 50, 88]; high-dose chemotherapy administered intravenously [82]; intrathecal chemotherapy [41]; adoptive immunotherapy [44]; and radiation [5, 7, 21, 53]. Every intervention is associated with some level of success, but the lack of structured clinical trials makes it difficult to discern the efficacy of any modality as published reports are biased toward successful outcomes. Furthermore, many of these interventions are administered in different combinations, making interpretation even more challenging. However, reports encompassing larger numbers of patients provide some indication of what therapies are associated with higher survival rates. Radiation therapy is associated with response rates ranging from 53% to 87% [5, 7, 21, 53] and antiviral therapy with AZT, ganciclovir, dexamethasone, and rituximab has demonstrated a response rate of 92% (95% CI, 64–100) in a series of 13 adult SOT recipients [18]. Based on these data and long-term neurological toxicity of whole brain radiotherapy, the German PTLD study group considers frontline therapy with AZT, ganciclovir, dexamethasone, and rituximab as a potential alternative to frontline whole brain radiation therapy plus rituximab as a first-line treatment standard in Germany.

Of note, despite the wide variety of therapies that have been utilized in this disease, there are virtually no reports utilizing conventional therapies for CNS lymphoma or lymphoma with CNS involvement. It is unclear whether such therapy would be tolerated in this population, and it is also unclear how effective such therapies would be in this clinical setting. However, reports of disease regression with simple immunosuppression reduction illustrate that CNS PTLD is not clinically identical to primary lymphoma. It is conceivable that disease management may require different approaches based on disease stratification that is risk based.

Unfortunately, clear prognostic risk factors that could be used to stratify patients and direct therapy currently do not exist in CNS PTLD. Thus, further advancement in this clinical area will only occur with the development of prospective clinical trials.

Monitoring Patients During Therapy

Conventional Monitoring of Graft and PTLD Status

Monitoring of tumor responses is performed by conventional methods appropriate to the site of disease. Computed tomography and magnetic resonance imaging are the most commonly used imaging techniques [93], though there is increasing interest in the use of positron emission tomography for evaluation and follow-up of PTLD [17]. Retrospective data from the PTLD-1 trials [72, 79] suggest that patients in PET-negative partial remission at the end of treatment share the same prognosis as patients in complete remission [90]. However, because of many FDG-positive foci due to cryptic infections or other malignancies, the positive predictive value of end-of-treatment PET in PTLD is low [90]. Regression of mass lesions often takes at least 2 weeks and frequently longer. Following reduction in immunosuppression, anti-EBV-CTL responses may recover more quickly, thus suggesting impending response to therapy or risk of development of rejection. Thus, there is considerable interest in immunological monitoring in combination with monitoring of clinical disease and status of the allograft.

The frequency and method of monitoring allograft status will depend on the clinical setting, including allograft type, prior rejection history, and time from transplantation. As discussed previously, rebound rejection is very common after reduction or cessation of immunosuppression for treatment of PTLD, and death due to allograft loss may be as common as death due to disease progression [86]. In contrast to lymphomas in the non-transplant setting, outcome of PTLD must consider the status of the allograft, and successful therapy should be defined in terms of complete response of PTLD without allograft loss and without development of chronic allograft dysfunction.

EBV Viral Load Monitoring

When EBV-PTLD is associated with high EBV viral load at presentation, serial monitoring appears to provide important information about response of disease after reduction in immunosuppression. This is probably just a simple indirect measure of EBV-CTL responses, and viral load may fall prior to clinical response. Most data on viral load monitoring in this setting is from pediatric centers, which predominantly see PTLD in the context of primary EBV infection and high viral loads. A decline in viral load suggests that the patient is responding and may identify the time when the patient is at risk for developing rejection. It is important to note that rituximab causes complete elimination of peripheral EBV viral load in almost all patients, and therefore viral load monitoring is not useful for evaluation of the effectiveness of treatment after rituximab. Furthermore, there have been reports of patients responding to treatment despite continuous high viral loads, and also of PTLD patients relapsing although EBV viral loads stayed low [47]. The topic of viral load monitoring is discussed in detail in Chap. 6.

Cellular Immune Responses

It would be beneficial to be able to monitor and accurately predict responses to therapy, especially if such techniques could allow for successful modification of ineffective treatments at an early stage. To this end, a number of groups have sought to develop laboratory monitoring techniques for EBV-associated PTLD. Such techniques would supplement, rather than supplant, EBV-viral load monitoring and careful clinical evaluation of the patient and allograft. Immunological techniques that have been employed include assessment of frequency of EBV-specific T-cell precursors by ELISPOT analysis [38], enumeration of EBV-specific CD8 T cells using HLA class I tetramers [64], intracellular cytokine staining for interferon-gamma-producing CD8+ T cells [29], and cytotoxicity assays [2]. A comprehensive immunological assessment might help predict response to therapy, to define the time of greatest risk of rejection, and also assess potential for relapse, for example, by monitoring persistence or loss of EBV-specific T cells following adoptive cellular immunotherapy [63]. However, these specialized tests of cellular immunity to EBV cannot be performed in routine clinical laboratories and remain the research tools at this time.

Conclusions

Treatment of PTLD has become more standardized in recent years. Rituximab monotherapy is used in almost all patients with CD20-positive B-cell PTLD not responding to an initial attempt of immunosuppression reduction. Among adults, patients with complete response after four doses of rituximab should receive four additional doses of rituximab monotherapy, while all others should generally receive CHOP-based chemotherapy. Pediatric recipients with primary EBV infection often respond to reductions in immunosuppression, though there is increasing evidence to support the use of rituximab monotherapy, as in adults. Many children not responding to rituximab have achieved responses with modified (and less toxic) chemotherapeutic regimens. Adoptive cellular immunotherapy with third-party EBV-CTLs is currently being evaluated in clinical phase III trials in patients with PTLD failing rituximab. Assessment of outcomes must include evaluation of the allograft and not just PTLD. Tumor behavior in the individual may vary depending on immunosuppression, type of transplant, EBV status, histology, tumor genetics, and treatment. Clinical risk factors such as the international prognostic index and response to rituximab monotherapy have been evaluated prospectively and can support clinical decision making, particularly in adult populations. New anti B-cell antibodies and oral medications interfering with the B-cell receptor and BCL-2 are currently being evaluated in the non-transplant lymphoma setting. Their low toxicity profiles make them interesting candidates for forthcoming clinical trials.

Take-Home Pearls
- Reduction of immunosuppression remains standard in the treatment of PTLD, while the extent of reduction and the question of how long to wait until further treatment is initiated depend on many factors including histology, stage of disease, other available treatment options, and type of transplant.
- Rebound rejection is common after reduction of immunosuppression, and death from graft loss and progressive disease both contribute to post-PTLD mortality.
- Four doses of weekly rituximab monotherapy have been evaluated in multiple phase II trials in CD20-positive B-cell PTLD and have become standard in patients not demonstrating complete response after reduction of immunosuppression.
- Adults with a complete response after 4 weekly doses of rituximab monotherapy should be treated with four additional doses of rituximab monotherapy in 3-week intervals. Adults not achieving complete response to four doses of rituximab monotherapy should receive four cycles of R-CHOP.
- Children with only partial response after 3–4 weekly doses of rituximab monotherapy should be treated with 3–4 additional doses of rituximab monotherapy. If complete response is not achieved, treatment with rituximab, prednisone plus cyclophosphamide, or rituximab combined with mCOMP (cyclophosphamide, vincristine, prednisone, low-dose MTX) should be evaluated.
- Infectious morbidity and mortality of chemotherapy remain high compared to non-transplant populations treated for lymphoma, but are significantly reduced when CHOP is applied sequentially to upfront rituximab monotherapy.
- Third-party EBV-specific CTLs are currently considered on clinical trials in children with EBV-associated PTLD who do not respond to standard therapies such as reduction of immunosuppression, rituximab, or chemotherapy, as well as in adults with EBV-associated PTLD who failed rituximab and CHOP.
- CNS PTLD may be primary or associated with extracranial disease. It is closely EBV-associated and restitution of normal immunosurveillance can be sufficient to cure the disease. However, prognosis is poor, and radiation and a combinational therapy of reduced immune suppression, followed by AZT, ganciclovir, dexamethasone, and rituximab are associated with the highest level of success though the latter was demonstrated in a small study of only 13 patients.

References

1. Aull MJ, Buell JF, Trofe J, First MR, Alloway RR, Hanaway MJ, Wagoner L, Gross TG, Beebe T, Woodle ES. Experience with 274 cardiac transplant recipients with posttransplant lymphoproliferative disorder: a report from the Israel Penn International Transplant Tumor Registry. Transplantation. 2004;78(11):1676–82.

2. Baudouin V, Dehee A, Pedron-Grossetete B, Ansart-Pirenne H, Haddad E, Maisin A, Loirat C, Sterkers G. Relationship between CD8+ T-cell phenotype and function, Epstein-Barr virus load, and clinical outcome in pediatric renal transplant recipients: a prospective study. Transplantation. 2004;77(11):1706–13.
3. Blaes AH, Peterson BA, Bartlett N, Dunn DL, Morrison VA. Rituximab therapy is effective for posttransplant lymphoproliferative disorders after solid organ transplantation: results of a phase II trial. Cancer. 2005;104(8):1661–7.
4. Buell JF, Gross TG, Hanaway MJ, Trofe J, Muthiak C, First MR, Alloway RR, Woodle ES. Chemotherapy for posttransplant lymphoproliferative disorder: the Israel Penn International Transplant Tumor Registry experience. Transplant Proc. 2005;37(2):956–7.
5. Buell JF, Gross TG, Hanaway MJ, Trofe J, Roy-Chaudhury P, First MR, Woodle ES. Posttransplant lymphoproliferative disorder: significance of central nervous system involvement. Transplant Proc. 2005;37(2):954–5.
6. Castellano-Sanchez AA, Li S, Qian J, Lagoo A, Weir E, Brat DJ. Primary central nervous system posttransplant lymphoproliferative disorders. Am J Clin Pathol. 2004;121(2):246–53.
7. Cavaliere R, Petroni G, Lopes MB, Schiff D. Primary central nervous system post-transplantation lymphoproliferative disorder: an International Primary Central Nervous System Lymphoma Collaborative Group Report. Cancer. 2010;116(4):863–70.
8. Chiou FK, Beath SV, Wilkie GM, Vickers MA, Morland B, Gupte GL. Cytotoxic T-lymphocyte therapy for post-transplant lymphoproliferative disorder after solid organ transplantation in children. Pediatr Transplant. 2018;22(2) https://doi.org/10.1111/petr.13133.
9. Choi M, Fink S, Prasad V, Anagnostopoulos I, Reinke P, Schmitt CA. T cell PTLD successfully treated with single-agent Brentuximab Vedotin first-line therapy. Transplantation. 2016;100(3):e8–e10.
10. Choquet S, Leblond V, Herbrecht R, Socié G, Stoppa A-M, Vandenberghe P, Fischer A, Morschhauser F, Salles G, Feremans W, et al. Efficacy and safety of rituximab in B-cell post-transplantation lymphoproliferative disorders: results of a prospective multicenter phase 2 study. Blood. 2006;107(8):3053–7.
11. Choquet S, Oertel S, LeBlond V, Riess H, Varoqueaux N, Dörken B, Trappe R. Rituximab in the management of post-transplantation lymphoproliferative disorder after solid organ transplantation: proceed with caution. Ann Hematol. 2007;86(8):599–607.
12. Choquet S, Trappe R, Leblond V, Jager U, Davi F, Oertel S. CHOP-21 for the treatment of post-transplant lymphoproliferative disorders (PTLD) following solid organ transplantation. Haematologica. 2007;92(2):273–4.
13. Comoli P, Maccario R, Locatelli F, Valente U, Basso S, Garaventa A, Toma P, Botti G, Melioli G, Baldanti F, et al. Treatment of EBV-related post-renal transplant lymphoproliferative disease with a tailored regimen including EBV-specific T cells. Am J Transplant. 2005;5(6):1415–22.
14. Czyzewski K, Styczynski J, Krenska A, Debski R, Zajac-Spychala O, Wachowiak J, Wysocki M. Intrathecal therapy with rituximab in central nervous system involvement of post-transplant lymphoproliferative disorder. Leuk Lymphoma. 2013;54(3):503–6.
15. Davis CL, Wood BL, Sabath DE, Joseph JS, Stehman-Breen C, Broudy VC. Interferon-alpha treatment of posttransplant lymphoproliferative disorder in recipients of solid organ transplants. Transplantation. 1998;66(12):1770–9.
16. Dierickx D, Habermann TM. Post-transplantation lymphoproliferative disorders in adults. N Engl J Med. 2018;378(6):549–62.
17. Dierickx D, Tousseyn T, Requilé A, Verscuren R, Sagaert X, Morscio J, Wlodarska I, Herreman A, Kuypers D, Van Cleemput J, et al. The accuracy of positron emission tomography in the detection of posttransplant lymphoproliferative disorder. Haematologica. 2013;98(5):771–5.
18. Dugan JP, Haverkos BM, Villagomez L, Martin LK, Lustberg M, Patton J, Martin M, Huang Y, Nuovo G, Yan F, et al. Complete and durable responses in primary central nervous system Posttransplant lymphoproliferative disorder with zidovudine, ganciclovir, rituximab, and dexamethasone. Clin Cancer Res. 2018;24(14):3273–81.
19. EBPG Expert Group on Renal Transplantation. European best practice guidelines for renal transplantation. Section IV: long-term management of the transplant recipient. IV.6.1. Cancer

risk after renal transplantation. Post-transplant lymphoproliferative disease (PTLD): prevention and treatment. Nephrol Dial Transplant. 2002;17(Suppl 4):31–3. 35–36

20. Elstrom RL, Andreadis C, Aqui NA, Ahya VN, Bloom RD, Brozena SC, Olthoff KM, Schuster SJ, Nasta SD, Stadtmauer EA, et al. Treatment of PTLD with rituximab or chemotherapy. Am J Transplant. 2006;6(3):569–76.
21. Evens AM, Choquet S, Kroll-Desrosiers AR, Jagadeesh D, Smith SM, Morschhauser F, Leblond V, Roy R, Barton B, Gordon LI, et al. Primary CNS Posttransplant Lymphoproliferative Disease (PTLD): an international report of 84 cases in the modern era. Am J Transplant. 2013;13(6):1512–22.
22. Fink SEK, Gandhi MK, Nourse JP, Keane C, Jones K, Crooks P, Jöhrens K, Korfel A, Schmidt H, Neumann S, et al. A comprehensive analysis of the cellular and EBV-specific microR-NAome in primary CNS PTLD identifies different patterns among EBV-associated tumors. Am J Transplant. 2014;14(11):2577–87.
23. Fischer A, Blanche S, Le Bidois J, Bordigoni P, Garnier JL, Niaudet P, Morinet F, Le Deist F, Fischer AM, Griscelli C, et al. Anti-B-cell monoclonal antibodies in the treatment of severe B-cell lymphoproliferative syndrome following bone marrow and organ transplantation. N Engl J Med. 1991;324(21):1451–6.
24. Fohrer C, Caillard S, Koumarianou A, Ellero B, Woehl-Jaegle ML, Meyer C, Epailly E, Chenard MP, Lioure B, Natarajan-Ame S, et al. Long-term survival in post-transplant lymphoproliferative disorders with a dose-adjusted ACVBP regimen. Br J Haematol. 2006;134(6):602–12.
25. Ghosh SK, Forman LW, Akinsheye I, Perrine SP, Faller DV. Short, discontinuous exposure to butyrate effectively sensitizes latently EBV-infected lymphoma cells to nucleoside analogue antiviral agents. Blood Cells Mol Dis. 2007;38(1):57–65.
26. Gonzalez-Barca E, Domingo-Domenech E, Capote FJ, Gomez-Codina J, Salar A, Bailen A, Ribera JM, Lopez A, Briones J, Munoz A, et al. Prospective phase II trial of extended treatment with rituximab in patients with B-cell post-transplant lymphoproliferative disease. Haematologica. 2007;92(11):1489–94.
27. Gross TG, Bucuvalas JC, Park JR, Greiner TC, Hinrich SH, Kaufman SS, Langnas AN, McDonald RA, Ryckman FC, Shaw BW, et al. Low-dose chemotherapy for Epstein-Barr virus-positive post-transplantation lymphoproliferative disease in children after solid organ transplantation. J Clin Oncol. 2005;23(27):6481–8.
28. Gross TG, Orjuela MA, Perkins SL, Park JR, Lynch JC, Cairo MS, Smith LM, Hayashi RJ. Low-dose chemotherapy and rituximab for posttransplant lymphoproliferative disease (PTLD): a Children's Oncology Group Report. Am J Transplant. 2012;12(11):3069–75.
29. Guppy AE, Rawlings E, Madrigal JA, Amlot PL, Barber LD. A quantitative assay for Epstein-Barr virus-specific immunity shows interferon-gamma producing CD8+ T cells increase during immunosuppression reduction to treat posttransplant lymphoproliferative disease. Transplantation. 2007;84(11):1534–9.
30. Haddad E, Paczesny S, Leblond V, Seigneurin JM, Stern M, Achkar A, Bauwens M, Delwail V, Debray D, Duvoux C, et al. Treatment of B-lymphoproliferative disorder with a monoclonal anti-interleukin-6 antibody in 12 patients: a multicenter phase 1-2 clinical trial. Blood. 2001;97(6):1590–7.
31. Hanto DW, Frizzera G, Gajl-Peczalska KJ, Sakamoto K, Purtilo DT, Balfour HH, Simmons RL, Najarian JS. Epstein-Barr virus-induced B-cell lymphoma after renal transplantation: acyclovir therapy and transition from polyclonal to monoclonal B-cell proliferation. N Engl J Med. 1982;306(15):913–8.
32. Haque T, Wilkie GM, Jones MM, Higgins CD, Urquhart G, Wingate P, Burns D, McAulay K, Turner M, Bellamy C, et al. Allogeneic cytotoxic T-cell therapy for EBV-positive posttransplantation lymphoproliferative disease: results of a phase 2 multicenter clinical trial. Blood. 2007;110(4):1123–31.
33. Herreman A, Dierickx D, Morscio J, Camps J, Bittoun E, Verhoef G, De Wolf-Peeters C, Sagaert X, Tousseyn T. Clinicopathological characteristics of posttransplant lymphoproliferative disorders of T-cell origin: single-center series of nine cases and meta-analysis of 147 reported cases. Leuk Lymphoma. 2013;54(10):2190–9.

34. Hurwitz M, Desai DM, Cox KL, Berquist WE, Esquivel CO, Millan MT. Complete immuno-suppressive withdrawal as a uniform approach to post-transplant lymphoproliferative disease in pediatric liver transplantation. Pediatr Transplant. 2004;8(3):267–72.
35. Jain AB, Marcos A, Pokharna R, Shapiro R, Fontes PA, Marsh W, Mohanka R, Fung JJ. Rituximab (chimeric anti-CD20 antibody) for posttransplant lymphoproliferative disorder after solid organ transplantation in adults: long-term experience from a single center. Transplantation. 2005;80(12):1692–8.
36. Kampers J, Orjuela-Grimm M, Schober T, Schulz TF, Stiefel M, Klein C, Körholz D, Mauz-Körholz C, Kreipe H, Beier R, et al. Classical Hodgkin lymphoma-type PTLD after solid organ transplantation in children: a report on 17 patients treated according to subsequent GPOH-HD treatment schedules. Leuk Lymphoma. 2017;58(3):633–8.
37. Knoop C, Kentos A, Remmelink M, Garbar C, Goldman S, Feremans W, Estenne M. Post-transplant lymphoproliferative disorders after lung transplantation: first-line treatment with rituximab may induce complete remission. Clin Transpl. 2006;20(2):179–87.
38. Macedo C, Donnenberg A, Popescu I, Reyes J, Abu-Elmagd K, Shapiro R, Zeevi A, Fung JJ, Storkus WJ, Metes D. EBV-specific memory CD8+ T cell phenotype and function in stable solid organ transplant patients. Transpl Immunol. 2005;14(2):109–16.
39. Maecker B, Jack T, Zimmermann M, Abdul-Khaliq H, Burdelski M, Fuchs A, Hoyer P, Koepf S, Kraemer U, Laube GF, et al. CNS or bone marrow involvement as risk factors for poor survival in post-transplantation lymphoproliferative disorders in children after solid organ transplantation. J Clin Oncol. 2007;25(31):4902–8.
40. Maecker-Kolhoff B, Beier R, Zimmermann M, Schlegelberger B, Baumann U, Mueller C, Pape L, Reiter A, Rossig C, Schubert S, et al. Response-adapted sequential Immuno-chemotherapy of post-transplant lymphoproliferative disorders in pediatric solid organ transplant recipients: results from the prospective Ped-PTLD 2005 trial. Blood. 2014;124(21):4468.
41. Mahapatra S, Chin CC, Iagaru A, Heerema-McKenney A, Twist CJ. Successful treatment of systemic and central nervous system post-transplant lymphoproliferative disorder without the use of high-dose methotrexate or radiation. Pediatr Blood Cancer. 2014;61(11):2107–9.
42. Mamzer-Bruneel MF, Lome C, Morelon E, Levy V, Bourquelot P, Jacobs F, Gessain A, Mac Intyre E, Brousse N, Kreis H, et al. Durable remission after aggressive chemotherapy for very late post-kidney transplant lymphoproliferation: a report of 16 cases observed in a single center. J Clin Oncol. 2000;18(21):3622–32.
43. Milpied N, Vasseur B, Parquet N, Garnier JL, Antoine C, Quartier P, Carret AS, Bouscary D, Faye A, Bourbigot B, et al. Humanized anti-CD20 monoclonal antibody (Rituximab) in post transplant B-lymphoproliferative disorder: a retrospective analysis on 32 patients. Ann Oncol. 2000;11(Suppl 1):113–6.
44. Morris J, Smith C, Streicher A, Magnuson A, Newman S, Bertoli R. A rare presentation of isolated CNS Posttransplantation lymphoproliferative disorder. Case Rep Oncol Med. 2017;2017:7269147.
45. Nepomuceno RR, Balatoni CE, Natkunam Y, Snow AL, Krams SM, Martinez OM. Rapamycin inhibits the interleukin 10 signal transduction pathway and the growth of Epstein Barr virus B-cell lymphomas. Cancer Res. 2003;63(15):4472–80.
46. Norin S, Kimby E, Ericzon BG, Christensson B, Sander B, Soderdahl G, Hagglund H. Posttransplant lymphoma–a single-center experience of 500 liver transplantations. Med Oncol. 2004;21(3):273–84.
47. Oertel S, Trappe RU, Zeidler K, Babel N, Reinke P, Hummel M, Jonas S, Papp-Vary M, Subklewe M, Dorken B, et al. Epstein-Barr viral load in whole blood of adults with posttransplant lymphoproliferative disorder after solid organ transplantation does not correlate with clinical course. Ann Hematol. 2006;85(7):478–84.
48. Oertel SH, Verschuuren E, Reinke P, Zeidler K, Papp-Vary M, Babel N, Trappe RU, Jonas S, Hummel M, Anagnostopoulos I, et al. Effect of anti-CD 20 antibody rituximab in patients with Post-Transplant Lymphoproliferative Disorder (PTLD). Am J Transplant. 2005;5(12):2901–6.
49. Parker A, Bowles K, Bradley JA, Emery V, Featherstone C, Gupte G, Marcus R, Parameshwar J, Ramsay A, Newstead C. Management of post-transplant lymphoproliferative disor-

der in adult solid organ transplant recipients – BCSH and BTS guidelines. Br J Haematol. 2010;149(5):693–705.

50. Patrick A, Wee A, Hedderman A, Wilson D, Weiss J, Govani M. High-dose intravenous rituximab for multifocal, monomorphic primary central nervous system posttransplant lymphoproliferative disorder. J Neuro-Oncol. 2011;103(3):739–43.

51. Paya CV, Fung JJ, Nalesnik MA, Kieff E, Green M, Gores G, Habermann TM, Wiesner PH, Swinnen JL, Woodle ES, et al. Epstein-Barr virus-induced posttransplant lymphoproliferative disorders. ASTS/ASTP EBV-PTLD task force and the Mayo Clinic organized international consensus development meeting. Transplantation. 1999;68(10):1517–25.

52. Pearse W, Pro B, Gordon LI, Karmali R, Winter JN, Ma S, Behdad A, Klein A, Petrich AM, Jovanovic B, et al. A phase I/II trial of Brentuximab Vedotin (BV) plus rituximab (R) as frontline therapy for patients with immunosuppression-associated CD30+ and/or EBV+ lymphomas. Blood. 2019;134(Supplement_1):351.

53. Penn I, Porat G. Central nervous system lymphomas in organ allograft recipients. Transplantation. 1995;59(2):240–4.

54. Perrine SP, Hermine O, Small T, Suarez F, O'Reilly R, Boulad F, Fingeroth J, Askin M, Levy A, Mentzer SJ, et al. A phase 1/2 trial of arginine butyrate and ganciclovir in patients with Epstein-Barr virus-associated lymphoid malignancies. Blood. 2007;109(6):2571–8.

55. Prichard MN, Hartline CB, Harden EA, Daily SL, Beadle JR, Valiaeva N, Kern ER, Hostetler KY. Inhibition of herpesvirus replication by hexadecyloxypropyl esters of purine- and pyrimidine-based phosphonomethoxyethyl nucleoside phosphonates. Antimicrob Agents Chemother. 2008;52(12):4326–30.

56. Prockop S, Doubrovina E, Suser S, Heller G, Barker J, Dahi P, Perales MA, Papadopoulos E, Sauter C, Castro-Malaspina H, et al. Off-the-shelf EBV-specific T cell immunotherapy for rituximab-refractory EBV-associated lymphoma following transplant. J Clin Invest. 2019; https://doi.org/10.1172/JCI121127.

57. Reshef R, Vardhanabhuti S, Luskin MR, Heitjan DF, Hadjiliadis D, Goral S, Krok KL, Goldberg LR, Porter DL, Stadtmauer EA, et al. Reduction of immunosuppression as initial therapy for posttransplantation lymphoproliferative disorder. Am J Transplant. 2011;11(2):336–47.

58. Riddler SA, Breinig MC, McKnight JL. Increased levels of circulating Epstein-Barr virus (EBV)-infected lymphocytes and decreased EBV nuclear antigen antibody responses are associated with the development of posttransplant lymphoproliferative disease in solid-organ transplant recipients. Blood. 1994;84(3):972–84.

59. Rooney CM, Smith CA, Ng CY, Loftin S, Li C, Krance RA, Brenner MK, Heslop HE. Use of gene-modified virus-specific T lymphocytes to control Epstein-Barr-virus-related lymphoproliferation. Lancet. 1995;345(8941):9–13.

60. Rosenberg AS, Klein AK, Ruthazer R, Evens AM. Hodgkin lymphoma post-transplant lymphoproliferative disorder: a comparative analysis of clinical characteristics, prognosis, and survival. Am J Hematol. 2016;91(6):560–5.

61. Rosenberg AS, Ruthazer R, Paulus JK, Kent DM, Evens AM, Klein AK. Survival analyses and prognosis of plasma-cell myeloma and Plasmacytoma-like Posttransplantation lymphoproliferative disorders. Clin Lymphoma Myeloma Leuk. 2016;16(12):684–692.e3.

62. Rossignol J, Terriou L, Robu D, Willekens C, Hivert B, Pascal L, Gueze R, Trappe R, Baillet C, Huglo D, et al. Radioimmunotherapy ((90) Y-Ibritumomab Tiuxetan) for Posttransplant lymphoproliferative disorders after prior exposure to rituximab. Am J Transplant. 2015; https://doi.org/10.1111/ajt.13244.

63. Savoldo B, Goss JA, Hammer MM, Zhang L, Lopez T, Gee AP, Lin Y-F, Quiros-Tejeira RE, Reinke P, Schubert S, et al. Treatment of solid organ transplant recipients with autologous Epstein Barr virus-specific cytotoxic T lymphocytes (CTLs). Blood. 2006;108(9):2942–9.

64. Sebelin-Wulf K, Nguyen TD, Oertel S, Papp-Vary M, Trappe RU, Schulzki A, Pezzutto A, Riess H, Subklewe M. Quantitative analysis of EBV-specific CD4/CD8 T cell numbers, absolute CD4/CD8 T cell numbers and EBV load in solid organ transplant recipients with PLTD. Transpl Immunol. 2007;17(3):203–10.

65. Shapiro RS, Chauvenet A, McGuire W, Pearson A, Craft AW, McGlave P, Filipovich A. Treatment of B-cell lymphoproliferative disorders with interferon alfa and intravenous gamma globulin. N Engl J Med. 1988;318(20):1334.
66. Starzl TE, Nalesnik MA, Porter KA, Ho M, Iwatsuki S, Griffith BP, Rosenthal JT, Hakala TR, Shaw BW, Hardesty RL, et al. Reversibility of lymphomas and lymphoproliferative lesions developing under cyclosporin-steroid therapy. Lancet. 1984;1(8377):583–7.
67. Swinnen LJ. Immune-cell treatment of Epstein–Barr-virus-associated lymphoproliferative disorders. Best Pract Res Clin Haematol. 2006;19(4):839–47.
68. Swinnen LJ, LeBlanc M, Grogan TM, Gordon LI, Stiff PJ, Miller AM, Kasamon Y, Miller TP, Fisher RI. Prospective study of sequential reduction in immunosuppression, interferon alpha-2B, and chemotherapy for posttransplantation lymphoproliferative disorder. Transplantation. 2008;86(2):215–22.
69. Swinnen LJ, Mullen GM, Carr TJ, Costanzo MR, Fisher RI. Aggressive treatment for postcardiac transplant lymphoproliferation. Blood. 1995;86(9):3333–40.
70. Tiede C, Maecker-Kolhoff B, Klein C, Kreipe H, Hussein K. Risk factors and prognosis in T-cell posttransplantation lymphoproliferative diseases: reevaluation of 163 cases. Transplantation. 2013;95(3):479–88.
71. Trappe R, Hinrichs C, Appel U, Babel N, Reinke P, Neumayer H-H, Budde K, Dreyling M, Dührsen U, Kliem V, et al. Treatment of PTLD with rituximab and CHOP reduces the risk of renal graft impairment after reduction of immunosuppression. Am J Transplant. 2009;9(10):2331–7.
72. Trappe R, Oertel S, Leblond V, Mollee P, Sender M, Reinke P, Neuhaus R, Lehmkuhl H, Horst HA, Salles G, et al. Sequential treatment with rituximab followed by CHOP chemotherapy in adult B-cell post-transplant lymphoproliferative disorder (PTLD): the prospective international multicentre phase 2 PTLD-1 trial. Lancet Oncol. 2012;13(2):196–206.
73. Trappe R, Riess H, Anagnostopoulos I, Neuhaus R, Gartner BC, Pohl H, Muller HP, Jonas S, Papp-Vary M, Oertel S. Efficiency of antiviral therapy plus IVIG in a case of primary EBV infection associated PTLD refractory to rituximab, chemotherapy, and antiviral therapy alone. Ann Hematol. 2009;88(2):167–72.
74. Trappe R, Riess H, Babel N, Hummel M, Lehmkuhl H, Jonas S, Anagnostopoulos I, Papp-Vary M, Reinke P, Hetzer R, et al. Salvage chemotherapy for refractory and relapsed post-transplant lymphoproliferative disorders (PTLD) after treatment with single-agent rituximab. Transplantation. 2007;83(7):912–8.
75. Trappe R, Zimmermann H, Fink S, Reinke P, Dreyling M, Pascher A, Lehmkuhl H, Gärtner B, Anagnostopoulos I, Riess H. Plasmacytoma-like post-transplant lymphoproliferative disorder, a rare subtype of monomorphic B-cell post-transplant lymphoproliferation, is associated with a favorable outcome in localized as well as in advanced disease – a prospective analysis of 8 cases. Haematologica. 2011;96(7):1067–71.
76. Trappe RU, Choquet S, Dierickx D, Mollee P, Zaucha JM, Dreyling MH, Dührsen U, Tarella C, Shpilberg O, Sender M, et al. International prognostic index, type of transplant and response to rituximab are key parameters to tailor treatment in adults with CD20-positive B cell PTLD: clues from the PTLD-1 trial. Am J Transplant. 2015;15(4):1091–100.
77. Trappe RU, Choquet S, Reinke P, Dreyling M, Mergenthaler HG, Jager U, Kebelmann-Betzing C, Jonas S, Lehmkuhl H, Anagnostopoulos I, et al. Salvage therapy for relapsed posttransplant lymphoproliferative disorders (PTLD) with a second progression of PTLD after upfront chemotherapy: the role of single-agent rituximab. Transplantation. 2007;84(12):1708–12.
78. Trappe RU, Dierickx D, Zimmermann H, Morschhauser F, Mollee P, Zaucha JM, Dreyling MH, Dührsen U, Reinke P, Verhoef G, et al. Response to rituximab induction is a predictive biomarker in Post-Transplant Lymphoproliferative Disorder (PTLD) and allows successful treatment stratification in an international phase II trial including 152 patients. Blood. 2015;126(23):816.
79. Trappe RU, Dierickx D, Zimmermann H, Morschhauser F, Mollee P, Zaucha JM, Dreyling MH, Dührsen U, Reinke P, Verhoef G, et al. Response to rituximab induction is a predictive

marker in B-cell post-transplant lymphoproliferative disorder and allows successful stratification into rituximab or R-CHOP consolidation in an international, prospective, multicenter phase II trial. J Clin Oncol. 2017;35(5):536–43.

80. Traum AZ, Rodig NM, Pilichowska ME, Somers MJG. Central nervous system lymphoproliferative disorder in pediatric kidney transplant recipients. Pediatr Transplant. 2006;10(4):505–12.

81. Tsai DE, Hardy CL, Tomaszewski JE, Kotloff RM, Oltoff KM, Somer BG, Schuster SJ, Porter DL, Montone KT, Stadtmauer EA. Reduction in immunosuppression as initial therapy for posttransplant lymphoproliferative disorder: analysis of prognostic variables and long-term follow-up of 42 adult patients. Transplantation. 2001;71(8):1076–88.

82. Twist CJ, Castillo RO. Treatment of recurrent posttransplant lymphoproliferative disorder of the central nervous system with high-dose methotrexate. Case Rep Transplant. 2013;2013:765230.

83. Valavoor SH, Ashraf Z, Narwal R, Ratnam S. Conservative management of post-transplant central nervous system lymphoma. Int Urol Nephrol. 2013;45(4):1219–22.

84. Vaysberg M, Balatoni CE, Nepomuceno RR, Krams SM, Martinez OM. Rapamycin inhibits proliferation of Epstein-Barr virus-positive B-cell lymphomas through modulation of cell-cycle protein expression. Transplantation. 2007;83(8):1114–21.

85. Webber S, Harmon W, Faro A, Green M, Sarwal M, Hayashi R, Canter C, Thomas D, Jaffe R, Fine R. Anti-CD20 monoclonal antibody (rituximab) for refractory PTLD after pediatric solid organ transplantation: multicenter experience from a registry and from a prospective clinical trial. Blood. 2004;104(11):746.

86. Webber SA, Naftel DC, Fricker FJ, Olesnevich P, Blume ED, Addonizio L, Kirklin JK, Canter CE. Lymphoproliferative disorders after paediatric heart transplantation: a multi-institutional study. Lancet. 2006;367(9506):233–9.

87. Williams-Aziz SL, Hartline CB, Harden EA, Daily SL, Prichard MN, Kushner NL, Beadle JR, Wan WB, Hostetler KY, Kern ER. Comparative activities of lipid esters of cidofovir and cyclic cidofovir against replication of herpesviruses in vitro. Antimicrob Agents Chemother. 2005;49(9):3724–33.

88. Wu M, Sun J, Zhang Y, Huang F, Zhou H, Fan Z, Xuan L, Yu G, Guo X, Dai M, et al. Intrathecal rituximab for EBV-associated post-transplant lymphoproliferative disorder with central nervous system involvement unresponsive to intravenous rituximab-based treatments: a prospective study. Bone Marrow Transplant. 2016;51(3):456–8.

89. Zimmermann H, Babel N, Dierickx D, Morschhauser F, Mollee P, Zaucha JM, Dreyling MH, Dührsen U, Reinke P, Verhoef G, et al. Immunosuppression is associated with clinical features and relapse risk of B cell Posttransplant lymphoproliferative disorder: a retrospective analysis based on the prospective, international, multicenter PTLD-1 trials. Transplantation. 2018;102(11):1914–23.

90. Zimmermann H, Denecke T, Dreyling MH, Franzius C, Reinke P, Subklewe M, Amthauer H, Kneba M, Riess H, Trappe RU. End-of-treatment positron emission tomography after uniform First-line therapy of B-cell Posttransplant lymphoproliferative disorder identifies patients at low risk of relapse in the prospective German PTLD registry. Transplantation. 2018;102(5):868–75.

91. Zimmermann H, Oschlies I, Fink S, Pott C, Neumayer HH, Lehmkuhl H, Hauser IA, Dreyling M, Kneba M, Gärtner B, et al. Plasmablastic Posttransplant lymphoma: cytogenetic aberrations and lack of Epstein-Barr virus association linked with poor outcome in the prospective German Posttransplant lymphoproliferative disorder registry. Transplantation. 2012;93(5):543–50.

92. Zimmermann H, Reinke P, Neuhaus R, Lehmkuhl H, Oertel S, Atta J, Planker M, Gärtner B, Lenze D, Anagnostopoulos I, et al. Burkitt post-transplantation lymphoma in adult solid organ transplant recipients: sequential immunochemotherapy with rituximab (R) followed by cyclophosphamide, doxorubicin, vincristine, and prednisone (CHOP) or R-CHOP is safe and effective in an analysis of 8 patients. Cancer. 2012;118(19):4715–24.

93. Zimmermann H, Trappe RU. EBV and posttransplantation lymphoproliferative disease: what to do? Hematology Am Soc Hematol Educ Program. 2013;2013:95–102.

Prevention of Epstein-Barr Virus Infection and PTLD following SOT

11

Michael Green and Sylvain Choquet

Introduction

The recognition of the importance of Epstein-Barr virus (EBV) infection in recipients of solid organ and stem cell transplantation has grown in parallel with the growth and success of these procedures. Despite an increasing understanding of EBV disease, the optimal management of this important complication remains unclear with ongoing concerns for morbidity and mortality attributable to pathogen [17, 35, 41, 46, 47]. Accordingly, attention has begun to focus on the prevention of EBV/PTLD in transplant recipients. As with the prevention of cytomegalovirus disease in SOT recipients, preventive strategies could include those provided to all patients at risk of developing disease (e.g., prophylactic therapy) or those focusing on individuals with subclinical infection to prevent progression to disease (e.g., preemptive therapy). Papers describing a variety of potential approaches to the prevention of EBV disease and PTLD have been published, including chemoprophylaxis using antiviral therapies, immunoprophylaxis (including adoptive immunotherapy), and viral load monitoring to inform preemptive strategies. This

M. Green (✉)
Departments of Pediatrics, University of Pittsburgh School of Medicine,
UPMC Children's Hospital of Pittsburgh, Pittsburgh, PA, USA

Departments of Surgery, University of Pittsburgh School of Medicine,
UPMC Children's Hospital of Pittsburgh, Pittsburgh, PA, USA

Division of Infectious Diseases, UPMC Children's Hospital of Pittsburgh,
Pittsburgh, PA, USA
e-mail: michael.green@chp.edu

S. Choquet (✉)
Department of Clinical Hematology, APHP-Sorbonne University, Pitié-Salpêtrière Hospital,
Paris, France
e-mail: sylvain.choquet@aphp.fr

© Springer Nature Switzerland AG 2021
V. R. Dharnidharka et al. (eds.), *Post-Transplant Lymphoproliferative Disorders*,
https://doi.org/10.1007/978-3-030-65403-0_11

chapter reviews the scientific rationale behind and clinical experience with these potential strategies for the prevention of EBV/PTLD in SOT recipients. The prevention of EBV and PTLD in HSCT recipients will be covered in Chap. 18.

Chemoprophylaxis Using Antiviral Therapy

Mechanisms of Action of Acyclovir, Ganciclovir, Foscarnet, and Cidofovir

Chemoprophylaxis using antiviral agents, such as acyclovir, ganciclovir (and their prodrugs valacyclovir and valganciclovir), foscarnet, and cidofovir, is one theoretical approach to the prevention of EBV disease and EBV-associated PTLD. Both acyclovir and ganciclovir (and their prodrugs valacyclovir and valganciclovir) are only active once they are phosphorylated by viral thymidine kinase which is only expressed during the lytic phase of viral replication. These agents actively inhibit lytic EBV replication in vitro [12, 22, 33] through inhibition of the late phase lytic replication without affecting the expression of immediate early or early lytic viral genes. Ganciclovir is phosphorylated to levels 100 times greater than acyclovir; it is approximately six times more potent against EBV [12] and has a prolonged effect in suppressing EBV genome replication in vitro compared to acyclovir [33]. However, while these antiviral agents suppress the lytic phase of EBV replication, they have no effect on EBV in its latent state or on the proliferation of EBV-transformed B-cells [12, 33, 46]. Analyses of pathologic specimens have shown that the vast majority of EBV-infected cells within PTLD lesions are transformed B-cells which are not undergoing lytic replication and thus their ongoing proliferation should not be inhibited by these agents [12, 17, 23, 28].

In contrast to these agents and their prodrugs, foscarnet activity is independent of viral thymidine kinase and directly inhibits viral DNA polymerase. Accordingly, the use of this agent may not be impacted by the presence or absence of lytic viral replication. However, since EBV proliferation in the setting of EBV-associated PTLD is felt to be accomplished through human replicative enzymes including human DNA polymerase, it is unclear that inhibition of viral DNA polymerase by foscarnet will have an impact on preventing the development of EBV disease including PTLD.

Cidofovir is a nucleotide analogue which undergoes cellular phosphorylation to its diphosphate form at which point it competitively inhibits the incorporation of deoxycytidine triphosphate into viral DNA by viral DNA polymerase which disrupts elongation and hence replication of viral DNA [30]. Unlike nucleoside analogues such as acyclovir or ganciclovir, cidofovir is not phosphorylated (and hence activated) by a viral kinase. While cidofovir (and its as-of-yet unlicensed prodrug brincidofovir) demonstrates in vitro activity against a number of DNA viruses including EBV, as with the other antiviral agents, the use of this agent will not inhibit EBV proliferation using human replicative enzymes associated with EBV proliferation in the setting of EBV-associated PTLD.

Studies have also been attempted evaluating the state of EBV infection in the steps leading up to the development of symptomatic EBV disease and PTLD. The correlation between EBV loads in the peripheral blood and the development of EBV disease and PTLD [18, 19, 27, 50, 52, 54, 56] suggests that characterization of the state of EBV infection in the blood of patients with elevated EBV loads could offer insight into the utility of antiviral therapy as prophylaxis against the EBV disease and PTLD. Babcock et al. characterized the state of EBV-infected B-cells from a small number of asymptomatic EBV-seropositive organ transplant recipients with elevated viral loads shortly after transplant [4]. These investigators found that the EBV load in the peripheral blood was maintained within resting memory B-cells and that although some patients only had episomal EBV DNA (characteristic of latently infected or immortalized B-cells), others had both episomal and linear EBV DNA (characteristic of active, lytic replication) [4]. Qu investigated the state of EBV gene expression in the peripheral blood of transplant recipients with elevated viral loads using RT-PCR, including some with active PTLD [49]. In this study, mRNA for ZEBRA (the immediate early transcriptional activator of EBV and a marker of entrance into the lytic cycle) was only detected in 6/40 specimens from 9 children with persistent high EBV load states who had serial samples available for evaluation and from only 3/8 specimens obtained from children at or near the time of PTLD. Further analyses suggested that even when positive, only a few EBV-infected B-cells in the peripheral blood expressed ZEBRA RNA at any given time. While both studies identify the presence of some components of lytic gene expression in SOT recipients with elevated EBV loads even in those who are EBV sero-positive at the time of transplant, neither study confirms the presence of lytic replication in these patients. Additional studies are necessary to confirm the state of EBV viral infection in patients at risk for development of EBV disease and PTLD.

Animal Models of Chemoprophylaxis

The potential role of acyclovir and ganciclovir in the prevention of EBV/PTLD has been explored in studies using the SCID mouse model of EBV/PTLD. Boyle demonstrated minimal activity for ganciclovir and none for acyclovir in reducing the frequency of EBV-associated B-cell lymphoma in the SCID mouse model of both active and latent infections [7]. Hong further evaluated the impact of acyclovir on development of EBV-lymphoproliferative disease (LPD) in a similar model [25]. In their system, EBV lymphoblastoid cell lines (LCLs) derived from an EBV wildtype strain, as well as two mutant EBV clones in which one or the other of the two immediate early (IE) genes (BZLF1 or BRLF1) had been knocked out, were infused into SCID mice. Growth of LPD was impaired in mice that had been infused with the two mutant strains of EBV. However, the use of acyclovir on SCID mice receiving wildtype EBV-derived LCL did not impact on the rate of growth of LPD. These results suggest that early lytic gene expression but not the release of infectious particles (which would be blocked by the presence of acyclovir) contributes to enhanced growth of LPD and raise doubts as to the likely effectiveness of acyclovir and ganciclovir to prevent development of PTLD. Data evaluating the potential role of foscarnet in the SCID mouse model is not available.

Clinical Studies of Chemoprophylaxis

Limited evidence is available to address the efficacy of antiviral therapy in the prevention of EBV/PTLD in humans. Two retrospective studies evaluated the rate of development of PTLD in adult organ transplant recipients who received acyclovir or ganciclovir as part of CMV prevention strategies [10, 11]. Although both studies appeared to demonstrate a beneficial effect of antiviral therapy against the development of EBV/PTLD, both were limited by the use of either historical [10] or, in the case of the latter study, no specific controls [11]. The difficulty in interpreting the results of such retrospective studies lacking concurrent controls is illustrated by a third study by Malouf which reported a drop in the incidence of PTLD from 4.2% to 1.34% after the introduction of ganciclovir prophylaxis in 1996 in lung transplant recipients [34]. Unfortunately, the introduction of ganciclovir was coincident with the elimination of anti-lymphocyte globulin as immunosuppression, an agent strongly associated with the development of PTLD. Accordingly, it is impossible to determine if the drop in incidence of EBV/PTLD was attributable to antiviral therapy or other changes in their management.

Funch and colleagues conducted a multicenter case-control study examining the impact of antiviral therapy on the development of PTLD in kidney transplant recipients [14]. Univariate analysis suggested a protective effect of antiviral treatment with ganciclovir or acyclovir. However, the study also showed that despite the fact that pretransplant EBV seronegativity was associated with developing PTLD (odds ratio 5.39), these patients were statistically less likely to receive antiviral therapy. To control for the possibility that the apparent protective effect of antiviral therapy might be a consequence of this confounding, additional analyses eliminating all individuals known to be EBV seronegative prior to transplant were performed which again demonstrated significant protective effect of ganciclovir and a trend towards protection with the use of acyclovir or both drugs. Unfortunately, a similar analysis was not carried out for those kidney transplant recipients who were EBV seronegative prior to transplant. In contrast to the results reported by Funch, a retrospective registry study of 44,828 kidney transplant recipients carried out by Opelz failed to identify any impact of antiviral prophylaxis with ganciclovir or acyclovir used for CMV prophylaxis on the incidence of lymphoma in the first year following transplantation (acyclovir $p = 0.28$, ganciclovir $p = 0.35$) [44]. The authors of this study concluded that the absence of an anti-lymphoma effect by the use of antiviral drugs was virtually proven. Hocker et al. carried out a small sub-analysis of a prospective trial in pediatric renal transplant recipients and observed a significant reduction of the 1-year incidence of EBV primary infection in 20 EBV D+/R patients on ganciclovir or valganciclovir prophylaxis compared with 8 patients without prophylaxis [24]. However, one patient each developed monomorphic

PTLD in both the treated and untreated cohorts and the authors concluded that no significant impact of ganciclovir or valganciclovir prophylaxis on PTLD occurrence could be derived from this study. More recently, Ostensen et al. carried out a retrospective study demonstrating a lack of effect of IV ganciclovir on the development of EBV-associated PTLD in pediatric patients [45]. One strength of this study was that the ganciclovir was used without the potential confounding effect of reduction of immune suppression.

To date, only a single randomized, controlled trial has been completed evaluating the role of antiviral agents in the prevention of EBV/PTLD [15]. This randomized trial compared 2 weeks of intravenous ganciclovir alone to 2 weeks of ganciclovir followed by 50 weeks of high-dose oral acyclovir in pediatric liver transplant recipients. PTLD developed in 8 of 24 patients who received ganciclovir followed by acyclovir compared to 5 cases of PTLD in 24 children who received the short course of ganciclovir alone (p = NS) [15]. This study suggested that the prolonged use of acyclovir did not prevent EBV/PTLD. However, it is possible that prolonged use of the more potent ganciclovir in lieu of acyclovir might have resulted in a different outcome. Another interpretation may simply be that ganciclovir has no protective role against PTLD, and as such development of PTLD in patients while receiving prolonged courses of intravenous ganciclovir has been reported [29]. A second prospective study of the use of IVIG and antiviral therapy with ganciclovir and/or acyclovir also failed to show the benefit of these therapies [26].

More recently, a 2016 meta-analysis showed that the use of antiviral drugs (ganciclovir, valganciclovir, acyclovir, and valacyclovir) in mismatched EBV transplant recipients (D+/R) had no effect on PTLD incidence [2]. No significant differences were seen across all types of solid organ transplants, age groups, or antiviral use as prophylaxis or preemptive strategy. The use of antivirals for prevention of EBV disease and PTLD was not recommended at the IPTA EBV Consensus Conference (2019, personal communication) and is also not currently recommended in the AST ID Guidelines [3].

As noted, foscarnet works by a different mechanism then acyclovir or ganciclovir. Accordingly, the absence of activity against lytic infection may not predict its potential impact for antiviral chemoprophylaxis. A potential therapeutic effect was suggested by a single case series of 3 adult SOT recipients with EBV-associated PTLD associated with the presence of EBV early antigen BZLF/ZEBRA protein which describes the potentially successful addition of foscarnet after failing to respond to a period of reduced immune suppression [43]. However, in two of the three patients the immune suppression had only been reduced for less than 2 weeks, and these reductions were continued throughout the time period that foscarnet was used. Accordingly, the initial period of reduced immune suppression might have been too short of a time period to observe a clinical impact, and the changes observed after starting foscarnet might have been attributable to ongoing reduction of immune suppression independent of an antiviral effect on the PTLD. The third case in this series showed an apparent response to foscarnet in a patient who could not undergo reduction of immune suppression due to a recent history of rejection. While this last case does suggest a potential therapeutic effect, the absence of additional published examples let alone prospective clinical trials leaves the impact of foscarnet unproven for treatment of the established EBV-associated PTLD in SOT recipients. Additionally, there is no published experience relating to the use of foscarnet for prevention, and the side effect profile of this drug makes this a suboptimal agent for a prevention strategy.

Because cidofovir has activity against EBV lytic infection in vitro, there is at least a theoretical role for its use for chemoprophylaxis against EBV disease including PTLD. The potential therapeutic role is raised by a case report of a 28-year-old liver transplant recipient with EBV-associated polymorphic PTLD involving his colon which was refractory to reduction of immune suppression followed by treatment with rituximab and subsequently CHOP-based chemotherapy [59]. For both rituximab and then chemotherapy, he initially appeared to respond but developed recurrent symptoms. He next received cidofovir to which he again appeared to initially respond but again developed recurrent symptoms prompting addition of IVIG with continued cidofovir. The patient seemed to improve on this regimen though he was switched to foscarnet due to persistent elevations of LDH and EBV load. He eventually experienced clinical improvement with resolution of EBV load in plasma but persistently elevated loads in PCR performed on whole blood. While the level of support that this report of a single case provides for the potential therapeutic role of cidofovir in the treatment of EBV-associated PTLD is debatable, there are no published data describing the use of cidofovir (or its as-of-yet unapproved prodrug brincidofovir) in the prevention of EBV disease or PTLD.

Immunoprophylaxis

Cellular Therapy

Cellular therapy has been considered both as a potential treatment and as a preventive strategy against EBV/PTLD. The rationale behind using cellular therapy is based on the critical role that EBV-specific cytotoxic T lymphocytes (CTLs) are known to play in the control of EBV infection in immunocompetent children and adults (see Chap. 5). EBV-specific CTLs may have several origins, either from the patient (autologous CTL) or from a healthy donor (allogeneic CTL). In the context of SOT, CTLs are usually obtained from donor libraries and are selected by their HLA compatibility. In the context of hematopoietic stem cell transplantation (HSCT), the CTLs come from the donor (if it is EBV positive), without selection, referred to as donor lymphocyte injection (DLI), or after selection and amplification of EBV-specific CTLs [21, 51]. The use of EBV-specific CTLs as a treatment for EBV/PTLD was first reported by Papadopoulos et al. in HSCT recipients using white blood cells from their EBV-seropositive donors (DLI) [42]. While successful in treating PTLD, this approach was associated with complications such as graft versus host disease and interstitial pulmonary infiltration which were attributed to the infusion of mature non-related lymphocytes. In an important modification of this approach, Rooney and colleagues used EBV-specific CTL derived from the actual stem cell donors of the affected HSCT recipients. Their initial efforts used these donor-derived EBV-specific CTLs to both treat PTLD and prevent development of EBV disease in patients with elevated EBV loads in their blood (preemptive treatment) [52]. Because of the requirement for HLA-matching for the effect of CTLs and the established observation that EBV/PTLD in HSCT recipients most often involves donor B-cells, this work involved the ex vivo stimulation and growth of pre-existing EBV-specific CTLs obtained from the HSCT donor. Given their initial successes, these investigators expanded their efforts and provided donor-derived EBV-specific CTLs as prophylaxis to 39 children who were at high risk for PTLD due to having undergone T-cell-depleted HSCT. None of these children developed PTLD; however, there was no control group [53]. Subsequently, others have also demonstrated the feasibility of this approach in the HSCT population.

While the use of cellular immunotherapy is clearly feasible for recipients of HSCT, implementation of this strategy for patients undergoing SOT has proven problematic. Unlike HSCT recipients, PTLDs developing in patients undergoing SOT typically involve B-cells of recipient origin and, in pediatric population, most commonly occur in patients who were immunologically naïve to EBV prior to transplantation. While EBV-seronegative adults are also at the greatest risk for development of EBV-associated PTLD, the disease may also uncommonly occur in EBV-seropositive SOT recipients when excessive immunosuppression inhibits the patient's immune response against the virus. Accordingly, patients most likely to benefit from prophylaxis using cellular immunotherapy will not have pre-existing EBV-specific CTLs available (EBV-seronegative SOT recipients), or very few, due to the immunosuppression (seropositive recipients), for ex vivo stimulation. However, Savoldo and colleagues demonstrated that autologous EBV-specific CTLs could be derived from patients at high risk for PTLD even before PTLD developed and given safely to prevent PTLD [57]. Twenty-three solid organ recipients with persistently high EBV-DNA viral load (but without evidence of PTLD) and four patients with early post-transplant EBV seroconversion were enrolled in an EBV-CTL generation protocol. Kinetics of CTL derivation were similar to healthy donors. None had recognized toxicity. The number of EBV-responsive cells increased after infusion. No PTLD developed within one year of the infusion although the viral load levels did not always fall substantially. More recently, Prockop and colleagues reported the use of third-party donors as the source of EBV-specific CTL therapy for both HSCT and SOT recipients [48]. In a recent publication, they achieved a 54% rate of complete or sustained partial remission from a cohort of 12 SOT recipients. However, data evaluating the use (for either prophylaxis or as preemptive therapy) of EBV-specific CTL for prevention of EBV disease and PTLD are not available.

Passive Immunization

Although CTL are thought to play the central role in the control of EBV infections, recent studies have raised questions regarding the role of antibodies in controlling the rapid proliferation of EBV-infected cells [36]. Several reports have documented an association between loss or absence of antibody against at least one of the Epstein-Barr nuclear antigens (EBNA) in EBV-seropositive organ transplant recipients and subsequent development of PTLD [50, 61]. It has also been recognized that many patients undergoing primary EBV infection following transplantation fail to develop anti-EBNA antibodies. Thus, the absence of antibodies against EBNA appears to correlate with an increased risk of developing PTLD. Riddler et al. further demonstrated a correlation between increasing levels of anti-EBNA antibodies, including those introduced through transfusions, with decreasing EBV load [50]. Taken together, these data suggest a potential role for antibody in controlling EBV-infected cells and therefore provide a potential rationale for the use of antibodies in the prevention and/or treatment of EBV/PTLD.

Several investigators have evaluated the potential of antibody treatment to prevent EBV/PTLD using the SCID mouse model. Abedi et al. demonstrated that weekly infusions of two different commercial gammaglobulin preparations as well as purified immunoglobulin from EBV-seropositive blood donors prevented development of PTLD in this model [1]. In contrast, these investigators found that infusion of purified immunoglobulin from EBV-seronegative blood donors, as well as rabbit anti-gp340 anti-serum (a potentially protective anti-EBV antibody), failed to protect SCID mice from development of PTLD. Nadal et al. also evaluated the ability of human immunoglobulin preparations to suppress the occurrence of Epstein-Barr virus-associated lymphoproliferation in this model [40]. These investigators found that the infusion of human immunoglobulin after reconstitution with human tonsillar mononuclear cells followed by infection with supernatant from B95-8 (a lytic replication-permissive cell line) delayed or prevented the development of EBV-associated lymphoma in their model.

The potential role of IVIG in the prevention of EBV/PTLD is further supported by the previously mentioned registry study carried out by Opelz [44]. As mentioned earlier, this international registry review of 44,824 kidney transplant recipients evaluated the impact of the use of strategies to prevent CMV infection on the subsequent development of post-transplant lymphoma. In contrast to the absence of any benefit at all for ganciclovir or acyclovir, these investigators found that none of 2103 kidney recipients, who received anti-CMV immunoglobulin during the 3 or 4 first months post-transplantation, developed lymphoma during the first year following kidney transplantation ($p = 0.012$). Of interest, the demographics of patients receiving CMV-IVIG did not appear to differ from those who had received ganciclovir or acyclovir as a method of preventing CMV. The protective effect of CMV-IVIG did not appear to persist beyond the first year as the rate of lymphoma development in the subsequent 5 years was similar for recipients of CMV-IVIG and antiviral therapy with ganciclovir or acyclovir and those kidney recipients who received no prophylaxis to prevent CMV.

The potential prophylactic benefit of intravenous immunoglobulin (IVIG) against the development of EBV/PTLD was evaluated in a randomized, multicentered, controlled trial of CMV-IVIG for prevention of EBV/PTLD in pediatric liver transplant recipients [16]. In a study of 82 evaluable patients, no significant differences were seen in the adjusted 2-year EBV disease-free rate (CMV-IVIG 79%, placebo 71%)

and PTLD-free rate (CMV-IVIG 91%, placebo 84%) between treatment and placebo groups at 2 years ($p > 0.20$). Although statistically significant differences were not observed, rates of EBV disease and PTLD were *somewhat* lower in recipients of CMV-IVIG than in those who received placebo. This was particularly true for children less than 1 year of age, where 25% of children receiving CMV-IVIG developed EBV disease compared with 38% receiving placebo. While differences in the rates of development of PTLD in the children <1 year of age were less dramatic, the advantage again favored the recipients of CMV-IVIG (12% vs. 19%). Of note, the use of EBV load monitoring to inform reductions in immune suppression occurred with increasing frequency during the latter part of the study and potentially confounded its ability to identify differences between the two treatment groups, and this contributed to the discontinuation of the study before adequate power to see a difference might have been achieved. In another prospective comparative study [26], 25 children and 9 adults at high risk of PTLD (EBV seronegative with EBV-positive donor) were treated with ganciclovir 3 months with or without IVIG 6 months. No difference in the incidence of primary EBV infection was noted and the only three PTLDs (all EBV associated) occurred in the ganciclovir + IVIG arm in pediatric recipients. These occurred at days 110, 128, and 289 post-transplant. Accordingly, one of the three was still on ganciclovir, while two were on oral acyclovir. Two of the three would still have received IVIG near the time of diagnosis.

Active Immunization

Active immunization would be another potential immunoprophylactic strategy. At present, there is no commercially available vaccine to prevent EBV infection or disease. Most efforts to develop an EBV vaccine have focused on the glycoprotein 350, which binds to CD21/CD35 to gain entry to B-lymphocytes and is the major target of serum-neutralizing antibody against EBV. A recombinant glycoprotein 350 ((gp350)/AS04) vaccine has been evaluated in clinical trials. Results of phase I and phase II trials using this candidate vaccine in both EBV-seropositive and EBV-seronegative healthy volunteers have been published [39, 58]. Use of this vaccine resulted in a reduction in symptomatic primary EBV infection and development of infectious mononucleosis but had little impact on EBV seroconversion rates. Of note, the vaccine had no reliable effect on the development of cell-mediated immunity. A second vaccine approach is to generate EBV-specific CD8+ T-cells that control the expansion of EBV-infected B-cells after infection. Results of a small phase I CD8+ T-cell epitope-based EBV vaccine trial in 14 previously healthy seronegative volunteers have recently been published [13]. The vaccine comprised the HLAB*0801-restricted CD8+ T-cell epitope FLRGRAYGL (FLR) from the latent EBNA3 using tetanus toxoid as a source of CD4+ T-cell help. The vaccine was well tolerated with no serious side effects recognized during the course of the study. All but one of eight volunteers receiving vaccine demonstrated production of FLR-specific T-cell response post-vaccination as measured by ELISPOT. More recent efforts have looked at using EBNA1/LMP2 as a potential immunogen for a vaccine aimed at augmenting immune response in patients with nasopharyngeal carcinoma. However, a review of clinical trials.com identifies that there are currently no active trials of EBV vaccines in any human population despite the clear rationale in support of having such a vaccine. Accordingly, active immunization is not a viable alternative to the prevention of EBV disease and PTLD in SOT recipients at this time.

Viral Load Monitoring and Preemptive Strategies of Prevention

The observation that EBV load in the peripheral blood rose prior to the development of overt PTLD and likewise fell with the resolution of disease (see Chap. 6) provided a model similar to CMV preemptive therapy for instituting prevention strategies [55]. However, the lack of impact of antiviral agents on EBV loads raised questions as to what is the most appropriate preemptive intervention. Potential strategies have included reduction or cessation of immunosuppression, use of antiviral medications such as ganciclovir or acyclovir alone or in combination with reduction of immune suppression, as well as the use of monoclonal anti-CD20 (rituximab) therapy. Each of these strategies is reviewed below.

McDiarmid and colleagues reported their experience using monitoring of EBV loads to inform the preemptive use of the combination of decreasing immunosuppression and intravenous ganciclovir (either reinitiation or continuation if patients were on it already) in pediatric liver transplant recipients [37]. EBV-seronegative children were classified as high risk and received 100 days of intravenous ganciclovir (followed by oral acyclovir) and were followed with frequent viral load measurement. Children who were EBV seropositive prior to transplantation were considered low risk; they received a shorter course of IV ganciclovir followed by oral acyclovir and were monitored less frequently. Elevated EBV viral loads were observed in most of the high-risk group while they were still on their initial course of ganciclovir prophylaxis. Accordingly, the only change made in their management in response to the elevated loads was a drop in immunosuppression. However, no PTLD occurred in this group. Interestingly, two children both under a year of age who had been seropositive pretransplant and hence classified as low risk developed PTLD. It is likely that EBV seropositivity was present on the basis of passive maternal antibody and that these infants were really at high risk. The overall rate of PTLD of 5% in this experience was lower than their previous rate of 10%. However, the investigators were unable to determine the relative impact of ganciclovir versus reduction of immunosuppression on the decreased rate of PTLD observed in this experience. Subsequently, Lee et al. evaluated 43 pediatric liver transplant recipients who underwent prospective EBV load monitoring with a rapid tapering of immunosuppression if their load reached a critically high threshold without addition of antiviral therapy [31]. The rates of PTLD and rejection were compared to 30 historical controls that had been consecutively transplanted just prior to the intervention group at their center. The rates of PTLD were 16% in the historical control compared with only 2% once the rapid weaning protocol was established. Only one patient received valganciclovir for concurrent CMV reactivation. Rejection occurred in one patient who required decreased immunosuppression and responded to steroid pulsing with cessation of tacrolimus tapering. These results are provocative but suffer from having a historic control in which EBV serologic status was not known before transplantation. Accordingly, it is possible that the differences observed in this experience could in part be due to a larger high-risk population.

In a similar approach, Bakker and colleagues used EBV load monitoring in 75 adult lung transplant recipients to inform reduction in immunosuppression with the hope of preventing PTLD [5]. This population differed somewhat from the experience in pediatric transplant recipients in that most of the patients were EBV seropositive prior to transplant. Thirty-five percent of patients in this study demonstrated reactivation of EBV as evidenced by elevated viral loads. However, immunosuppression was only able to be reduced in 19 of 26 patients with an elevated EBV load. Overall, no patient developed and EBV-associated PTLD regardless of the inability to modify immune suppression in 7 of the patients, though one of the 75 subjects did develop an EBV-negative PTLD. Importantly there was no accelerated rejection of the graft or worse survival in the patients who had immunosuppression reduced due to EBV viral load monitoring [5].

Because of concerns for EBV load having low-positive predictive value for development of PTLD particularly in a previously immune population [6], some investigators sought to ascertain if viral load monitoring combined with evaluation of cellular immune response to phytohemagglutinin (PHA) would improve the safety of intervening with decreased immunosuppression [32]. Eighteen children undergoing liver transplantation were followed in this fashion; those children with moderate to high levels of EBV viremia were also found to have a decreased response to PHA, suggesting a state of over-immunosuppression. Three of the patients had immunosuppression lowered in response to EBV viral load; all had increase PHA responses and no development of PTLD. EBV viral load monitoring failed to predict the development of PTLD in one child whose EBV load remained low; however, his PHA response had also been low, suggesting he was over-immunosuppressed. It is possible that by reducing immune suppression in response to either an elevated EBV load or a low PHA, his episode of PTLD could have been prevented. As the cellular response to PHA has not shown any advantage over the monitoring of the viral load and this technique is much less available than the second, the monitoring of EBV viral load is currently the best technique to propose preemptive treatments.

A final approach that has been considered is the use of the anti-B-cell monoclonal antibody, rituximab, as a preemptive therapy in response to an elevated EBV load. Rituximab was used as a preemptive therapy with successful outcome in high-risk hematopoietic transplant recipients [26, 60]. Seventeen prospectively monitored HSCT recipients showed a high level of EBV reactivation; 15 of the 17 were given rituximab preemptively. Only one of the 15 developed PTLD but ultimately responded to two further doses of rituximab [60]. A similar approach was taken by Gruhn and colleagues in three children at high risk for PTLD after T-cell-depleted HSCT. The children received rituximab when they were found to have critically high viral loads for EBV; all remained PTLD-free 7–9 months after HSCT [20]. Meerbach and colleagues took it one step further and used a single dose of rituximab in combination with two doses of intravenous cidofovir a week apart in four HSCT recipients who had persistently elevated EBV viral loads [38]. The viral load fell in all cases and no PTLD developed. Although these studies are small, they favor the use of preemptive rituximab after HSCT (Chap. 18), especially since the treatment of PTLD in this context is more limited and has a poorer prognosis than after SOT.

With regard to SOT, a large prospective study has recently been published [9]. Nearly 300 adult cardiac transplant patients treated by the same team with the same immunosuppression were systematically followed up on their EBV viral load during the first year after the transplant. At a viral load $>10^5$ copies/mL, immunosuppression was lowered and viral load was monitored weekly; if the viral load increased or was stable at 4 weeks, patients received rituximab. In the case of viral load $>10^6$ copies/mL, rituximab was immediately injected in combination with the decrease of immunosuppression. Of the six EBV-seronegative patients at the time of transplantation, all presented a primary infection during the follow-up; among the other patients, 31 developed reactivation above the treatment threshold, all patients preemptively treated by the proposed algorithm responded by lowering their viral load, and none has a PTLD. Compared with 820 cardiac transplant patients in the same department, with the same immunosuppression, for whom 24 PTLDs had been diagnosed, including 13 early positive EBV PTLDs, the difference was significant ($p = 0.033$). It should be noted that no toxicity and in particular no rejection have been described.

One potential concern with the preemptive use of rituximab is the potential development of persistent hypogammaglobulinemia after treatment with this monoclonal antibody in at least the pediatric SOT population. Chiou et al. reported that two-thirds of a cohort of 18 pediatric SOT recipients developed persistent (>2 years) hypogammaglobulinemia after exposure to rituximab as treatment for PTLD [8]. The authors also attributed an increase in significant bacterial infection in those with hypogammaglobulinemia. Accordingly, studies that determine the frequency, duration, and sequelae of this potential complication as well as the comparative benefits compared to reduction of immune suppression are needed to define which SOT recipients with elevated EBV loads may be the appropriate candidates for this approach. It may be that a sequential approach of an initial reduction of immune suppression followed by the use of rituximab for SOT recipients with persistently highly elevated EBV loads despite this intervention will be the optimal strategy for the prevention of EBV disease and PTLD.

Take-Home Pearls
- Increasing attention on EBV disease and PTLD is being focused on prevention strategies prompting some centers to routinely use antiviral and/or immunoglobulin agents as standard prophylaxis against the development of EBV/PTLD despite the absence of strong data in support of these approaches.
- At present, the use of serial monitoring of the EBV viral load as a stimulus to reduce immunosuppression (for solid organ transplant recipients or for stem cell

transplant recipients) appears to be the most promising strategy for the prevention of EBV disease and PTLD in SOT recipients.

- The preemptive use of rituximab may also be an effective strategy in the prevention of EBV disease in SOT recipients, but studies are needed to define the optimal time, population, risks (particularly hypogammaglobulinemia), and benefits of this approach compared to reduction of immune suppression.
- Well-designed clinical trials are necessary to evaluate the potential role of both antiviral and immunoglobulin agents in the prevention of EBV/PTLD in organ transplant recipients.
- Finally, the development of an effective EBV vaccine to provide to EBV-naïve transplant candidates would likely prove to be an extremely effective strategy in the prevention of this complication though efforts to date have failed to identify an effective vaccine candidate against EBV.

References

1. Abedi MR, Linde A, Christensson B, Mackett M, Hammarstrom L, Smith C. Preventive effect of IgG from EBV-seropositive donors on the development of human lymphoproliferative disease in SCID mice. Int J Cancer. 1997;71:624–9.
2. Aldabbagh MA, Gitman MR, Kumar D, et al. The role of antiviral prophylaxis for the prevention of Epstein-Barr virus-associated Posttransplant lymphoproliferative disease in solid organ transplant recipients: a systematic review. Am J Transplant. 2017;17:770–81.
3. Allen UD, Preiksaitis JK, Practice ASTIDCo. Post-transplant lymphoproliferative disorders, EBV infection and disease in solid organ transplantation: guidelines from the American Society of Transplantation Infectious Diseases Community of Practice. Clin Transpl. 2019;33 (9):e13652. https://doi.org/10.1111/ctr.13652. Epub 2019 Jul 23.
4. Babcock GJ, Decker L, Freeman RB, Thorley-Dawon DA. Epstein-Barr virus-infected resting memory B-cells, not proliferating lymphoblasts, accumulate in the peripheral blood of immunosuppressed patients. J Exp Med. 1999;190:567–76.
5. Bakker NA, Verschuuren EAM, Erasmus ME, Hepkema BG, Veeger NJGM, Kallenberg CGM, van der Bij W. Epstein-Barr virus DNA load monitoring late after lung transplantation: a surrogate marker of the degree of immunosuppression and a safe guide to reduce immunosuppression. Transplantation. 2007;83:433–8.
6. Benden C, Aurora P, Burch M, Cubitt D, Lloyd C, Whitmore P, Neligan S, Elliot MJ. Monitoring of Epstein-Barr viral load in pediatric heart and lung transplant recipients by real-time polymerase chain reaction. J Heart Lung Transplant. 2005;24:2103–8.
7. Boyle TJ, Tamburini M, Berend KR, Kizilbash AM, Borowitz MJ, Lyerly HK. Human B-cell lymphoma in severe combined immunodeficient mice after active infection with Epstein-Barr virus. Surgery. 1992;112:378–86.
8. Chiou FK, Beath SV, Patel M, Gupte GL. Hypogammaglobulinemia and bacterial infection follow pediatric post-transplant lymphoproliferative disorder in the rituximab era. Pediatr Transplant. 2019;23(6):e13519. https://doi.org/10.1111/petr.13519. Epub 2019 Jun 17
9. Choquet S, Varnous S, Deback C, Golmard JL, Leblond V. Adapted treatment of Epstein–Barr virus infection to prevent post-transplant lymphoproliferative disorder after heart transplantation. Am J Transplant. 2014;14:857–66.
10. Darenkov IA, Marcarelli MA, Basadonna GP, Friedman AL, Lorber KM, Howe JG, Crouch J, Bia MJ, Kliger AS, Lorber MI. Reduced incidence of Epstein-Barr virus-associated posttransplant lymphoproliferative disorder using preemptive antiviral therapy. Transplantation. 1997;64:848–52.

11. Davis CL, Harrison KL, McVicar JP, Forg P, Bronner M, Marsh CL. Antiviral prophylaxis and the Epstein Barr virus-related post-transplant lymphoproliferative disorder. Clin Transpl. 1995;9:53–9.
12. Davis CL. The antiviral prophylaxis of post-transplant lymphoproliferative disorder. Springer Sem Immunopathol. 1998;20:437–53.
13. Elliott SL, Suhrbier A, Miles JJ, Lawrence G, Pye SJ, Le TT, Rosenstengel A, Nguyen T, Allworth A, Burrows SR, Cox J, Pye D, Moss DJ, Bharadwaj M. Phase I trial of CD8+ T-cell peptide epitope-based vaccine for infectious mononucleosis. J Virol. 2008;82:14481457.
14. Funch DP, Walker AM, Schneider G, Ziyadeh NJ, Pescovitz MD. Ganciclovir and acyclovir reduce the risk of post-transplant lymphoproliferative disorder in renal transplant recipients. Am J Transplant. 2005;5:2894–900.
15. Green M, Kaufmann M, Wilson J, Reyes J. Comparison of intravenous ganciclovir followed by oral acyclovir with intravenous ganciclovir alone for the prevention of cytomegalovirus and Epstein-Barr virus after liver transplantation in children. Clin Infect Dis. 1997;25:1344–9.
16. Green M, Michaels MG, Katz BZ, Burroughs M, Gerber D, Shneider BL, Newell K, Rowe D, Reyes J. CMV-IVIG for prevention of Epstein-Barr virus disease and posttransplant lymphoproliferative disease in pediatric liver transplant recipients. Am J Transplant. 2006;6:1906–12.
17. Green M, Michaels MG, Webber SA, Rowe D, Reyes J. The management of Epstein-Barr virus associated post-transplant lymphoproliferative disorders in pediatric solid-organ transplant recipients. Pediatr Transpl. 1999;3:271–81.
18. Green M, Reyes J, Webber S, Michaels MG, Rowe D. The role of viral load in the diagnosis, management and possible prevention of Epstein-Barr virus-associated posttransplant lymphoproliferative disease following solid organ transplantation. Curr Opin Organ Transplant. 1999;4:292–6.
19. Green M, Bueno J, Rowe D, et al. Predictive negative value of persistent low Epstein-Barr virus viral load after intestinal transplantation in children. Transplantation. 2000;70:593–6.
20. Gruhn B, Meerbach A, Häfer R, Zell R, Wutzler P, Zintl F. Pre-emptive therapy with rituximab for prevention of Epstein-Barr virus-associated lymphoproliferative disease after hematopoietic stem cell transplantation. Bone Marrow Transplant. 2003;31:1023–5.
21. Gustafsson A, Levitsky V, Zou J, Frisan T, Daliani TS, Ljungman P, Ringden O, Winiarsk JI, Ernberg I, Masucci MG. Epstein-Barr virus (EBV) load in bone marrow transplant recipients at risk to develop posttransplant lymphoproliferative disease: prophylactic infusion of EBV-specific cytotoxic. T Cells Blood. 2000;95(3):807–14.
22. Hanto DW, Frizzera G, Gajl-Peczalska KJ, et al. Epstein-Barr virus induced B-cell lymphoma after renal transplantation. N Engl J Med. 1982;306:913–8.
23. Haque T, Crawford DH. Role of donor versus recipient Epstein-Barr virus in post-transplant lymphoproliferative disorders. Springer Semin Immunopathol. 1998;20:375–87.
24. Hocker B, Fickenscher H, Delecluse HJ, et al. Epidemiology and morbidity of Epstein-Barr virus infection in pediatric renal transplant recipients: a multicenter, prospective study. Clin Infect Dis. 2013;56:84–92.
25. Hong GK, Gulley ML, Feng WH, Delecluse HJ, Holley-Guthrie E, Kenney SC. Epstein-Barr virus lytic infection contributes to lymphoproliferative disease in a SCID mouse model. J Virol. 2005;79:1393–403.
26. Humar A, Hébert D, Davies HD, Humar A, Stephens D, O'Doherty B, Allen U. A randomized trial of ganciclovir versus ganciclovir plus immune globulin for prophylaxis against Epstein-Barr virus related posttransplant lymphoproliferative disorder. Transplantation. 2006;81:856–61.
27. Kenagy DN, Schlesinger Y, Weck K, Ritter JH, Gaudreault-Keener MM, Storch GA. Epstein-Barr virus DNA in peripheral blood leukocytes of patients with posttransplant lymphoproliferative disease. Transplantation. 1995;19:547–54.
28. Knowles DM, Cesarmen E, Chadburn A, et al. Correlative morphologic and molecular genetic analysis demonstrates three distinct categories of posttransplantation lymphoproliferative disorders. Blood. 1995;85:552–65.
29. Kuo PC, Dafoe DC, Alfrey EJ, Sibley RK, Scandling JD. Posttransplant lymphoproliferative disorders and Epstein-Barr virus prophylaxis. Transplantation. 1995;59:135–8.

30. Lea AP, Bryson HM. Cidofovir. Drugs. 1996;52:225. https://doi.org/10.2165/00003495-199652020-00006.
31. Lee TC, Savoldo B, Rooney CM, Heslop HE, Gee AP, Caldwell Y, Barshes NR, Scott JD, Bristow LJ, O'Mahony CA, Goss JA. Quantitative EBV viral loads and immunosuppression alterations can decrease PTLD incidence in pediatric liver transplant recipients. Am J Transplant. 2005;5:2222–8.
32. Lee TC, Goss JA, Rooney CM, Heslop HE, Barshes NR, Caldwell YM, Gee AP, Scott JD, Savoldo B. Quantification of a low cellular immune response to aid in identification of pediatric liver transplant recipients at high-risk for EBV infection. Clin Transpl. 2006;20:689–94.
33. Lin JC, Smith MC, Pagano JS. Prolonged inhibitory effect of 9-(1,3-dihydroxy-2-propoxymethyl)guanine against replication of Epstein-Barr virus. J Virol. 1984;50:50–5.
34. Malouf MA, Chhajed PN, Hopkins P, Plit M, Turner J, Glanville AR. Anti-viral prophylaxis reduces the incidence of lymphoproliferative disease in lung transplant recipients. J Heart Lung Transplant. 2002;21:547–54.
35. Manez R, Breinig MC, Linden P, et al. Posttransplant lymphoproliferative disease in primary Epstein-Barr virus infection after liver transplantation: the role of cytomegalovirus disease. J Infect Dis. 1997;176:1462–7.
36. McKnight JLC, Cen H, Riddler SA, Breinig MC, Williams PA, Ho M, Joseph PS. EBV gene expression, EBNA antibody responses and EBV+ peripheral blood lymphocytes in posttransplant lymphoproliferative disease. Leuk Lymphoma. 1994;15:9–16.
37. McDiarmid SV, Jordan S, Lee GS, et al. Prevention and preemptive therapy of posttransplant lymphoproliferative disease in pediatric liver recipients. Transplantation. 1998;66:1604–11.
38. Meerbach A, Wutzler P, Häfer R, Zintl F, Gruhn B. Monitoring of Epstein-Barr virus load after hematopoietic stem cell transplantation for early intervention in post-transplant lymphoproliferative disease. J Med Virol. 2008;80:441–54.
39. Moutschen M, Leonard P, Sokal EM, Smets F, Haumont M, Mazzu P, Bollen A, Denamur F, Peeters P, Dubin G, Denis M. Phase I/II studies to evaluate safety and immunogenicity of a recombinant gp350 Epstein-Barr virus vaccine in healthy adults. Vaccine. 2007;25:4697–705.
40. Nadal D, Guzman J, Frohlich S, Braun DG. Human immunoglobulin preparations suppress the occurrence of Epstein-Barr virus-associated lymphoproliferation. Exp Hematol. 1997;25:223–31.
41. Newell KA, Alonso EM, Whitingdon PF, et al. Post-transplant lymphoproliferative disease in pediatric liver transplantation. Transplantation. 1996;62:370–5.
42. Papadopoulos EB, Ladanyi M, Emanuel D, Mackinnon S, Boulad F, Carabasi MH, Castro-Malaspina H, Childs BH, Gillio AP, Small TN, Young JW, Kernan NA, O'Reilly RJ. Infusions of donor leukocytes to treat Epstein-Barr virus-associated lymphoproliferative disorders after allogeneic bone marrow transplantation. New Eng J Med. 1994;330:1185–91.
43. Oertel SH, Anagnostopoulos I, Hummel MW, Jonas S, Riess HB. Identification of early antigen BZLF1/ZEBRA protein of Epstein-Barr virus can predict the effectiveness of antiviral treatment in patients with post-transplant lymphoproliferative disease. British J Haematol. 2002;118:1120–3.
44. Opelz G, Daniel V, Naujokat C, Fickenscher H, Dohler B. Effect of cytomegalovirus prophylaxis with immunoglobulin or with antiviral drugs on post-transplant non-Hodgkin lymphoma: a multicentre retrospective analysis. [see comment] [erratum appears in Lancet Oncol. 2007 Mar;8(3):191]. [Journal Article. Multicenter study. Research Support, Non-U.S. Gov't]. Lancet Oncol. 2007;8(3):212–8.
45. Ostensen AB, Sanengen T, Holter E, Pal-Dag L, Almaas R. No effect of treatment with intravenous ganciclovir on Epstein-Barr virus viremia demonstrated after pediatric liver transplantation. Pediatr Transplant. 2017;21:e13010. wileyonlinelibrary.com/journal/petr 11 of 8. https://doi.org/10.1111/petr.13010.
46. Paya CV, Fung JJ, Nalesnik MA, Kieff E, Green M, Gores G, Habermann TH, Wiesner RH, Swinnnen L, Woodle ES, Bromberg JS. Epstein-Barr virus-induced posttransplant lymphoproliferative disorders. Transplantation. 1999;68:1517–25.

47. Preiksaitis JK. New developments in the diagnosis and management of posttransplantation lymphoproliferative disorders in solid organ transplant recipients. Clin Infect Dis. 2004;39:1016–23.

48. Prockop S, Doubrovina E, Suser S, Heller G, Barker J, Dahi P, Perales MA, Papadopoulos E, Sauter C, Castro-Malaspina H, Boulad F, Curran KJ, Giralt S, Gyurkocza B, Hsu KC, Jakubowski A, Hanash AM, Kernan NA, Kobos R, Koehne G, Landau H, Ponce D, Spitzer B, Young JW, Behr G, Dunphy M, Haque S, Teruya-Feldstein J, Arcila M, Moung C, Hsu S, Hasan A, O'Reilly RJ. Off-the-shelf EBV-specific T cell immunotherapy for rituximab-refractory EBV-associated lymphoma following transplant. J Clin Invest. 2019; https://doi.org/10.1172/JCI121127.

49. Qu L, Green M, Webber S, Reyes J, Ellis D, Rowe D. Epstein-Barr virus gene expression in the peripheral blood of transplant recipients with persistent circulating viral loads. J Inf Dis. 2000;182:1013–21.

50. Riddler SA, Breinig MC, McKnight JLC. Increased levels of circulating Epstein-Barr virus-infected lymphocytes and decreased EBV nuclear antigen antibody responses are associated with the development of posttransplant lymphoproliferative disease in solid-organ transplant recipients. Blood. 1994;84:972–84.

51. Rooney CM, Loftin SK, Holladay MS, Brenner MK, Krance RA, Heslop HB. Early identification of Epstein-Barr virus-associated post-transplant lymphoproliferative disease. Br J Haematol. 1995;89:98–103.

52. Rooney CM, Smith CA, Ng CYC, Loftin S, Li C, Krance RA, Brenner MK, Heslop HE. Use of gene-modified virus-specific T lymphocytes to control Epstein-Barr virus-related lymphoproliferation. Lancet. 1995;345:9–13.

53. Rooney CM, Smith CA, Ng CYC, Loftin SK, Sixbey JW, Gan Y, Srivastava DK, Bowman LC, Krance RA, Brenner MK, Heslop HE. Infusion of cytotoxic T cells for the prevention and treatment of Epstein-Barr virus-induced lymphoma in allogeneic transplant recipients. Blood. 1998;92:1549–55.

54. Rowe DT, Qu L, Reyes J, Jabbour N, Yunis E, Putnam P, Todo S, Green M. Use of quantitative competitive PCR to measure Epstein-Barr virus genome load in peripheral blood of pediatric transplant recipients with lymphoproliferative disorders. J Clin Microbiol. 1997;35:1612–5.

55. Rubin RH. Preemptive therapy in immunocompromised hosts. N Engl J Med. 1991;324:1057–9.

56. Savoie A, Perpete C, Carpentier L, Joncas K, Alfieri C. Direct correlation between the load of Epstein-Barr virus-infected lymphocytes in the peripheral blood of pediatric transplant patients and risk of lymphoproliferative disease. Blood. 1994;83:2715–22.

57. Savoldo B, Goss JA, Hammer MM, Zhang L, Lopez T, Gee AP, Lin YF, Quiros-Tejeira RE, Reinke P, Schubert S, Gottschalk S, Finegold MJ, Brenner MK, Rooney CM, Heslop HE. Treatment of solid organ transplant recipients with autologous Epstein Barr virus–specific cytotoxic T lymphocytes (CTLs). Blood. 2006;108:2942–9.

58. Sokal EM, Hoppenbrouwers K, Vandermeulen C, Moutschen M, Leonard P, Moreels A, Haumont M, Bollen A, Smets F, Denis M. Recombinant gp350 vaccine for infectious mononucleosis: a phase 2, randomized double-blind, placebo-controlled trial to evaluate the safety, immunogenicity and efficacy of an Epstein-Barr virus vaccine in healthy young adults. J Inf Dis. 2007;196:1749–53.

59. Trappe R, Riess H, Anagnostopoulos I, Neuhaus R, Gartner BC, Pohl H, Muller HP, Jonas S, Papp-Vary M, Oertal S. Efficiency of antiviral therapy plus IVIG in a case of primary EBV infection associated PTLD refractory to rituximab, chemotherapy and antiviral therapy alone. Ann Hematol. 2008; https://doi.org/10.1007/s00277-008-0538-0.

60. van Esser JWJ, Niesters HGM, van der Holt B, Meijer E, Osterhaus ADME, Gratama JW, Verdonck LF, Löwenberg B, Cornelissen JJ. Prevention of Epstein-Barr virus-lymphoproliferative disease by molecular monitoring and preemptive rituximab in high-risk patients after allogeneic stem cell transplantation. Blood. 2002;99:4364–9.

61. Walker RC, Marshall WF, Strickler JG, Wiesner RH, Velosa JA, Habermann TM, McGregor CGA, Paya CV. Pretransplantation assessment of the risk of lymphoproliferative disorder. Clin Infect Dis. 1995;20:1346–53.

Part III

Clinical Considerations in Hematopoietic Stem Cell Transplant (HSCT)

Epidemiology and Prognosis of PTLD After HSCT

12

Vikas R. Dharnidharka and Thomas G. Gross

Introduction

This chapter is devoted to a detailed discussion of (1) the incidence of PTLD after HSCT and over time period eras, (2) the time to PTLD development after HSCT, (3) the different risk factors involved, and (4) prognostic factors and mortality rates after PTLD. The equivalent epidemiologic aspects of PTLD after solid organ transplant (SOT) are discussed in Chap. 7 and prognostic factors in Chap. 9. For purposes of this chapter, HSCT includes all types of bone marrow, peripheral blood stem cell, or umbilical cord blood transplants.

PTLDs after HSCT are classified using the same WHO classification as used by SOT. The latest 2016 classification is provided in Chap. 2 [1]. The main sources of epidemiologic information on PTLD after HSCT are by collaborative registries [2–4] such as the Center for International Blood and Marrow Transplant Research (CIBMTR) or the Japanese national bone marrow transplant registry. In addition, major epidemiologic publications [3, 5–10] have arisen from multicenter data (the Spanish group of blood and bone marrow transplantation GETH) or large single center data (e.g., University of Minnesota in Minneapolis, USA; Fred Hutchinson Cancer Research Center in Seattle, USA; the Karolinska Institute in Stockholm, Sweden; Medical Center Hamburg in Germany; Helsinki University Central Hospital in Finland; or Vancouver General Hospital in Canada). Combined series of recent PTLDs after either SOT or HSCT have been published by Romero et al. [11] and Bishnoi

V. R. Dharnidharka (✉)
Division of Pediatric Nephrology, Hypertension and Pheresis, Washington University School of Medicine, St. Louis, MO, USA
e-mail: vikasd@wustl.edu

T. G. Gross
Department of Pediatrics, University of Colorado School of Medicine, Center for Cancer and Blood Diseases, Children's Hospital Colorado, Aurora, CO, USA
e-mail: THOMAS.GROSS@CUANSCHUTZ.EDU

© Springer Nature Switzerland AG 2021
V. R. Dharnidharka et al. (eds.), *Post-Transplant Lymphoproliferative Disorders*,
https://doi.org/10.1007/978-3-030-65403-0_12

et al. [12], and a major review of both was published by Dierickx and Habermann [13]. Major recent reviews on the topic of PTLD that are limited to after HSCT (not including SOT) have been published by Al Hamed et al. [14] and Ru et al. [15].

Incidence of PTLD

The incidence of PTLD has been reported in the 0.5–17% range of all patients who receive an HSCT [7, 8, 10, 14]. As with any rare disease, the incidence is best expressed as an incidence density or a cumulative incidence by a certain time post-transplant. Thus, Romero et al. [11] found a 2% incidence and Fujimoto et al. [2] found a 0.79% incidence by 2 years post-transplant. Pagliuca et al. [16] found a 6.3% incidence at 2 years if a patient developed EBV DNAemia and received at least one dose rituximab [16]. The incidence appears to have increased in more recent eras. Fujimoto et al. [2] reported an increase to 1.24% at 2 years post-transplant by 2010, and Uhlin et al. [5] reported an increase from <2% before 1998 to >6% after 2011, both groups attributing the increase to greater HLA mismatch and higher intensity of immunosuppression in more recent periods.

Time to PTLD

In HSCT, the complication of PTLD is generally an early event. Landgren et al. calculated the incidence rates at various time periods post-transplant [3]. The highest rates were in the first few months post-transplant, with the rates dropping to very low levels beyond the first year (Fig. 12.1). Cumulative incidence Kaplan-Meier

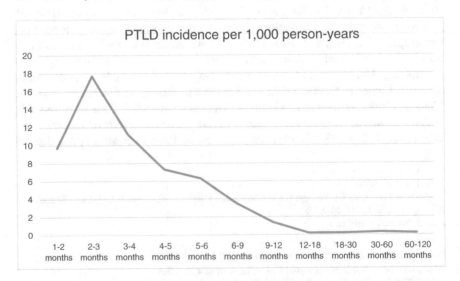

Fig. 12.1 This line chart shows that the risk of PTLD is very high in the first few months post-HSCT and drops to negligible rates after the first year (This figure was created from data published by Landgren et al. [3])

curves or data by the other groups [2, 5, 7, 10, 16] have shown similar trends, with steep upward slopes in the first few months, followed by a flattening of the curve, indicating a very small incidence after the first year. This pattern is in contrast to the incidence after SOT, where both EBV + PTLD and EBV-negative PTLD show steady increases in incidence over time (see Chap. 7). This pattern of PTLD after HSCT is attributed to the fact that most PTLDs after HSCT are EBV + PTLD, >80% in most series [11, 17], and EBV infection is generally an early event after HSCT. In contrast, up to 50% of PTLDs after SOT are EBV negative.

Risk Factors for PTLD

Several studies have reported a variety of risk factors for PTLD after HSCT. Some factors are unique to HSCT, such as acute graft versus host disease (GVHD) or its treatment. Some risk factors seem to be consistent across several studies, such as the use of unrelated or more highly HLA-mismatched donors [3, 5, 16], acute GVHD [2, 5, 18], more intense induction of immunosuppression [8] (especially T-cell-depleting conditioning or as therapy for acute GVHD) [2, 3, 8, 18], EBV seromismatch (where donor is EBV seropositive and recipient is negative) [5], and higher EBV DNA loads post-transplant [18]. Other risk factors such as reduced intensity conditioning, splenectomy, mesenchymal stromal cell infusion [5], or primary disease chronic myeloid leukemia [9] or aplastic anemia [2] have only been reported in specific studies. The different risk factors for PTLD after HSCT show partial overlap with those for PTLD after SOT (Table 12.1). The magnitude of risk has been represented in the different studies as adjusted hazard ratios (aHR) or relative risk (RR) or relative hazard (RH). The different risk factors and the fold higher risk across studies of several types of HSCTs are shown in Table 12.2 and Fig. 12.2.

Table 12.1 Comparison of risk factors for PTLD after either solid organ transplant (SOT) or hematopoietic stem cell transplant (HSCT)

	After SOT	After HSCT
Unique to either SOT or HSCT	Intestinal or thoracic organ transplants	Reduced intensity conditioning
	Sirolimus use de novo	Umbilical cord blood transplant
	Caucasian race	Splenectomy
		Graft versus host disease
		More highly HLA-mismatched donor
		Mesenchymal stromal cell infusion
Common to both SOT and HSCT, consistently reported	High EBV DNAemia	High EBV DNAemia
	Higher overall immunosuppression	Higher overall immunosuppression
	Age <20 or >60 at transplant	Age <20 or >50 at transplant
	EBV seromismatch (D+/R−)	EBV seromismatch (D+/R−)

(continued)

Table 12.1 (continued)

	After SOT	After HSCT
Common to both SOT and HSCT, but inconsistently reported	CMV infection	CMV infection
	Alemtuzumab induction	Alemtuzumab induction
	Anti-thymocyte globulins induction	Anti-thymocyte globulin induction
	Underlying diseases such as cystic fibrosis	Underlying diseases such as aplastic anemia, chronic myeloid leukemia

Table 12.2 The different risk factors reported for PTLD after HSCT and the magnitude of risk (either relative risk RR, hazard ratio HR, or relative hazard RH in multivariable analyses)

Study	Risk factor	Fold higher risk
Micallef et al. 1998	T cell depletion	3.05
	Anti-T cell therapy for GVHD	12.7
	Acute GVHD grades 3–4	7.7
Gross et al. 1999	T cell depletion	5.4
	Immune deficiency	3.8
	Higher donor age (per year)	1.04
Uhlin et al. 1999	EBV D+/R−	4.97
	Reduced intensity conditioning	3.25
	Acute GVHD grades 2–4	2.65
	Splenectomy	4.81
	Mesenchymal stromal cell infusion	3.05
	Higher HLA mismatch	5.89
Landgren et al. 2009	HLA-mismatched or unrelated donor	3.8
	Recipient >50 years age	5.1
	Second HSCT	3.5
	ATG use	3.8
Fujimoto et al. 2019	2010–2015 era (versus prior)	1.87
	Aplastic anemia	5.19
	Non-matched related donor	Vary, depending on type
	2 or more allogeneic HSCT	1.5
	ATG preconditioning	6.13
	ATG treatment for GVHD	2.04
	Acute GVHD	1.93
Pagliuca et al. 2019	Unrelated donor	2.11
	Recipient HLA DRB*11:01 allele	4.85
	Fever at diagnosis of EBV infection	6.12
	Donor-recipient sex mismatch	4.69

ATG anti-thymocyte globulin, *EBV* Epstein-Barr virus, *GVHD* graft versus host disease, *HSCT* hematopoietic stem cell transplant

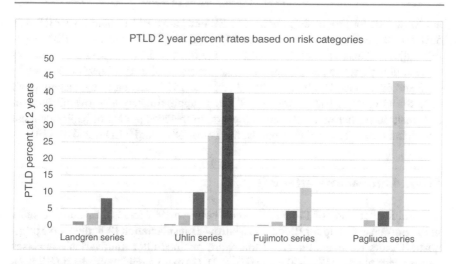

Fig. 12.2 Bar graph of PTLD percent rate after HSCT, based on risk categories from studies by (a) Landgren et al., which list 4 risk categories (0 risk factor, 1 risk factor, 2 or greater than 3); (b) Uhlin et al. [5], which list 1–5 cumulative risk factors; (c) Fujimoto et al. [2], which list 4 risk categories – low risk 0–1 points, intermediate risk 2 points, high risk 3 points, very high risk 4–5 points; (d) Pagliuca et al. [16], which list 3 risk categories – low risk 0–1 risk factors, intermediate risk 2 risk factors, very high risk 3–4 risk factors. See Table 12.2 for further descriptions of the individual risk factors

Only Landgren et al. reported any risk *reducing* factors: alemtuzumab use or elutriation. In addition, Gao et al. [19] studied a specific subgroup, those receiving matched sibling or haplo-identical peripheral blood stem cell transplants. In this group of 200 subjects, the risk factors identified were fludarabine containing conditioning regimens (HR 3.8), CMV DNAemia (HR 11.6), and age <40 years (HR 2.5).

Survival After PTLD

In general, survival when PTLD develops after an HSCT is poor. Curtis et al. [4] and Gross et al. [9], both in 1999, reported an 84% or 92% mortality and the rates have not improved much in more recent eras. Uhlin et al. [5] reported in 2014 a 1-year overall survival (OS) of 28% and 3-year overall survival of 20%, compared to a 3-year OS of 62% if HSCT recipients did not develop PTLD. In the series by Ocheni et al., 9 of 11 patients with PTLD had died within 84 days, the remaining 2 surviving to more than 2000 days [7]. More recently, Romero et al. [11] reported a 1-year OS of 19% and 4-year OS of just 10%. Of their 21 cases, 18 (86%) died, of which 94% of deaths were related to the PTLD itself. This was despite complete remission rates of 50%, stable disease 10%, and progressive disease only 40%. Garcia-Cadenas et al. from the Spanish GETH group reported a 2-year OS of 33% and a PTLD-related mortality of 45% [10]. When comparing 222 EBV + PTLD to 45 EBV-negative PTLDs, Naik et al. [17] reported that EBV positivity of the PTLD did not show a better prognosis compared to EBV-negative PTLD. The 1-year OS was 53% for their entire cohort, stratified as 55% if EBV + PTLD and 44% if EBV negative (adjusted hazard ratio 1.42, $p = 0.097$). Pagliuca et al. [16] reported a 2-year OS of 63% in their entire cohort, but complete remission after PTLD was only seen in 46% and 69% died [16]. In a combined series of 141 PTLD cases by Bishnoi et al. [12], the 11 cases of PTLD after HSCT had an approximately 45% overall survival at 1 year, no further mortality out to 5 years. In matched sibling or haplo-identical peripheral blood stem cell transplants, the 1-year OS after PTLD was 44% [19].

Prognostic Factors After PTLD

In a multicenter study of 144 PTLD events between 1999 and 2011 from 19 centers in the European Group for Blood and Marrow Transplantation [20], the worse prognostic factors for overall survival that were retained after multivariable analyses were (1) age at transplant >30 years (HR 2.2), (2) extranodal involvement (HR 3.2), (3) acute GVHD ≥ grade II at PTLD diagnosis (HR 3.6), and (4) no reduction of immunosuppression at PTLD diagnosis (HR 0.6 if reduction performed). Separately, a decrease of EBV DNAemia improved the PTLD prognosis, whereas an increase of EBV DNAemia after 1 or 2 weeks of therapy was a predictor of poor response [20].

The Spanish GETH group recently published their comprehensive study of prognostic factors. In their multivariable analyses of 102 PTLDs across 14 centers between 2000 and 2015, (a) age >40 years (HR 1.9, $P = 0.02$), (b) malignant underlying disease (HR 2.1, $P = 0.03$), (c) non-response to rituximab (HR 2.1, $P = 0.03$), and (d) severe thrombocytopenia (HR 2.3, $P = 0.004$) or (e) lymphocytopenia (HR 9.7, $P = 0.003$) at PTLD diagnosis were associated with worse overall survival [10].

The most impactful intervention in reducing mortality due to PTLD following HSCT has been the monitoring of patients at risk for EBV DNAemia and preemptive therapy, usually with rituximab or with EBV-CTL. Even in the setting of T cell depletion, this approach not only reduces the incidence of PTLD but has almost eliminated mortality due to PTLD [21]. This approach is now recommended as the standard practice [22].

Take-Home Messages

1. The risk for PTLD after HSCT is highest in the first few months post-transplant, with low risk beyond the first year.
2. The incidence of PTLD varies with several, transplant and immunosuppression-related risk factors; highest risk is seen in EBV-seronegative very young or very old recipients receiving umbilical cord blood or highly HLA-mismatched transplant organs and a high overall level of immunosuppression, especially at induction.
3. Most PTLDs after HSCT are Epstein-Barr virus positive.

4. The mortality after PTLD is very high in HSCT recipients.
5. Monitoring for EBV DNAemia and pre-emptive therapy has had the greatest impact on reducing PTLD mortality after HSCT.

References

1. Swerdlow SH, Campo E, Pileri SA, Harris NL, Stein H, Siebert R, et al. The 2016 revision of the World Health Organization classification of lymphoid neoplasms. Blood. 2016;127(20):2375–90.
2. Fujimoto A, Hiramoto N, Yamasaki S, Inamoto Y, Uchida N, Maeda T, et al. Risk factors and predictive scoring system for post-transplant lymphoproliferative disorder after hematopoietic stem cell transplantation. Biol Blood Marrow Transplant. 2019;25(7):1441–9.
3. Landgren O, Gilbert ES, Rizzo JD, Socie G, Banks PM, Sobocinski KA, et al. Risk factors for lymphoproliferative disorders after allogeneic hematopoietic cell transplantation. Blood. 2009;113(20):4992–5001.
4. Curtis RE, Travis LB, Rowlings PA, Socie G, Kingma DW, Banks PM, et al. Risk of lymphoproliferative disorders after bone marrow transplantation: a multi-institutional study. Blood. 1999;94(7):2208–16.
5. Uhlin M, Wikell H, Sundin M, Blennow O, Maeurer M, Ringden O, et al. Risk factors for Epstein-Barr virus-related post-transplant lymphoproliferative disease after allogeneic hematopoietic stem cell transplantation. Haematologica. 2014;99(2):346–52.
6. Micallef IN, Chhanabhai M, Gascoyne RD, Shepherd JD, Fung HC, Nantel SH, et al. Lymphoproliferative disorders following allogeneic bone marrow transplantation: the Vancouver experience. Bone Marrow Transplant. 1998;22(10):981–7.
7. Ocheni S, Kroeger N, Zabelina T, Sobottka I, Ayuk F, Wolschke C, et al. EBV reactivation and post transplant lymphoproliferative disorders following allogeneic SCT. Bone Marrow Transplant. 2008;42(3):181–6.
8. Juvonen E, Aalto SM, Tarkkanen J, Volin L, Mattila PS, Knuutila S, et al. High incidence of PTLD after non-T-cell-depleted allogeneic haematopoietic stem cell transplantation as a consequence of intensive immunosuppressive treatment. Bone Marrow Transplant. 2003;32(1):97–102.
9. Gross TG, Steinbuch M, DeFor T, Shapiro RS, McGlave P, Ramsay NK, et al. B cell lymphoproliferative disorders following hematopoietic stem cell transplantation: risk factors, treatment and outcome. Bone Marrow Transplant. 1999;23(3):251–8.
10. Garcia-Cadenas I, Yanez L, Jarque I, Martino R, Perez-Simon JA, Valcarcel D, et al. Frequency, characteristics, and outcome of PTLD after allo-SCT: a multicenter study from the Spanish group of blood and marrow transplantation (GETH). Eur J Haematol. 2019;102(6):465–71.
11. Romero S, Montoro J, Guinot M, Almenar L, Andreu R, Balaguer A, et al. Post-transplant lymphoproliferative disorders after solid organ and hematopoietic stem cell transplantation. Leuk Lymphoma. 2019;60(1):142–50.
12. Bishnoi R, Bajwa R, Franke AJ, Skelton WPT, Wang Y, Patel NM, et al. Post-transplant lymphoproliferative disorder (PTLD): single institutional experience of 141 patients. Exp Hematol Oncol. 2017;6:26.
13. Dierickx D, Habermann TM. Post-transplantation lymphoproliferative disorders in adults. N Engl J Med. 2018;378(6):549–62.
14. Al Hamed R, Bazarbachi AH, Mohty M. Epstein-Barr virus-related post-transplant lymphoproliferative disease (EBV-PTLD) in the setting of allogeneic stem cell transplantation: a comprehensive review from pathogenesis to forthcoming treatment modalities. Bone Marrow Transplant. 2020;55(1):25–39.
15. Ru Y, Chen J, Wu D. Epstein-Barr virus post-transplant lymphoproliferative disease (PTLD) after hematopoietic stem cell transplantation. Eur J Haematol. 2018;101(3):283–90.

16. Pagliuca S, Bommier C, Michonneau D, Meignin V, Salmona M, Robin M, et al. Epstein-Barr virus-associated post-transplantation lymphoproliferative disease in patients who received anti-CD20 after hematopoietic stem cell transplantation. Biol Blood Marrow Transplant. 2019;25(12):2490–500.
17. Naik S, Riches M, Hari P, Kim S, Chen M, Bachier C, et al. Survival outcomes of allogeneic hematopoietic cell transplants with EBV-positive or EBV-negative post-transplant lymphoproliferative disorder, A CIBMTR study. Transplant Infect Dis. 2019;21(5):e13145.
18. Wareham NE, Mocroft A, Sengelov H, Da Cunha-Bang C, Gustafsson F, Heilmann C, et al. The value of EBV DNA in early detection of post-transplant lymphoproliferative disorders among solid organ and hematopoietic stem cell transplant recipients. J Cancer Res Clin Oncol. 2018;144(8):1569–80.
19. Gao XN, Lin J, Wang LJ, Li F, Li HH, Wang SH, et al. Risk factors and clinical outcomes of Epstein-Barr virus DNAemia and post-transplant lymphoproliferative disorders after hap-loidentical and matched-sibling PBSCT in patients with hematologic malignancies. Ann Hematol. 2019;98(9):2163–77.
20. Styczynski J, Gil L, Tridello G, Ljungman P, Donnelly JP, van der Velden W, et al. Response to rituximab-based therapy and risk factor analysis in Epstein Barr virus-related lymphoproliferative disorder after hematopoietic stem cell transplant in children and adults: a study from the Infectious Diseases Working Party of the European Group for Blood and Marrow Transplantation. Clin Infect Dis. 2013;57(6):794–802.
21. van Esser JW, Niesters HG, van der Holt B, Meijer E, Osterhaus AD, Gratama JW, et al. Prevention of Epstein-Barr virus-lymphoproliferative disease by molecular monitoring and preemptive rituximab in high-risk patients after allogeneic stem cell transplantation. Blood. 2002;99(12):4364–9.
22. Styczynski J, van der Velden W, Fox CP, Engelhard D, de la Camara R, Cordonnier C, et al. Management of Epstein-Barr Virus infections and post-transplant lymphoproliferative disorders in patients after allogeneic hematopoietic stem cell transplantation: sixth European Conference on Infections in Leukemia (ECIL-6) guidelines. Haematologica. 2016;101(7):803–11.

Clinical Presentations and Features of PTLD After HSCT

13

Britta Maecker-Kolhoff and Daan Dierickx

In contrast to lymphomas in immune-competent patients, presentation of PTLD in general is associated with a higher number of extranodal involvement and central nervous system invasion. In addition allograft localization is a peculiar finding in solid organ transplantation (SOT)-related PTLD, but seems to be observed less frequently in allogeneic hematopoietic stem cell transplantation (HSCT)-related PTLD. In allogeneic HSCT recipients, risk factors for PTLD development mainly include the degree of HLA matching and, hence, the need for T-cell depletion protocols before transplantation. In addition higher recipient age and underlying primary immunodeficiency disorders are also considered risk factors. PTLD following allogeneic HSCT typically is donor lymphocyte-derived, whereas SOT-related PTLD in most cases is recipient-derived [1].

Presentation of patients with PTLD after allogeneic HSCT may be highly variable due to the organs and structures involved [2, 3]. Often cases are preceded by a mainly asymptomatic phase of EBV reactivation or primary infection in peripheral blood. The lack of symptoms in these early stages may be attributable to the depletion of T cells, preventing typical symptoms of fever and enlarged lymph nodes. However, if left untreated, rapid disease progression finally leading to organ involvement may occur, causing a huge variety of organ-specific symptoms. Late onset PTLD has been described in a minority of patients and almost always results from ongoing immune-suppressive therapy for chronic graft versus host disease (GVHD) [2].

B. Maecker-Kolhoff (✉)
Hannover Medical School, Pediatric Hematology and Oncology, Hannover, Germany
e-mail: Maecker.Britta@mh-hannover.de

D. Dierickx
Department of Hematology, University Hospitals Leuven, Leuven, Belgium
e-mail: daan.dierickx@uzleuven.be

© Springer Nature Switzerland AG 2021
V. R. Dharnidharka et al. (eds.), *Post-Transplant Lymphoproliferative Disorders*,
https://doi.org/10.1007/978-3-030-65403-0_13

Based on this concept, there are mainly two forms of clinical presentation: a more classical nodal presentation with frequent involvement of Waldeyer's ring, lymph nodes, liver, and spleen. Patients often present with lymph node, liver, or spleen enlargement or difficulties in swallowing and breathing. Involvement of lung is common and may represent a risk organ, and patients may suffer from gastrointestinal symptoms like abdominal pain, mucocutaneous ulcers, or diarrhea [3–7].

On the other hand patients may present with a fulminant course, resembling primary EBV-mononucleosis infectiosa or even hemophagocytic syndrome with high fevers, cytopenias, and organ dysfunction up to multi-organ failure. The latter is associated with high risk of fatal outcome [8]. Bone marrow examination should be done at least in all patients with blood count abnormalities [9]. A minority of patients (10–15%) presents with involvement of the central nervous system (CNS), which may be suspected in the case of neurological symptoms (headache, seizures, neurologic deficits) [8]. A lumbar puncture and, if symptoms are present, MRI imaging of the brain are advisable in all patients. Recently a new entity, EBV-positive mucocutaneous ulcer, was added to the revised WHO 2016 classification; thus, a thorough inspection of the oral cavity is mandatory in all patients [10].

As symptoms of PTLD are often unspecific, the clinician is challenged by sorting out several differential diagnoses (pathogen-induced sepsis, graft versus host disease, recurrence of the underlying disease, toxic organ failure). A biopsy and histologic evaluation are mandatory whenever deemed possible.

Few studies have compared the clinical presentation of PTLD following allogeneic HSCT and SOT. In a recent retrospective analysis, Romero et al. compared 82 cases of SOT-PTLD with 21 cases of HSCT-PTLD, showing differences in presentation. HSCT-PTLD was associated with a higher incidence of B symptoms and more advanced stage and of specific nodal (Waldeyer's ring), splenic and extranodal (liver and CNS) involvement. In this series 91% of the cases had an early onset presentation [11]. In a large retrospective European Society for Blood and Marrow Transplantation (EBMT) study, extranodal involvement was seen in 42% of the patients [12].

Although most cases of PTLD following allogeneic HSCT are EBV-associated, a recent retrospective analysis of the Center for International Blood and Marrow Transplant Research (CIBMTR) showed 17% of PTLD cases were EBV-negative. Time of occurrence following transplantation, clinical features, and histology were not significantly different between EBV-positive and EBV-negative PTLD. Outcome was poor in both subtypes [13].

In conclusion, clinical presentation of PTLD following allogeneic HSCT may be very variable, often confronting transplant physicians with difficult but important differential diagnoses including several early and life-threatening transplant-related complications. In contrast to SOT-related PTLD, less information is available on clinical presentation, which is probably due to the relative limited number of transplantations (and hence cases) compared to SOT and to the widespread use of pre-emptive administration of rituximab following allogeneic HSCT.

References

1. Dierickx D, Habermann TM. Post-transplantation lymphoproliferative disorders in adults. N Engl J Med. 2018;378(6):549–62.
2. Landgren O, Gilbert ES, Rizzo JD, et al. Risk factors for lymphoproliferative disorders after allogeneic hematopoietic cell transplantation. Blood. 2009;113(20):4992–5001.
3. Rasche L, Kapp M, Einsele H, Mielke S. EBV-induced post transplant lymphoproliferative disorders: a persisting challenge in allogeneic hematopoietic SCT. Bone Marrow Transplant. 2014;49(2):163–7.
4. Sanz J, Andreu R. Epstein-Barr virus-associated posttransplant lymphoproliferative disorder after allogeneic stem cell transplantation. Curr Opin Oncol. 2014;26(6):677–83.
5. Chen DB, Song QJ, Chen YX, Chen YH, Shen DH. Clinicopathologic spectrum and EBV status of post-transplant lymphoproliferative disorders after allogeneic hematopoietic stem cell transplantation. Int J Hematol. 2013;97(1):117–24.
6. Hou HA, Yao M, Tang JL, et al. Poor outcome in post transplant lymphoproliferative disorder with pulmonary involvement after allogeneic hematopoietic SCT: 13 years' experience in a single institute. Bone Marrow Transplant. 2009;43(4):315–21.
7. Deeg HJ, Socie G. Malignancies after hematopoietic stem cell transplantation: many questions, some answers. Blood. 1998;91(6):1833–44.
8. Sanz J, Arango M, Senent L, et al. EBV-associated post-transplant lymphoproliferative disorder after umbilical cord blood transplantation in adults with hematological diseases. Bone Marrow Transplant. 2014;49(3):397–402.
9. Llaurador G, McLaughlin L, Wistinghausen B. Management of post-transplant lymphoproliferative disorders. Curr Opin Pediatr. 2017;29(1):34–40.
10. Swerdlow SH, Webber SA, Chadburn A, Ferry JA. Post-transplant lymphoproliferative disorders. In: Swerdlow SH, Campo E, Harris NL, et al., editors. WHO classification of tumours of haematopoietic and lymphoid tissues. 4th ed. Lyon: IARC Press; 2017. p. 453–62.
11. Romero S, Montoro J, Guinot M, et al. Post-transplant lymphoproliferative disorders after solid organ and hematopoietic stem cell transplantation. Leuk Lymphoma. 2019;60(1):142–50.
12. Styczynski J, Gil L, Tridello G, et al. Response to rituximab-based therapy and risk factor analysis in Epstein Barr Virus-related lymphoproliferative disorder after hematopoietic stem transplant in children and adults: a study from the Infectious Diseases Working Party of the European Group for Blood and Marrow Transplantation. Clin Infect Dis. 2013;57(6):794–802.
13. Naik S, Riches M, Hari P, et al. Survival outcomes of allogeneic hematopoietic cell transplants with EBV-positive or EBV-negative post-transplant lymphoproliferative disorder, a CIBMTR study. Transpl Infect Dis. 2019;21(5):e13145.

Management of PTLD After HSCT

14

Patrizia Comoli and Jan Styczynski

Introduction

Post-transplant lymphoproliferative disorders (PTLDs) constitute a heterogeneous group of lymphoproliferative diseases and result from the uncontrolled neoplastic proliferation of lymphoid or plasmacytic cells in the context of extrinsic immuno-suppression after transplantation [1, 2]. PTLDs in the HSCT setting are mainly of donor origin; more often develop between 3 and 6 months post-transplant, when virus-specific T-cell immunity has not yet reconstituted; and are almost exclusively EBV-related, although rare cases of non-EBV-associated PTLD also exist in this setting.

Diagnosis of PTLD

The diagnosis of EBV-associated PTLD is based on symptoms and/or signs consistent with PTLD, together with detection of EBV by an appropriate method applied to a specimen from the involved tissue [1, 3]. Diagnosis of EBV-associated PTLD requires non-invasive and invasive techniques. Non-invasive diagnostic methods include the quantitative determination of EBV-DNAemia and computed tomography (CT) or positron emission tomography CT (PET-CT). Invasive methods include

P. Comoli (✉)
Pediatric Hematology/Oncology and Cell Factory, IRCCS Fondazione Policlinico San Matteo, Pavia, Italy
e-mail: pcomoli@smatteo.pv.it

J. Styczynski
Department of Pediatric Hematology and Oncology, Collegium Medicum, Nicolaus Copernicus University Torun, Jurasz University Hospital, Bydgoszcz, Poland
e-mail: jstyczynski@cm.umk.pl

© Springer Nature Switzerland AG 2021
V. R. Dharnidharka et al. (eds.), *Post-Transplant Lymphoproliferative Disorders*,
https://doi.org/10.1007/978-3-030-65403-0_14

biopsy of lymph nodes and/or other sites suspected for EBV disease. Definitive diagnosis of EBV-associated PTLD requires biopsy and histological examination, including immunohistochemistry or flow cytometry for B-cell, T-cell, and plasma cell lineage-specific antigens. EBV detection requires detection of viral antigens or in situ hybridization for the EBER transcripts. Histological WHO 2016 classification includes six types of morphological PTLD: plasmacytic hyperplasia, infectious mononucleosis-like, florid follicular hyperplasia, polymorphic, monomorphic (B-cell or T-/NK-cell types), and classical Hodgkin lymphoma PTLD [4].

In contrast to PTLD following SOT, EBV-associated PTLD following HSCT can be diagnosed at the probable or proven level [5]. Probable EBV disease is defined as the presence of symptoms and/or signs of lymphoproliferative disease in the absence of tissue biopsy, but without other documented cause, together with significant EBV DNAemia. Diagnosis of proven EBV-associated PTLD requires detection of EBV nucleic acids or EBV-encoded proteins in a tissue specimen [5].

Treatment of PTLD After HSCT

Since PTLDs developing after HSCT are mainly EBV-positive B-cell lymphoproliferations occurring in a heavily immunosuppressed setting, therapeutic options include strategies aimed at either targeting B cells, such as anti-CD20 monoclonal antibody rituximab and chemotherapy, or enhancing EBV-specific cytotoxic T-lymphocyte (CTL) response, through reduction of immunosuppression (RIS) and/or cellular therapy [6–14].

Therapeutic Agents

Rituximab

Rituximab is the treatment of choice for post-HSCT EBV-associated PTLD, with positive outcome observed in 50–80% of patients, according to the different clinical settings (reviewed by [1, 3, 7]). Rituximab is most often administered for up to 4 weekly doses, together with simultaneous monitoring of EBV viral load. More prolonged treatment was also used successfully [15, 16]. The European Ped-PTLD-2005 study for pediatric SOT recipients with PTLD observed a 64% complete or partial response to three doses of rituximab as single agent and showed how 84% remained in remission after three additional doses [17]. However, it should be noted that additional doses of rituximab might lead to down-regulation of CD20 expression and thereby possibly decreasing its efficacy [18, 19]. Rituximab was shown to be effective also when administered intrathecally in CNS involvement [20].

Rituximab treatment is associated with limited toxicity; however, resistance can be induced by down-regulation of CD20 on lymphoma cells [18, 21]. Although rituximab is considered to be a relatively safe drug for the majority of patients, its use, alone or in combination with chemotherapy, may bring a number of toxicities, including allergy, late-onset neutropenia [22], hypogammaglobulinemia leading to an increased risk for infections [23], decreased effectiveness of post-transplant vaccinations, and progressive multifocal leukoencephalopathy [24]. Although allergy to rituximab is the only absolute contraindication for the use of this agent, still it should not be confused with infusion-related reactions. Early post-transplant use of rituximab in association with chemotherapy is often accompanied by prolonged neutropenia with the risk of graft failure or graft loss necessitating a stem cell boost. There are no clear data on the role of growth factors in preventing neutropenia: the use of hematopoietic growth factors might be considered, according to the current European Organisation for Research and Treatment of Cancer (EORTC) guidelines [25]. Rituximab causes significant hypogammaglobulinemia and increases the incidence of bacterial infections [23]. Therefore, close monitoring of Ig levels in order to help in decision making on immunoglobulin replacement therapy, or other strategies to limit infectious-related mortality, should be implemented following its use.

Reduction of Immunosuppression (RIS)

In many cases, RIS is the first intervention performed in patients diagnosed with PTLD, in an attempt to restore tumor-specific immune responses. RIS is usually defined as a sustained decrease of at least 20% of the daily dose of immunosuppressive drugs with the exception of low-dose corticosteroid therapy [15]. Generally, EBV-positive PTLDs respond much better to RIS than EBV-negative PTLDs [14].

RIS remains the gold standard for first-line PTLD therapy after SOT [26], while it is rarely successful as the sole intervention in PTLD following HSCT [27]. In the latter setting, the major defect consists in a delayed recovery of EBV-specific cellular immune surveillance, and the time delay required for RIS to induce immune reconstitution does not allow to counteract malignant cell outgrowth. Recent data show that RIS, when feasible and applied in combination with rituximab, significantly improves the outcome of PTLD after HSCT [15]. In detail, RIS was associated with a lower PTLD mortality (16% vs. 39%) and a decrease of EBV DNAemia in peripheral blood during therapy, being predictive of better survival.

The use of RIS might be an obvious factor for an increased risk of rejection or GVHD [28, 29]. An amenable alternative to RIS is the switch from conventional IS to regimens including immunosuppressive agents with antitumor activity, such as inhibitors of the mTOR pathway, that is central to B-cell proliferation in PTLD [30]. In SOT recipients with PTLD, replacement of calcineurin inhibitors with the mTOR inhibitor sirolimus has been associated with good outcome [31], but data are conflicting and the effect probably is small, if any [32]. There is so far no evidence that the SOT experience may be extrapolated to the HSCT setting.

Cellular Therapy

The simplest form of cellular therapy for PTLD occurring after HSCT, when the stem cell donor is EBV-seropositive, is administration of unmanipulated donor lymphocyte infusions (DLI). This strategy has proven curative in a good proportion of patients, but has been associated with the development of clinically relevant GVHD, mediated by the alloreactive T lymphocytes present in the cell product [33]. An elegant strategy to reduce the risk of inducing GVHD consists of manipulating DLI to introduce a suicide gene, to induce susceptibility to drug-mediated lysis in case of development of alloreactive response [34, 35].

An alternative to overcome the problem of alloreactivity is adoptive cell therapy with EBV-specific CTLs, reactivated from the peripheral blood of HSCT donors and infused as EBV-associated PTLD prophylaxis or treatment in recipients of T-cell-depleted, HLA-disparate, unrelated or haploidentical HSCT [21, 36–38]. CTLs proved safe and effective in the prevention of PTLD and in patients with aggressive disease induced stable complete remissions. Literature data, reviewed in [39], indicate an overall response rate of 80% in established PTLD, with 1% GVHD. In the case of an EBV-negative donor, or when the donor is not easily available, third-party, HLA partially matched EBV-CTLs may be employed. These cells, which have the advantage of being banked and, thus, readily available, showed a complete response rate of 42% at 6 months in patients who failed conventional treatment and were treated in a phase II multicenter clinical trial [40]. The response correlated with closer HLA matching between recipient and cell donor [40]. These results have been recently confirmed by two phase II trials with third-party EBV-CTLs in EBV-associated PTLDs refractory to rituximab, which demonstrated a rate of 60% long-lasting remissions [41]. Among the possible caveats of third-party CTL treatment was the theoretical risk of inducing acute GVHD, but only 1 of 33 HSCT recipients developed grade I acute skin GVHD, compared to a GVHD rate of 17% observed after DLI [42].

Chemotherapy

Chemotherapy has traditionally been reserved for the refractory and/or relapsing PTLD cases [13, 28]. Chemotherapy for PTLDs after HSCT is not recommended and should not be used as first-line therapy, due to its poor tolerability in patients who have already received intensive chemotherapy and because of the risk of inducing neutropenia and graft failure [43].

The current approach in solid organ transplantation is to limit the use of chemotherapy only to those patients who fail rituximab [17, 44], or to combine chemotherapy with the application of rituximab [44–46]. The experience with the use of chemotherapy for PTLD after HSCT is limited to anecdotal cases unresponsive to anti-CD20 monoclonal antibody or cellular therapy.

Chemotherapy regimens similar to those used in the SOT setting can be considered for initial use in monomorphic PTLD occurring late in the post-transplant course. CHOP, originally designed for the treatment of non-Hodgkin lymphoma, is the most commonly used chemotherapeutic regimen after SOT and is administered at 3-week intervals, usually combined with rituximab (R-CHOP) [47].

Antiviral Therapy

Currently, a relatively wide range of antiviral drugs is available. Although ganciclovir, foscarnet, and cidofovir show some in vitro activity against replicating EBV [48], treatment of established EBV-associated PTLD has been unsuccessful [49], since these agents, except foscarnet, require thymidine kinase for activation, and latently infected B cells do not express the EBV-specific enzyme. Taking advantage of antiviral compound efficacy against cells in the lytic phase of viral infection, studies have focused on the possibility to induce the lytic cycle in PTLD cells. A phase I/II trial of histone deacetylase inhibitor arginine butyrate in combination with ganciclovir demonstrated overall response rates in 10 of 15 patients with EBV+ lymphoid malignancies, including patients with PTLD [50]. Unfortunately this agent is no longer available for clinical use.

A new antiviral agent, maribavir, has shown in vitro activity against EBV [51, 52]. However this drug failed clinical trial for CMV prophylaxis and is not currently available [53]. Another new unlicensed antiviral agent, brincidofovir, has excellent antiviral activity against EBV in vitro [54], but there are no clinical studies in patients with EBV-DNAemia/PTLD, and, as for maribavir, the drug is currently unavailable.

Other Therapies

There are no data to support the use of intravenous immunoglobulins (IVIG), or immunomodulatory agents, such as interferons or anti-interleukin 6 monoclonal antibodies, in the treatment of EBV-DNAemia or PTLD after HSCT. Interferons have been employed in the past in SOT recipients, mostly in combination with RIS and/or antiviral therapy, and the relatively low anti-tumor activity observed was coupled with toxicity, including allograft rejection.

Since PTLD is mostly a disseminated lymphoproliferative disease, surgical therapy and radiotherapy are of limited benefit after SOT, and they are not usually employed in HSCT patients, unless required to manage local complications, such as vital organ compression by the tumor [1, 13].

Novel Therapeutic Agents

Future therapeutics for PTLD include new monoclonal antibodies, small molecules, and cellular therapies. The rarity of the disease is a major obstacle in testing these strategies within clinical trials.

New anti-CD20 monoclonal antibodies, such as ofatumumab and obinutuzumab, that showed enhanced ADCC activity and higher ability to evoke apoptosis are being tested in the treatment of rituximab-refractory B-cell lymphomas, in combination with other agents, with good results [55].

Other new possibilities, being already successfully used in clinical practice in resistant cases, include (i) the immunomodulatory agent lenalidomide [56, 57], that, in addition to being used in monotherapy, has been shown to increase ADCC activity of rituximab when used in combination; (ii) the anti-PD1 checkpoint inhibitor nivolumab [58], preferred to anti-CTLA-4 blockers for the lower risk of rejection; (iii) the proteasome inhibitor bortezomib [59]; (iv) the CD19 chimeric antigen receptor-modified T cells (CD19-CAR-T cells); and v) the anti-CD30 monoclonal antibody brentuximab vedotin [60]. The rationale for the use of brentuximab vedotin is based on high expression of CD30 on EBV-infected B cells, reaching 85% of cases in EBV-associated PTLD [55, 61, 62]. The use of this compound gives significantly low risk of neutropenia and graft failure or graft loss. CD30 targeting might also eventually be beneficial on theoretical grounds for patients with GVHD [63]. All these products are not yet approved in PTLD.

Currently ongoing clinical trials for PTLD treatment aiming at elucidating treatment regimens for patients after HSCT include also combination therapy with mTOR inhibitor everolimus, histone deacetylase inhibitor panobinostat, and valganciclovir used with phenylbutyrate (reviewed in [7, 55]).

First- and Second-Line Therapy for PTLD After HSCT

In the setting of HSCT, in the case of both proven and probable EBV-associated PTLD, therapy should be started as soon as practicable, due to the risk of a rapidly growing high-grade lymphoid tumor, together with the risk of EBV causing the development of multi-organ impairment.

First-Line Therapy Rituximab monotherapy is the treatment of choice for EBV-associated PTLD (Table 14.1). RIS should be combined with rituximab administration, when feasible, as results with the combined approach are more favorable [15].

Second-Line Therapy In the setting of rituximab failure, second-line therapy options include cellular therapy (DLI or CTLs) or chemotherapy ± rituximab. Unselected DLI from an EBV-positive donor are employed to restore broad T-cell reactivity, including EBV-specific responses; however, unselected DLI can be associated with severe GVHD [33], and thus, previous GVHD is usually a contraindication to DLI. ECIL's (European Conference on Infections in Leukemia) preferred approach is specific cellular therapy. As donor EBV-specific CTLs are not readily available for all centers, third-party banked CTLs could be a more feasible option.

Table 14.1 Recommended first- and second-line therapy for PTLD after HSCT

Type of recommendation for clinical use	Therapy
First-line therapy	1. Anti-CD20 monoclonal antibodies: rituximab 2. Reduction of immunosuppression
Second-line therapy	1. EBV-CTL 2. DLI (donor lymphocyte infusions) 3. Chemotherapy
Not recommended	1. Antivirals 2. IVIG 3. Interferon 4. Surgery
Experimental	1. Anti-CD30 monoclonal antibodies 2. Anti-PD1 antibodies 3. Lenalidomide 4. Bortezomib 5. Everolimus 6. Panobinostat 7. CD19-CAR-T cells

Data on the efficacy of second-line treatments in the HSCT setting are limited. A number of novel agents, potentially effective and with better toxicity profile than chemotherapy, are being evaluated in prospective clinical trials (Table 14.1).

Response to Therapy

The treatment goal is resolution of all signs and symptoms of PTLD, including a negative viral load. Response to rituximab therapy can be identified by a decrease in EBV DNAemia of at least 1 $\log_{10}$ in the first week of treatment. Peripheral blood viral load monitoring after PTLD treatment, particularly when anti-CD20 monoclonal antibodies have been employed, has limitations, as EBV-DNAemia may decrease and remain low even in the presence of disease progression [65]. The use of plasma as a monitoring compartment seems to have a better correlation with response [66].

Younger age is a favorable factor predicting outcome to rituximab-based therapy. Two prognostic models for outcome of PTLD after HSCT are available (Table 14.2). In one study favorable prognostic factors for outcome to rituximab therapy included age below 30 years, underlying non-malignant disease, no acute GVHD, RIS at EBV-associated PTLD diagnosis, and decrease of EBV DNAemia after initial therapy [15]. In the study of Garcia-Cadenas et al. [64], positive factors involved: age <40 years, non-malignant underlying disease, response to rituximab, and lack of severe thrombocytopenia or lymphocytopenia.

The response to therapy can be confirmed by achievement of a PET-negative complete remission for avid lymphomas and CT/MRI for non-avid histologies or CNS localization [67, 68]. Partial response requires a decrease by more than 50% in the sum of the product of the perpendicular diameters (PPDs) of up to six representative nodes or extranodal lesions. Progressive disease is diagnosed with an increase in the PPDs of a single node by $\geq$50% [67].

Current Results and Outcome
Pooled results from published studies in HSCT recipients reveal that administration of rituximab results in a positive outcome for over 90% of patients treated preemptively and over 65% when it is used as targeted therapy for EBV-associated PTLD

Table 14.2 Prognostic models for outcome of EBV-associated PTLD

References	Population	Prognostic model: poor predictive factors
Styczynski et al. [15]	144 PTLD (54 children and 90 adults); international	Age $\geq$30 years Involvement of extralymphoid tissue Acute GVHD Lack of reduction of immunosuppression upon PTLD diagnosis
Garcia-Cadenas et al. [64]	102 PTLD (children and adults); national	Age $\geq$40 years Malignant underlying disease Non-response to rituximab Severe thrombocytopenia or lymphocytopenia

Table 14.3 Results of anti-EBV-associated PTLD therapy

Treatment strategy	Therapy of PTLD	References
Rituximab	65%	[15, 43, 79–86]
Rituximab + RIS	78%	[15, 16, 93–95]
EBV-CTL	71–75%	[21, 38, 40–43, 87–90]
RIS	61%	[16, 96–99]
DLI	58%[a]	[15, 16, 42, 43, 91, 92]
Chemotherapy (±rituximab)	26–35%[a]	[15, 16, 43, 81, 82]
Antivirals (cidofovir)	34%[a]	[42]

[a]Usually used with other therapies (in second-line therapy)

RIS reduction of immunosuppression, *DLI* donor lymphocyte infusions, *CTL* cytotoxic T lymphocyte

(Table 14.3) [15, 43, 69–86]. Recent data demonstrate that RIS, when applied in combination with rituximab, appears to improve the outcome to 80% success rate [15]. The use of EBV-CTLs gives a positive outcome for >90% of patients treated preemptively and for approximately 75% of subjects receiving therapy for established disease [21, 38, 40–43, 87–90].

There are no studies directly comparing the efficacy of rituximab ± RIS vs. EBV-CTL in either prophylaxis, preemptive, or targeted therapy. Thus, there is insufficient evidence to support a recommendation for one treatment modality over another as a first-line approach for centers with access to both therapies.

Worse results were obtained in the treatment of EBV-associated PTLD with other agents, which are nowadays not recommended and should be regarded as historical (Table 14.1). The use of DLI gave improvement in 57% of patients with PTLD; however, patients' numbers were low [15, 16, 42, 43, 91, 92]. Chemotherapy applied usually as a second-line therapy, together with other treatment modalities, was successful in less than 35% of the patients [15, 16, 43, 81, 82]. Antivirals, mainly cidofovir, often used in combination with other treatment modalities, also had a success rate lower than 35% [43].

Outcome of Treatment: Children Versus Adults

Younger age has a positive prognostic value for outcome after rituximab-based therapy. In the IDWP-EBMT study, risk factor analysis for outcome of PTLD therapy with rituximab was performed in 55 children (<18 years) and 89 adults after HSCT: response to therapy was 78% in pediatric patients vs. 64% in adults, with children showing a twofold lower hazard ratio of mortality from PTLD than adults ($p = 0.04$) [15, 100]. Multivariate analysis identified variables predictive for good outcome in children and in adults. In children early response after 1 week of therapy and RIS at PTLD diagnosis were associated with a good prognosis, while involvement of extra-lymphoid tissue, initial plasma EBV-DNAemia >10^5 copies/mL, and increase of EBV-DNAemia during therapy by 1 log were predictors of poor outcome. In adults, good prognosis factors were the same observed for children, while age >30 years, initial plasma EBV-DNAemia >10^4 copies/mL, and increase of EBV-DNAemia during therapy by 1 log predicted poor outcome [15, 100].

Refractory and Relapsed PTLD

Refractory PTLD is diagnosed when no complete or partial response is observed after 4 weeks of therapy, or no complete remission is observed after 8 weeks of therapy.

Refractory and recurrent PTLD following first-line treatment in HSCT recipients represents a particularly difficult therapeutic challenge. Therapeutic choice should be based on a number of factors including PTLD histology and the type of PTLD treatment previously received. Patients with a history of previous treatment of EBV-associated PTLD, and undergoing a second transplant, should possibly receive prophylactic rituximab after stem cell infusion.

Treatment of Central Nervous System (CNS) Disease

Central nervous system localization of PTLD is a special form of the disease, due to the risk of neurological consequences even in the case of successful eradication of EBV from the CNS. No standard therapy has been accepted up to date. Although no clear recommendations exist for therapy of CNS disease, possible therapeutic options include (a) rituximab, either systemic [15, 94] or intrathecal [20]; in the latter case, dose of rituximab was 10–30 mg in 3–10 mL saline administered weekly [20]; (b) T-cell therapy with EBV-CTLs [37, 101]; (c) radiotherapy [102]; and (d) chemotherapy ± rituximab according to primary CNS lymphoma protocols based on high dose of methotrexate ± cytarabine [103, 104], CHOP protocol [102], or hydroxyurea [105].

Treatment of Atypical Forms of PTLD

EBV-Negative PTLD

More than 90% of B-cell PTLD after HSCT are associated with EBV. However, a growing number of EBV-negative B-cell PTLD cases have been reported, presenting late (>5 years) after transplant. Several observations point toward the fact that EBV-positive PTLDs are different from EBV-negative PTLDs. In EBV-positive cases immune responses play an important role, and genomic aberrations are less complex in comparison with EBV-negative PTLDs [14, 106].

EBV-negative PTLD following HSCT is biologically similar to EBV-negative lymphoma occurring in the general population; however, the different immune status of the host should be taken into account in the treatment plan. Biological and clinical differences between EBV-positive and EBV-negative PTLDs suggest that these are different entities that should be analyzed and treated separately. Currently, the prognostic impact of EBV is not clear, but several data point toward a positive prognostic significance of the presence of EBV on the outcome of lymphoma patients [14]. According to ECIL-6, these cases should be regarded as malignant lymphoma rather than PTLD [1]. Consequently, in the post-HSCT setting, EBV-negative PTLDs developing at more than 5 years from the cessation of immunosuppressive therapy should be treated using protocols for malignant lymphoma [1].

Treatment of T-/NK-PTLD

T- and NK-PTLDs are extremely rare after HSCT. So far, only 10 cases of T-PTLD after HSCT were described in the literature, almost exclusively EBV-negative [107–113]. In comparison to B-cell PTLD, T-PTLDs present usually later following transplant. Prolonged immunosuppression is the most important risk factors for T-PTLD development [114, 115]. For the majority of B-cell PTLD, a putative role of EBV has been known, whereas no direct role for EBV has been confirmed in T-PTLD. Mature T lymphocytes do not express the EBV receptor CD21; however, some T-PTLDs might display aberrant expression of CD21 and EBV [116]. Late cases should be regarded as malignant lymphoma rather than as PTLD [1], have a poor outcome, and should therefore be treated using protocols for malignant lymphoma. Genetic and molecular studies should confirm the differences.

Some T-/NK-cell PTLDs occur shortly after transplantation, and of those, almost 40% are EBV+ and have a better prognosis than their EBV-negative counterpart [117]. EBV-positive cases may benefit from donor or third-party EBV-CTL treatment, in association, when feasible, with RIS [101]. Composite B-cell and T-cell lineage PTLDs, harboring both B- and T-cell clones either concurrently or successively in the same patient, are extremely rare and only a few cases have been reported in the literature, exclusively after SOT, with poor outcome.

Conclusions

PTLD is one of the most severe complications associated with transplantation. The last 15 years dramatically changed the clinical picture of EBV-associated PTLD after HSCT and caused a shift from deadly disease to considerable improvement, with a positive outcome currently reached in about 70% of cases.

This progress was made possible by the introduction of new key diagnostic and therapeutic approaches in PTLD, including the use of quantitative monitoring for EBV-DNAemia by PCR, preemptive therapy, and timely treatment with rituximab. Novel therapeutic strategies that are being tested in clinical trials will likely further improve results, hopefully contributing to ameliorate outcome for those PTLD entities that are still burdened by poor prognosis.

References

1. Styczynski J, van der Velden W, Fox CP, Engelhard D, de la Camara R, Cordonnier C, Ljungman P. Management of Epstein-Barr virus infections and post-transplant lymphoproliferative disorders in patients after allogeneic hematopoietic stem cell transplantation:

Sixth European Conference on Infections in Leukemia (ECIL-6) guidelines. Haematologica. 2016;101:803–11.
2. Dharnidharka VR, Webster AC, Martinez OM, Preiksaitis JK, Leblond V, Choquet S. Post-transplant lymphoproliferative disorders. Nat Rev Dis Primers. 2016;2:15088.
3. Styczynski J. Managing post-transplant lymphoproliferative disorder. Expert Opin Orphan Drugs. 2017;5:19–35.
4. Swerdlow SH, Campo E, Pileri SA, Harris NL, Stein H, Siebert R, et al. The 2016 revision of the World Health Organization classification of lymphoid neoplasms. Blood. 2016;127:2375–90.
5. Styczynski J, Reusser P, Einsele H, de la Camara R, Cordonnier C, Ward KN, et al. Management of HSV, VZV and EBV infections in patients with hematological malignancies and after SCT: guidelines from the Second European Conference on Infections in Leukemia. Bone Marrow Transplant. 2009;43:757–70.
6. Dierickx D, Habermann TM. Post-transplantation lymphoproliferative disorders in adults. N Engl J Med. 2018;378:549–62.
7. Al Hamed R, Bazarbachi AH, Mohty M. Epstein-Barr virus-related post-transplant lymphoproliferative disease (EBV-associated PTLD) in the setting of allogeneic stem cell transplantation: a comprehensive review from pathogenesis to forthcoming treatment modalities. Bone Marrow Transplant. 2019;55(1):25–39. https://doi.org/10.1038/s41409-019-0548-7.
8. Locatelli F, Merli P, Pagliara D, et al. Outcome of children with acute leukemia given HLA-haploidentical HSCT after αβ T-cell and B-cell depletion. Blood. 2017;130:677–85.
9. Sundin M, Le Blanc K, Ringden O, Barkholt L, Omazic B, Lergin C, et al. The role of HLA mismatch, splenectomy and recipient Epstein-Barr virus seronegativity as risk factors in post-transplant lymphoproliferative disorder following allogeneic hematopoietic stem cell transplantation. Haematologica. 2006;91:1059–67.
10. Uhlin M, Wikell H, Sundin M, Blennow O, Maeurer M, Ringden O, et al. Risk factors for Epstein-Barr virus-related post-transplant lymphoproliferative disease after allogeneic hematopoietic stem cell transplantation. Haematologica. 2014;99:346–52.
11. Loren AW, Porter DL, Stadtmauer EA, Tsai DE. Post-transplant lymphoproliferative disorder: a review. Bone Marrow Transplant. 2003;31:145–55.
12. Comoli P, Rooney CM. Treatment of Epstein-Barr virus infections. In: Jenson HB, Tselis A, editors. Epstein-Barr virus (EBV). New York: Taylor & Francis Publishers; 2006. p. 351–72.
13. Heslop HE. How I treat EBV lymphoproliferation. Blood. 2009;114:4002–8.
14. Morscio J, Tousseyn T. The role of the Epstein-Barr virus in the pathogenesis of post-transplant lymphoproliferative disorders. In: Styczynski J, editor. Epstein-Barr virus (EBV): transmission, diagnosis and role in the development of cancers. New York: Nova Science Publishers; 2014. p. 73–152.
15. Styczynski J, Gil L, Tridello G, Ljungman P, Donnelly JP, van der Velden W, et al. Response to rituximab-based therapy and risk factor analysis in Epstein Barr Virus-related lymphoproliferative disorder after hematopoietic stem cell transplant in children and adults: a study from the Infectious Diseases Working Party of the European Group for Blood and Marrow Transplantation. Clin Infect Dis. 2013;57:794–802.
16. Fox CP, Burns D, Parker AN, Peggs KS, Harvey CM, Natarajan S, et al. EBV-associated post-transplant lymphoproliferative disorder following in vivo T-cell-depleted allogeneic transplantation: clinical features, viral load correlates and prognostic factors in the rituximab era. Bone Marrow Transplant. 2014;49:280–6.
17. Maecker-Kolhoff B, Zimmermann M, Schlegelberger B, et al. Response-adapted sequential immune-chemotherapy of post-transplant lymphoproliferative disorders in pediatric solid organ transplant recipients: results from the prospective Ped-PTLD 2005 trial. Blood. 2014;124:4468.
18. Hiraga J, Tomita A, Sugimoto T, Shimada K, Ito M, Nakamura S, et al. Down-regulation of CD20 expression in B-cell lymphoma cells after treatment with rituximab-containing combination chemotherapies: its prevalence and clinical significance. Blood. 2009;113:4885–93.

19. Stolz C, Schuler M. Molecular mechanisms of resistance to rituximab and pharmacologic strategies for its circumvention. Leuk Lymphoma. 2009;50:873–85.
20. Czyzewski K, Styczynski J, Krenska A, Debski R, Zajac-Spychala O, Wachowiak J, et al. Intrathecal therapy with rituximab in central nervous system involvement of post-transplant lymphoproliferative disorder. Leuk Lymphoma. 2013;54:503–6.
21. Comoli P, Basso S, Zecca M, Pagliara D, Baldanti F, Bernardo ME, et al. Preemptive therapy of EBV-related lymphoproliferative disease after pediatric haploidentical stem cell transplantation. Am J Transplant. 2007;7:1648–55.
22. Lemieux B, Tartas S, Traulle C, Espinouse D, Thieblemont C, Bouafia F, et al. Rituximab-related late-onset neutropenia after autologous stem cell transplantation for aggressive non-Hodgkin's lymphoma. Bone Marrow Transplant. 2004;33:921–3.
23. Petropoulou AD, Porcher R, de Latour RP, Xhaard A, Weisdorf D, Ribaud P, et al. Increased infection rate after preemptive rituximab treatment for Epstein-Barr virus reactivation after allogeneic hematopoietic stem-cell transplantation. Transplantation. 2012;94:879–83.
24. Carson KR, Evens AM, Richey EA, Habermann TM, Focosi D, Seymour JF, et al. Progressive multifocal leukoencephalopathy after rituximab therapy in HIV-negative patients: a report of 57 cases from the Research on Adverse Drug Events and Reports project. Blood. 2009;113:4834–40.
25. Aapro MS, Bohlius J, Cameron DA, Dal Lago L, Donnelly JP, Kearney N, et al. 2010 update of EORTC guidelines for the use of granulocyte-colony stimulating factor to reduce the incidence of chemotherapy-induced febrile neutropenia in adult patients with lymphoproliferative disorders and solid tumours. Eur J Cancer. 2011;47:8–32.
26. Paya CV, Fung JJ, Nalesnik MA, Kieff E, Green M, Gores G, et al. Epstein-Barr virus-induced posttransplant lymphoproliferative disorders. ASTS/ASTP EBV-associated PTLD Task Force and The Mayo Clinic Organized International Consensus Development Meeting. Transplantation. 1999;68:1517–25.
27. Cesaro S, Pegoraro A, Tridello G, Calore E, Pillon M, Varotto S, et al. A prospective study on modulation of immunosuppression for Epstein-Barr virus reactivation in pediatric patients who underwent unrelated hematopoietic stem-cell transplantation. Transplantation. 2010;89:1533–40.
28. Gross TG. Treatment for Epstein-Barr virus-associated PTLD. Herpes. 2009;15:64–7.
29. Bishnoi R, Bajwa R, Franke AJ, Skelton WP 4th, Wang Y, Patel NM, et al. Post-transplant lymphoproliferative disorder (PTLD): single institutional experience of 141 patients. Exp Hematol Oncol. 2017;6:26.
30. El-Salem M, Raghunath PN, Marzec M, Wlodarski P, Tsai D, Hsi E, Wasik MA. Constitutive activation of mTOR signaling pathway in post-transplant lymphoproliferative disorders. Lab Investig. 2007;87:29–39.
31. Gibelli NE, Tannuri U, Pinho-Apezzato ML, Tannuri AC, Maksoud-Filho JG, Andrade WC, et al. Sirolimus in pediatric liver transplantation: a single-center experience. Transplant Proc. 2009;41:901–3.
32. Zimmermann H, Babel N, Dierickx D, Morschhauser F, Mollee P, Zaucha JM, et al. Immunosuppression is associated with clinical features and relapse risk of B cell posttransplant lymphoproliferative disorder: a retrospective analysis based on the prospective, international, multicenter PTLD-1 Trials. Transplantation. 2018;102:1914–23.
33. Papadopoulos EB, Ladanyi M, Emanuel D, et al. Infusions of donor leukocytes as treatment of Epstein–Barr virus associated lymphoproliferative disorders complicating allogeneic marrow transplantation. N Engl J Med. 1994;330:1185–91.
34. Ciceri F, Bonini C, Stanghellini MT, Bondanza A, Traversari C, Salomoni M, et al. Infusion of suicide-gene-engineered donor lymphocytes after family haploidentical haemopoietic stem-cell transplantation for leukaemia (the TK007 trial): a non-randomised phase I–II study. Lancet Oncol. 2009;10:489–500.
35. Di Stasi A, Tey SK, Dotti G, Fujita Y, Kennedy-Nasser A, Martinez C, et al. Inducible apoptosis as a safety switch for adoptive cell therapy. N Engl J Med. 2011;365(18):1673–83.

36. Rooney CM, Smith CA, Ng CY, et al. Use of gene-modified virus-specific T lymphocytes to control Epstein–Barr-virus-related lymphoproliferation. Lancet. 1995;345:9–12.
37. Gustafsson A, Levitsky V, Zou JZ, et al. Epstein–Barr virus (EBV) load in bone marrow transplant recipients at risk to develop posttransplant lymphoproliferative disease: prophylactic infusion of EBV-specific cytotoxic T cells. Blood. 2000;95:807–14.
38. Heslop HE, Slobod KS, Pule MA, et al. Long-term outcome of EBV-specific T-cell infusions to prevent or treat EBV-related lymphoproliferative disease in transplant recipients. Blood. 2010;115:925–35.
39. Bollard CM, Heslop HE. T cells for viral infections after allogeneic hematopoietic stem cell transplant. Blood. 2016;127:3331–40.
40. Haque T, Wilkie GM, Jones MM, et al. Allogeneic cytotoxic T-cell therapy for EBV-positive posttransplantation lymphoproliferative disease: results of a phase 2 multicenter clinical trial. Blood. 2007;110:1123–31.
41. Prockop S, Doubrovina E, Suser S, et al. Off-the-shelf EBV-specific T cell immunotherapy for rituximab-refractory EBV-associated lymphoma following transplant. J Clin Invest. 2019;130:733. https://doi.org/10.1172/JCI121127.
42. Doubrovina E, Oflaz-Sozmen B, Prockop SE, Kernan NA, Abramson S, Teruya-Feldstein J, et al. Adoptive immunotherapy with unselected or EBV-specific T cells for biopsy-proven EBV+ lymphomas after allogeneic hematopoietic cell transplantation. Blood. 2012;119:2644–56.
43. Styczynski J, Einsele H, Gil L, Ljungman P. Outcome of treatment of Epstein-Barr virus-related post-transplant lymphoproliferative disorder in hematopoietic stem cell recipients: a comprehensive review of reported cases. Transpl Infect Dis. 2009;11:383–92.
44. Trappe RU, Dierickx D, Zimmermann H, et al. Response to rituximab induction is a predictive marker in B-cell post-transplant lymphoproliferative disorder and allows successful stratification into rituximab or R-CHOP consolidation in an international, prospective, multicenter phase II trial. J Clin Oncol. 2017;35:536–43.
45. Gross TG, Orjuela MA, Perkins SL, et al. Low–dose chemotherapy and rituximab for post-transplant lymphoproliferative disease (PTLD): a Children's Oncology Group report. Am J Transplant. 2012;12:3069–75.
46. Knight JS, Tsodikov A, Cibrik DM, Ross CW, Kaminski MS, Blayney DW. Lymphoma after solid organ transplantation: risk, response to therapy, and survival at a transplantation center. J Clin Oncol. 2009;27:3354–62.
47. Choquet S, Trappe R, Leblond V, Jager U, Davi F, Oertel S. CHOP-21 for the treatment of post-transplant lymphoproliferative disorders (PTLD) following solid organ transplantation. Haematologica. 2007;92:273–4.
48. Williams-Aziz SL, Hartline CB, Harden EA, Daily SL, Prichard MN, Kushner NL, et al. Comparative activities of lipid esters of cidofovir and cyclic cidofovir against replication of herpesviruses in vitro. Antimicrob Agents Chemother. 2005;49:3724–33.
49. Green M. Management of Epstein-Barr virus-induced posttransplant lymphoproliferative disease in recipients of solid organ transplantation. Am J Transplant. 2001;1:103–8.
50. Perrine SP, Hermine O, Small T, Suarez F, O'Reilly R, Boulad F, et al. A phase 1/2 trial of arginine butyrate and ganciclovir in patients with Epstein-Barr virus-associated lymphoid malignancies. Blood. 2007;109:2571–8.
51. Wang FZ, Roy D, Gershburg E, Whitehurst CB, Dittmer DP, Pagano JS. Maribavir inhibits Epstein-Barr virus transcription in addition to viral DNA replication. J Virol. 2009;83:12108–17.
52. Whitehurst CB, Sanders MK, Law M, Wang FZ, Xiong J, Dittmer DP, et al. Maribavir inhibits Epstein-Barr virus transcription through the EBV protein kinase. J Virol. 2013;87:5311–5.
53. Marty FM, Ljungman P, Papanicolaou GA, Winston DJ, Chemaly RF, Strasfeld L, et al. Maribavir prophylaxis for prevention of cytomegalovirus disease in recipients of allogeneic stem-cell transplants: a phase 3, double-blind, placebo-controlled, randomised trial. Lancet Infect Dis. 2011;11:284–92.

54. Hostetler KY. Synthesis and early development of hexadecyloxypropylcidofovir: an oral anti-poxvirus nucleoside phosphonate. Viruses. 2010;2:2213–25.
55. Cheah CY, Fowler NH. Novel agents for relapsed and refractory follicular lymphoma. Best Pract Res Clin Haematol. 2018;31:41–8.
56. Portell C, Nand S. Single agent lenalidomide induces a response in refractory T-cell post-transplantation lymphoproliferative disorder. Blood. 2008;111:4416–7.
57. Laubli H, Tzankov A, Juskevicius D, Degen L, Rochlitz C, Stenner-Liewen F. Lenalidomide monotherapy leads to a complete remission in refractory B-cell post-transplant lymphopro-liferative disorder. Leuk Lymphoma. 2016;57:945–8.
58. Kassa C, Remenyi P, Sinko J, Kallay K, Kertesz G, Krivan G. Successful nivolumab therapy in an allogeneic stem cell transplant child with post-transplant lymphoproliferative disorder. Pediatr Transplant. 2018;22:e13302.
59. Plant AS, Venick RS, Farmer DG, Upadhyay S, Said J, Kempert P. Plasmacytoma-like post-transplant lymphoproliferative disorder seen in pediatric combined liver and intestinal trans-plant recipients. Pediatr Blood Cancer. 2013;60:E137–9.
60. Choi M, Fink S, Prasad V, Anagnostopoulos I, Reinke P, Schmitt CA. T cell PTLD suc-cessfully treated with single-agent brentuximab vedotin first-line therapy. Transplantation. 2016;100:e8–e10.
61. Vase MO, Maksten EF, Bendix K, Hamilton-Dutoit S, Andersen C, Moller MB, et al. Occurrence and prognostic relevance of CD30 expression in post-transplant lymphoprolif-erative disorders. Leuk Lymphoma. 2015;56:1677–85.
62. Hill BT, Tubbs RR, Smith MR. Complete remission of CD30-positive diffuse large B-cell lymphoma in a patient with post-transplant lymphoproliferative disorder and end-stage renal disease treated with single-agent brentuximab vedotin. Leuk Lymphoma. 2015;56:1552–3.
63. Blazar BR, Levy RB, Mak TW, Panoskaltsis-Mortari A, Muta H, Jones M, et al. CD30/CD30 ligand (CD153) interaction regulates CD4+ T cell-mediated graft-versus-host disease. J Immunol. 2004;173:2933–41.
64. Garcia-Cadenas I, Yanez L, Jarque I, Martino R, Perez-Simon JA, Valcarcel D, et al. Frequency, characteristics and outcome of PTLD after allo-SCT: a multicenter study from the Spanish group of blood and marrow transplantation (GETH). Eur J Haematol. 2019;102:465–71.
65. Yang J, Tao Q, Flinn IW, et al. Characterization of Epstein-Barr virus-infected B cells in patients with posttransplantation lymphoproliferative disease: disappearance after rituximab therapy does not predict clinical response. Blood. 2000;96:4055–406.
66. Kanakry J, Hegde A, Durand C, et al. The clinical significance of EBV DNA in the plasma and peripheral blood mononuclear cells of patients with or without EBV diseases. Blood. 2016;127:2007–10.
67. Cheson BD, Fisher RI, Barrington SF, Cavalli F, Schwartz LH, Zucca E, et al. Recommendations for initial evaluation, staging, and response assessment of Hodgkin and non-Hodgkin lymphoma: the Lugano classification. J Clin Oncol. 2014;32:3059–68.
68. Barrington SF, Mikhaeel NG, Kostakoglu L, Meignan M, Hutchings M, Mueller SP, et al. Role of imaging in the staging and response assessment of lymphoma: consensus of the International Conference on Malignant Lymphomas Imaging Working Group. J Clin Oncol. 2014;32:3048–58.
69. Ahmad I, Cau NV, Kwan J, Maaroufi Y, Meuleman N, Aoun M, et al. Preemptive man-agement of Epstein-Barr virus reactivation after hematopoietic stem-cell transplantation. Transplantation. 2009;87:1240–5.
70. Carpenter B, Haque T, Dimopoulou M, Atkinson C, Roughton M, Grace S, et al. Incidence and dynamics of Epstein-Barr virus reactivation after alemtuzumab-based conditioning for allogeneic hematopoietic stem-cell transplantation. Transplantation. 2010;90:564–70.
71. Blaes AH, Cao Q, Wagner JE, Young JA, Weisdorf DJ, Brunstein CG. Monitoring and pre-emptive rituximab therapy for Epstein-Barr virus reactivation after antithymocyte globulin containing nonmyeloablative conditioning for umbilical cord blood transplantation. Biol Blood Marrow Transplant. 2010;16:287–91.

72. Coppoletta S, Tedone E, Galano B, Soracco M, Raiola AM, Lamparelli T, et al. Rituximab treatment for Epstein-Barr virus DNAemia after alternative-donor hematopoietic stem cell transplantation. Biol Blood Marrow Transplant. 2011;17:901–7.
73. Worth A, Conyers R, Cohen J, Jagani M, Chiesa R, Rao K, et al. Pre-emptive rituximab based on viraemia and T cell reconstitution: a highly effective strategy for the prevention of Epstein-Barr virus-associated lymphoproliferative disease following stem cell transplantation. Br J Haematol. 2011;155:377–85.
74. van der Velden WJ, Mori T, Stevens WB, de Haan AF, Stelma FF, Blijlevens NM, Donnelly JP. Reduced PTLD-related mortality in patients experiencing EBV infection following allo-SCT after the introduction of a protocol incorporating pre-emptive rituximab. Bone Marrow Transplant. 2013;48:1465–71.
75. Garcia-Cadenas I, Castillo N, Martino R, Barba P, Esquirol A, Novelli S, et al. Impact of Epstein Barr virus-related complications after high-risk allo-SCT in the era of pre-emptive rituximab. Bone Marrow Transplant. 2015;50:579–84.
76. D'Aveni M, Aissi-Rothe L, Venard V, Salmon A, Falenga A, Decot V, et al. The clinical value of concomitant Epstein Barr virus (EBV)-DNA load and specific immune reconstitution monitoring after allogeneic hematopoietic stem cell transplantation. Transpl Immunol. 2011;24:224–32.
77. Muramatsu H, Takahashi Y, Shimoyama Y, Doisaki S, Nishio N, Ito Y, et al. CD20-negative Epstein-Barr virus-associated post-transplant lymphoproliferative disease refractory to rituximab in a patient with severe aplastic anemia. Int J Hematol. 2011;93:779–81.
78. Bordon V, Padalko E, Benoit Y, Dhooge C, Laureys G. Incidence, kinetics, and risk factors of Epstein-Barr virus viremia in pediatric patients after allogeneic stem cell transplantation. Pediatr Transplant. 2012;16:144–50.
79. Patriarca F, Medeot M, Isola M, Battista ML, Sperotto A, Pipan C, et al. Prognostic factors and outcome of Epstein-Barr virus DNAemia in high-risk recipients of allogeneic stem cell transplantation treated with preemptive rituximab. Transpl Infect Dis. 2013;15:259–67.
80. Pinana JL, Sanz J, Esquirol A, Martino R, Picardi A, Barba P, et al. Umbilical cord blood transplantation in adults with advanced Hodgkin's disease: high incidence of post-transplant lymphoproliferative disease. Eur J Haematol. 2015;96(2):128–35.
81. Sanz J, Arango M, Senent L, Jarque I, Montesinos P, Sempere A, et al. EBV-associated post-transplant lymphoproliferative disorder after umbilical cord blood transplantation in adults with hematological diseases. Bone Marrow Transplant. 2014;49:397–402.
82. Kuriyama T, Kawano N, Yamashita K, Ueda A. Successful treatment of Rituximab-resistant Epstein-Barr virus-associated post-transplant lymphoproliferative disorder using R-CHOP. J Clin Exp Hematop. 2014;54:149–53.
83. Meyer SC, Medinger M, Halter JP, Baldomero H, Hirsch HH, Tzankov A, et al. Heterogeneity in clinical course of EBV-associated lymphoproliferative disorder after allogeneic stem cell transplantation. Hematology. 2014;19:280–5.
84. Han SB, Bae EY, Lee JW, Jang PS, Lee DG, Chung NG, et al. Features of Epstein-Barr virus reactivation after allogeneic hematopoietic cell transplantation in Korean children living in an area of high seroprevalence against Epstein-Barr virus. Int J Hematol. 2014;100:188–99.
85. Helgestad J, Rosthoj S, Pedersen MH, Johansen P, Iyer V, Ostergaard E, Heilmann C. Very late relapse of PTLD 10 yr after allogeneic HSCT and nine yr after stopping immunosuppressive therapy. Pediatr Transplant. 2014;18:E35–9.
86. Weber T, Wickenhauser C, Monecke A, Glaser C, Stadler M, Desole M, et al. Treatment of rare co-occurrence of Epstein-Barr virus-driven post-transplant lymphoproliferative disorder and hemophagocytic lymphohistiocytosis after allogeneic stem cell transplantation. Transpl Infect Dis. 2014;16:988–92.
87. Barker JN, Doubrovina E, Sauter C, Jaroscak JJ, Perales MA, Doubrovin M, et al. Successful treatment of EBV-associated posttransplantation lymphoma after cord blood transplantation using third-party EBV-specific cytotoxic T lymphocytes. Blood. 2010;116:5045–9.

88. Moosmann A, Bigalke I, Tischer J, Schirrmann L, Kasten J, Tippmer S, et al. Effective and long-term control of EBV PTLD after transfer of peptide-selected T cells. Blood. 2010;115:2960–70.
89. Leen AM, Bollard CM, Mendizabal AM, Shpall EJ, Szabolcs P, Antin JH, et al. Multicenter study of banked third-party virus-specific T cells to treat severe viral infections after hematopoietic stem cell transplantation. Blood. 2013;121:5113–23.
90. Bollard CM, Rooney CM, Heslop HE. T-cell therapy in the treatment of post-transplant lymphoproliferative disease. Nat Rev Clin Oncol. 2012;9:510–9.
91. Kawaguchi T, Tsukamoto S, Ohwada C, Takeuchi M, Muto T, Tanaka S, et al. Successful treatment with rituximab and donor lymphocyte infusions for fulminant EBV-associated lymphoproliferative disorder that developed 14 years after unrelated BMT. Bone Marrow Transplant. 2011;46:1583–5.
92. Kittan NA, Beier F, Kurz K, Niller HH, Egger L, Jilg W, et al. Isolated cerebral manifestation of Epstein-Barr virus-associated post-transplant lymphoproliferative disorder after allogeneic hematopoietic stem cell transplantation: a case of clinical and diagnostic challenges. Transpl Infect Dis. 2011;13:524–30.
93. Li X, Li N, Yang T, Chen Z, Hu J. Lymph node flow cytometry as a prompt recognition of ultra early onset PTLD: a successful case of rituximab treatment. Case Rep Hematol. 2015;2015:430623.
94. Cheng FW, Lee V, To KF, Chan KC, Shing MK, Li CK. Post-transplant EBV-related lymphoproliferative disorder complicating umbilical cord blood transplantation in patients of adrenoleukodystrophy. Pediatr Blood Cancer. 2009;53:1329–31.
95. Wroblewska M, Gil LA, Komarnicki MA. Successful treatment of Epstein-Barr virus-related post-transplant lymphoproliferative disease with central nervous system involvement following allogeneic haematopoietic stem cell transplantation – a case study. Cent Eur J Immunol. 2015;40:122–5.
96. Gu Z, Cai B, Yuan L, Li H, Huang W, Jing Y, et al. Successful treatment of polymorphic post-transplant lymphoproliferative disorder after allo-HSCT with reduction of immunosuppression. Int J Clin Exp Med. 2014;7:1904–9.
97. Luo L, Zhang L, Cai B, Li H, Huang W, Jing Y, et al. Post-transplant lymphoproliferative disease after allogeneic hematopoietic stem cell transplantation: a single-center experience. Ann Transplant. 2014;19:6–12.
98. Chen DB, Song QJ, Chen YX, Chen YH, Shen DH. Clinicopathologic spectrum and EBV status of post-transplant lymphoproliferative disorders after allogeneic hematopoietic stem cell transplantation. Int J Hematol. 2013;97:117–24.
99. Krenauer A, Moll A, Ponisch W, Schmitz N, Niedobitek G, Niederwieser D, Aigner T. EBV-associated post-transplantation B-cell lymphoproliferative disorder following allogenic stem cell transplantation for acute lymphoblastic leukaemia: tumor regression after reduction of immunosuppression – a case report. Diagn Pathol. 2010;5:21.
100. Styczynski J. Results of therapy of EBV-associated post-transplant lymphoproliferative disorder in children and adults with anti-CD20 antibodies after hematopoietic stem cell transplantation. In: Styczynski J, editor. Epstein-Barr virus (EBV): transmission, diagnosis and role in the development of cancers. New York: Nova Science Publishers; 2014. p. 239–68.
101. Vickers MA, Wilkie GM, Robinson N, Rivera N, Haque T, Crawford DH, et al. Establishment and operation of a Good Manufacturing Practice-compliant allogeneic Epstein-Barr virus (EBV)-specific cytotoxic cell bank for the treatment of EBV-associated lymphoproliferative disease. Br J Haematol. 2014;167:402–10.
102. Valencia-Sanchez C, Steenerson KK, Kelemen K, Orenstein R, Kusne S, Grill MF. Post-transplant primary central nervous system lymphoma after Epstein-Barr virus cerebellitis. J Neurovirol. 2019;25:280–3.
103. Evens AM, Choquet S, Kroll-Desrosiers AR, Jagadeesh D, Smith SM, Morschhauser F, et al. Primary CNS posttransplant lymphoproliferative disease (PTLD): an international report of 84 cases in the modern era. Am J Transplant. 2013;13:1512–22.

104. Mahapatra S, Chin CC, Iagaru A, Heerema-McKenney A, Twist CJ. Successful treatment of systemic and central nervous system post-transplant lymphoproliferative disorder without the use of high-dose methotrexate or radiation. Pediatr Blood Cancer. 2014;61:2107–9.
105. Pakakasama S, Eames GM, Morriss MC, Huls MH, Rooney CM, Heslop HE, Krance RA. Treatment of Epstein-Barr virus lymphoproliferative disease after hematopoietic stem-cell transplantation with hydroxyurea and cytotoxic T-cell lymphocytes. Transplantation. 2004;78:755–7.
106. Ferreiro JF, Morscio J, Dierickx D, Vandenberghe P, Gheysens O, Verhoef G, et al. EBV-positive and EBV-negative posttransplant diffuse large B cell lymphomas have distinct genomic and transcriptomic features. Am J Transplant. 2016;16:414–25.
107. Zutter MM, Durnam DM, Hackman RC, Loughran TP Jr, Kidd PG, Ashley RL, et al. Secondary T-cell lymphoproliferation after marrow transplantation. Am J Clin Pathol. 1990;94:714–21.
108. Wang LC, Lu MY, Yu J, Jou ST, Chiang IP, Lin KH, et al. T cell lymphoproliferative disorder following bone marrow transplantation for severe aplastic anemia. Bone Marrow Transplant. 2000;26:893–7.
109. Au WY, Lam CC, Lie AK, Pang A, Kwong YL. T-cell large granular lymphocyte leukemia of donor origin after allogeneic bone marrow transplantation. Am J Clin Pathol. 2003;120:626–30.
110. Chang H, Kamel-Reid S, Hussain N, Lipton J, Messner HA. T-cell large granular lymphocytic leukemia of donor origin occurring after allogeneic bone marrow transplantation for B-cell lymphoproliferative disorders. Am J Clin Pathol. 2005;123:196–9.
111. Santos-Briz A, Romo A, Antunez P, Roman C, Alcoceba M, Garcia JL, et al. Primary cutaneous T-cell lymphoproliferative disorder of donor origin after allogeneic haematopoietic stem-cell transplantation. Clin Exp Dermatol. 2009;34:e778–81.
112. Nishida A, Yamamoto H, Ohta Y, Karasawa M, Kato D, Uchida N, et al. T-cell post-transplant lymphoproliferative disorder in a patient with chronic idiopathic myelofibrosis following allogeneic PBSC transplantation. Bone Marrow Transplant. 2010;45:1372–4.
113. Tanaka T, Takizawa J, Miyakoshi S, Kozakai T, Fuse K, Shibasaki Y, et al. Manifestations of fulminant CD8 T-cell post-transplant lymphoproliferative disorder following the administration of rituximab for lymphadenopathy with a high level of Epstein-Barr virus (EBV) replication after allogeneic hematopoietic stem cell transplantation. Intern Med. 2014;53:2115–9.
114. Herreman A, Dierickx D, Morscio J, Camps J, Bittoun E, Verhoef G, et al. Clinicopathological characteristics of posttransplant lymphoproliferative disorders of T-cell origin: single-center series of nine cases and meta-analysis of 147 reported cases. Leuk Lymphoma. 2013;54:2190–9.
115. Tiede C, Maecker-Kolhoff B, Klein C, Kreipe H, Hussein K. Risk factors and prognosis in T-cell posttransplantation lymphoproliferative diseases: reevaluation of 163 cases. Transplantation. 2013;95:479–88.
116. Roncella S, Cutrona G, Truini M, Airoldi I, Pezzolo A, Valetto A, et al. Late Epstein-Barr virus infection of a hepatosplenic gamma delta T-cell lymphoma arising in a kidney transplant recipient. Haematologica. 2000;85:256–62.
117. Swerdlow SH. T-cell and NK-cell posttransplantation lymphoproliferative disorders. Am J Clin Pathol. 2007;127:887–95.

Preventative and Preemptive Strategies for EBV Infection and PTLD After HSCT

15

Rayne H. Rouce, Lauren P. McLaughlin, Cliona M. Rooney, and Catherine M. Bollard

R. H. Rouce
Center for Cell and Gene Therapy, Baylor College of Medicine, Houston Methodist Hospital and Texas Children's Hospital, Houston, TX, USA

Dan L. Duncan Comprehensive Cancer Center, Children's National Health System, Washington, DC, USA
e-mail: rhrouce@texaschildrens.org

L. P. McLaughlin
Center for Cancer and Immunology Research, Children's National Health System, Washington, DC, USA

Department of Pediatrics, George Washington University School of Medicine, Washington, DC, USA

C. M. Rooney
Center for Cell and Gene Therapy, Baylor College of Medicine, Houston Methodist Hospital and Texas Children's Hospital, Houston, TX, USA

Dan L. Duncan Comprehensive Cancer Center, Children's National Health System, Washington, DC, USA

Department of Pediatrics, Baylor College of Medicine, Houston, TX, USA

Department of Immunology, Baylor College of Medicine, Houston, TX, USA

Department of Virology, Baylor College of Medicine, Houston, TX, USA
e-mail: CMROONEY@texaschildrens.org

C. M. Bollard (✉)
Center for Cancer and Immunology Research, Children's National Health System, Washington, DC, USA

Department of Pediatrics, George Washington University School of Medicine, Washington, DC, USA

Department of Microbiology, Immunology and Tropical Medicine, George Washington University School of Medicine, Washington, DC, USA
e-mail: CBollard@childrensnational.org

© Springer Nature Switzerland AG 2021
V. R. Dharnidharka et al. (eds.), *Post-Transplant Lymphoproliferative Disorders*,
https://doi.org/10.1007/978-3-030-65403-0_15

Introduction

After hematopoietic stem cell transplantation (HSCT), posttransplant lymphoproliferative disorder (PTLD) arises due to impaired immune surveillance of Epstein-
Barr virus (EBV). EBV is a human gamma-herpesvirus that establishes lifelong
persistence in oral epithelial cells and B lymphocytes. In a healthy person, EBV
causes a mild to moderate viral illness and induces potent cell-mediated immunity
by EBV-specific T cells that control the pool of latently infected cells [1]. However,
during the period of severe immune suppression after HSCT, particularly T-cell-
depleted HSCT, patients are at risk for EBV-driven PTLD.

While the incidence of PTLD after HSCT is less than 5% and remains unchanged
in recent years, frequencies of up to 20% have been reported in patients with established high-risk features [2, 3]. Despite the introduction of regular surveillance, the
incidence of PTLD is not decreasing, a finding that relates at least in part to (i) an
increase in the number and complexity of transplants performed, in particular haploidentical transplants, (ii) the use of T-cell depletion, and (iii) improved awareness
and diagnosis of PTLD [4]. PTLD after HSCT is often more disseminated and
aggressive with a worse prognosis than after solid organ transplantation (SOT) [5].
Twenty years ago, the mortality rate of patients with PTLD after HSCT was as high
as 84% [6], with reduction of immunosuppression being the only effective treatment. The introduction of the anti-CD20 antibody rituximab targeting EBV-infected
B cells dramatically improved survival to around 70% [4, 5, 7]. However, current
rituximab and chemotherapy-based treatments carry significant morbidity from
B-cell immune suppression and organ toxicity in an already vulnerable patient population. Preventive approaches, especially in patients at high risk of developing
PTLD after HSCT, are therefore needed to avoid later treatment complications.

Biology of PTLD After HSCT

Subtypes

PTLD is a heterogeneous disease that is most commonly of B-cell origin, regardless
of subtype. It is currently subdivided as classified by the World Health Organization
(see Chap. 2). Several key features distinguish PTLD that occurs following HSCT
from that occurring post-SOT. PTLD most commonly occurs in the first 6–12 months
after HSCT during the time of most substantial immune compromise, and before
reconstitution of the EBV-specific immune response has occurred [8, 9]. PTLD after
HSCT is almost always donor-derived as the immune-compromised setting allows
for uncontrolled proliferation of donor-derived EBV-infected B cells [10–12].
PTLD can occur many years after SOT due to continued immune suppression, and
in cases occurring over 2 years from SOT, up to 33% are EBV-negative PTLD,
which is rare post-HSCT. Reports detailing a high incidence of PTLD in pediatric
patients receiving reduced intensity conditioning including ATG and alemtuzumab
highlight the likely contribution of residual recipient B cells in the development of
PTLD [13, 14].

EBV Gene Expression in PTLD Post-HSCT

All EBV-associated malignancies, including PTLD, are associated with the virus' latent cycle [15], which makes antiviral agents that generally target the lytic cycle highly ineffective [16]. Viral gene expression defines the pattern of latency and the pathogenicity of the PTLD [17]. Type III latency, in which B cells express all EBV latency proteins, is highly immunogenic and is seen in most polymorphic, polyclonal PTLD that develops after HSCT. Importantly, this Type III latency profile is identical to that seen in EBV-transformed B lymphoblastoid cell lines (LCLs), the in vitro use of which has been instrumental not only in the study of EBV but also for the manufacture of T-cell-based therapies for PTLD. More aggressive, monomorphic forms of PTLD, which are more commonly seen in recipients of SOT, generally resemble Hodgkin or non-Hodgkin lymphoma (Burkitt, diffuse large B cell, etc.) and express a more restricted pattern of latency genes, typically known as Type I and Type II latency, respectively [8]. These types of latency are less immunogenic and more difficult to target with T cells.

Risks Factors for PTLD After HSCT

PTLD most commonly occurs within 12 months of HSCT, while patients may still be receiving immunosuppression to prevent or treat graft-versus-host disease (GVHD) and before immune reconstitution occurs. Risk factors for the development of PTLD have been well established, with increased T-cell depletion leading to uncontrolled proliferation of EBV-infected B cells as the most substantial contributor. Hence, preparative regimens that include selective T-cell-depleting agents such as antithymocyte globulin (ATG) and to a lesser degree broader depleting agents that target both T and B cells such as Campath (commonly used in HLA-mismatched HSCT settings) are more likely to cause PTLD [3, 12]. Donor/recipient EBV serology status mismatch, while more common in the SOT setting, remains a major risk factor for PTLD after HSCT [2]. For example, recipients of cord blood donor grafts are at higher risk of PTLD because of the seronegative (naïve) donor source, coupled with slow antigen-specific T-cell immune reconstitution following umbilical cord blood transplantation [18]. By contrast the risk of PTLD following SOT is higher when an EBV-negative recipient receives a graft from an EBV-positive donor, resulting from uncontrolled infection of recipient B cells by virus carried in by the graft [19].

Scoring systems based on established risk factors (described in Chap. 12) have been designed to predict the risk of PTLD. These can be used to determine the appropriateness of preemptive interventions. One such scoring system, created by Fujimoto et al., was based on three pre-transplant risk factors identified in a nationwide retrospective analysis of EBV+ PTLD in patients undergoing transplant between 1990 and 2016: ATG use in a conditioning regimen (high dose, 2 points; low dose, 1 point), donor type (mismatched related donor, 1 point; unrelated donor, 1 point; cord blood, 2 points), and aplastic anemia (1 point). Patients were classified into 4 risk groups according to the total score: low risk (0 or 1 point), intermediate risk (2 points), high risk (3 points), and very high risk (4 or 5 points), with probabilities at 2 years of 0.3%, 1.3%, 4.6%, and 11.5%, respectively [20]. It is worth noting that increased use of ATG and of mismatched (unrelated and CB) donor sources, as well as second transplants after 2010, likely contributed to the rising incidence of PTLD. While the overall rate of PTLD in this population was lower than in similar smaller reports (likely due to diminished use of ATG in the earlier vs. later years studied and exclusion of haploidentical donors), this sort of scoring system is of potential use in predicting patients at highest risk for PTLD. Importantly, while the incidence varies, the risk factors for PTLD are clear and should be incorporated into surveillance and preemptive therapy algorithms.

Prevention Strategies

Surveillance After HSCT

Measuring EBV DNA load by quantitative PCR is the mainstay for monitoring for EBV after HSCT, but should not supplant biopsy as the "gold standard" to definitively diagnose PTLD [21]. Elevated and rising EBV DNA loads are the hallmarks of PTLD development, but differences in EBV DNA assays between different laboratories and hospitals and a lack of consensus regarding threshold values that indicate the need to search for PTLD hinder the utility of viral load as an indicator for PTLD. The reported positive and negative predictive values vary widely for the use of EBV DNAemia to diagnose PTLD following HSCT, ranging from 25% to 40% and 67% to 86%, respectively [4, 22–24].

EBV DNAemia can be measured in plasma, in whole blood, or in blood mononuclear cells (PBMC). The relative advantages and disadvantages of measurement of each of these compartments are discussed in Chap. 6. Hakim et al. found that quantitative PCR using whole blood or PBMC was more sensitive than using plasma in the pediatric HSCT setting, and thus, many transplant centers prefer to use whole blood detection over plasma [25]. EBV DNA in blood can represent cell-free virus, killed virus-infected cells, or circulating EBV-infected cells. Hence, for the purpose of prevention, measurement of EBV load in whole blood is more sensitive and likely to be positive prior to detection in plasma and thus is likely the preferable compartment to follow EBV loads.

Reduction of Immune Suppression

Reduction of immune suppression (RIS), if possible, should be considered with rising EBV levels of DNAemia. Liu et al. used a preemptive intervention protocol combining antiviral agents with RIS when EBV DNA was detected in two consecutive samples. This approach resulted in complete responses (CR), as defined by resolution of EBV DNA loads in plasma, without signs or symptoms of EBV-associated disease in 22 of 48 patients with EBV DNAemia after HSCT when treated with antiviral agents with RIS, but in only 2 out of 16 treated with antiviral agents alone [26]. However, RIS may increase the risk of GVHD, and the potential risk and benefit must be weighed on an individual patient basis [23].

Preemptive Treatment with Rituximab

Because PTLD carries a high risk of mortality, many practitioners elect to use rituximab, a monoclonal antibody targeting CD20+ cells, as preemptive therapy prior to the development of PTLD for patients with EBV DNAemia after HSCT. However, there is no consensus for the threshold of EBV load appropriate to initiate preemptive rituximab, with recommendations ranging from 1000 to 40,000 EBV copies/ml of blood [27–30]. Moreover, a specific value may be of less importance than a rapid rate of increase in EBV copy number [23]. In one study of 70 children receiving reduced intensity conditioning with alemtuzumab, 20 were treated preemptively with rituximab due to elevated EBV DNA loads. These patients had a significantly lower incidence of PTLD than historical cohorts (1.4% vs. 21.7%, $p = 0.003$) [29]. In the study of Liu et al. mentioned earlier [26], 15 patients required preemptive rituximab after failing antiviral agents and RIS, and of these 14 subsequently achieved a CR. However, as rituximab causes an increased risk of infection from prolonged hypogammaglobulinemia and neutropenia, the risks of preemptive rituximab should be carefully weighed against its benefits [23, 31, 32]. The Sixth European Conference on Infections in Leukemia (ECIL-6) guidelines recommend a weekly rituximab dose of 375 mg/m² until EBV DNAemia has resolved, with 1–4 doses usually being sufficient in the post-HSCT setting [23].

Prophylaxis or Preemptive Therapy with T Cells

Donor lymphocyte infusion (DLI) to increase EBV-specific immunity was the first form of cellular therapy for PTLD with initial reports published almost 30 years ago [33, 34]. In 1994, Papadopoulos et al. demonstrated complete responses in all of five PTLD patients treated with DLI from their seropositive donors [35]. In 2012, Doubrovina et al. induced sustained complete remissions in over 70% of 30 patients treated with DLI. However, this approach carries the risk of GVHD, with DLI recipients having a 14% cumulative incidence of acute GVHD within 1 year after DLI [36].

Donor-derived EBV-specific T cells (EBVSTs) were therefore developed to increase EBV immunity through cellular therapy while minimizing the risk of GVHD [37, 38]. Donor-derived EBVSTs have been used not only to treat PTLD but also as a preventative measure to reduce high EBV DNA loads and as prophylaxis for patients at high risk for developing PTLD. Rooney et al. treated 39 patients who were at high risk for developing PTLD with donor-derived EBVSTs, and none developed PTLD compared to 7 of 61 in a historical control group. Notably, 6 of the 39 patients who received prophylactic T-cell infusions had high EBV viral loads at the time of infusion, and substantial decreases in viral load were obtained in all. Two additional patients who did not receive prophylactic T cells developed PTLD and received EBVSTs as treatment. Both patients achieved CRs [37]. In an extension of these studies, Heslop et al. used donor-derived EBVSTs to treat 101 patients at high risk of developing PTLD after HSCT, and none developed PTLD [39]. These results were compared to a historical incidence of 11% in patients undergoing similar transplants. Twelve of the 101 patients had EBV DNAemia at the time of prophylactic infusion, and EBV viral load decreased after infusion in 11 of these patients. No patient in this cohort developed de novo acute GVHD.

To evaluate whether virus-specific T-cell (VST) products that target multiple viral antigens in a single product can control EBV DNAemia, Leen et al. infused 11 patients with multivirus-specific T cells targeting CMV, EBV, and adenovirus; 10 of the 11showed an increase in the frequency of EBV-responsive T cells by 4 weeks after infusion. Three of the 11 patients had PTLD or EBV DNAemia at time of infusion, and all showed a clinical response to infusion, including complete resolution of PTLD [38]. Leen et al. also demonstrated clearance of EBV DNA in the blood of 3 of 3 patients treated with donor-derived, bivirus (EBV and adenovirus) T cells [40]. In 2014, Papadopoulos et al. treated 11 patients with donor-derived VSTs targeting five viruses (including EBV) of whom three had either EBV DNAemia ($n = 2$) or PTLD ($n = 1$) post-HSCT, and all patients with EBV-related disease achieved a CR [41]. Overall, EBV-specific T-cell infusions are well tolerated, have a low risk of GVHD, and provide a safe and effective strategy to treat PTLD and to prevent PTLD by eradicating EBV DNAemia.

Advances in Manufacturing of EBV-Specific T Cells

The initial successes of donor-derived EBVSTs were hindered by the lengthy manufacture process. More recently, several "rapid manufacturing" strategies have improved upon the complex procedures classically used to generate EBVSTs. Newer approaches replace lymphoblastoid cell lines or viral vector-transduced antigen-presenting cells (APC) with APCs pulsed with overlapping peptide libraries covering the entire protein sequence of selected viral antigens to stimulate and expand EBVSTs. This technique shortens the manufacturing process to as little as 10 days and is used in current clinical trials of VSTs [42].

To further shorten the time of VST manufacture, several groups have selected VSTs directly from donor blood, either by selection of multimer (HLA-peptide complex)-positive cells or by IFN-γ capture selecting cells that secrete IFN-γ in response to antigen stimulation (IFN-γ capture). Icheva et al. infused donor-derived EBNA-1-directed VSTs into ten patients with EBV viremia or PTLD [43]. Donor PBMCs were first stimulated overnight with EBNA-1 protein ($n = 7$) or overlapping peptide libraries ($n = 3$), then isolated by IFN-γ capture using the CliniMACS (Miltenyi Biotec) immunomagnetic device, and infused directly. The therapy was well tolerated, though one patient experienced Grade 1–2 acute skin GVHD. Clinical response was correlated with in vivo EBNA1 VST expansion. Seven of eight patients with T-cell expansion exhibited a decrease in viral load and/or some improvement in disease (despite the small doses used). In contrast, the two patients without T-cell expansion did not respond to the therapy [43]. Multimer selection uses magnetically labeled peptide multimers to isolate T cells specific for pertinent peptide/MHC multimers [44]. While both of these methods can selectively isolate EBVSTs in less than 48 hours without ex vivo expansion, they both require considerable amounts of donor blood, since the EBV-specific T-cell precursor frequency is low, and donors that are available and willing [43–47].

Alternative VST Cell Donor Sources

A limitation of donor-derived T cells is the need for a seropositive donor. However, recent studies from Hanley et al. demonstrated that multivirus (CMV, EBV, and AdV)-specific T cells can be generated from umbilical cord and from virus-naïve adult donors [48]. Cord blood-derived multivirus-specific T cells targeting CMV, EBV, and adenovirus have proved feasible to generate and safe and efficacious in patients. In two related clinical trials, investigators were able to manufacture an eligible T-cell product from cord blood (CB) in 18 out of 21 cases. Fourteen patients received cord blood-derived T-cell products: seven for treatment of DNAemia and seven as prophylaxis [49]. All patients with active DNAemia (including two with EBV) who received CB-VSTs had decreases in viral load with complete clearance occurring in five patients. There were no infusion-related adverse events and no cases of Grade 3 or 4 acute GVHD. As patients receiving umbilical cord transplantation are at a higher risk for developing PTLD due to delayed immune reconstitution, the ability to generate virus-specific T cells from CB for either prophylaxis or treatment is a significant advance in the field of adoptive immune therapy. However, CB-derived VSTs still take several weeks to manufacture and undergo release testing and thus are not readily available for a patient with quickly rising EBV load or PTLD, which has prompted the development of third-party VST banks.

Third-Party EBV-Specific T Cells

Despite its promise, prophylaxis of PTLD with HSCT donor-derived EBVSTs has challenges. The procurement and manufacture of EBVSTs may be prolonged when the donor is unrelated and/or EBV seronegative. Immediate selection strategies require a large amount of blood and are limited by the precursor frequency of EBVSTs in patient blood, and HSCT donors are not always willing or available. An "off-the-shelf" T-cell product is therefore an attractive option and, once such banks are commercially available, should enable more widespread use of EBVSTs.

Several groups have generated banked, cryopreserved "off-the-shelf" or "third-party" EBVSTs to treat patients with relapsed or refractory PTLD as well as EBV

DNAemia. These immediately available third-party banks are generated from the peripheral blood of blood bank-eligible, EBV-seropositive healthy donors [36, 42, 50–53]. These banks may be manufactured using the rapid expansion strategies discussed above and are designed to yield T cells with high EBV antigen specificity and effector function. Third-party EBVST banks allow the selection of EBVST lines with potent virus specificity through shared HLA alleles. Since each EBVST line may recognize EBV proteins through only one or two alleles, the lines should ideally be characterized for their HLA restricting alleles to ensure the best choice of line. However, the degree of characterization varies depending on the VST bank [36, 42, 50–53], but at a minimum, third-party EBVSTs are HLA typed to allow product selection based on the degree of HLA match with the recipient. Early studies found that the majority of patients who did not respond to therapy received a product with EBV-specific activity through an HLA allele not shared by the recipient's EBV PTLD [36]. Hence, later studies determined the HLA restriction of each line using banks of EBV-LCLs matched at a single HLA allele in cytotoxicity or other immunoassays [36, 42, 50–53]. Strategic bank design to maximize HLA coverage based on the most commonly encountered HLA types has enabled smaller banks, often specific to one geographic region, to cover the majority (>90%) of referred patients [34, 35].

To date, none of the abovementioned studies has reported de novo acute or chronic GVHD or flares of preexisting GVHD. The absence of GVHD relates to the fact that the manufacturing process reduces or eliminates the number of alloreactive T cells in the infusion product. The disadvantage of third-party EBVSTs is their short persistence compared to patient-specific VSTs. Since they are mismatched at a number of HLA class I and II alleles, they are vulnerable to rejection and clearance even in immunocompromised hosts. This may limit the efficacy of third-party EBVST as prophylaxis in patients without EBV DNAemia as EBV-specific immunity may not persist long-term. However, third-party EBVSTs may still be an effective preemptive strategy due to their ability to eradicate EBV DNAemia in patients with high viral loads who are at high risk for developing PTLD.

The feasibility, remarkable clinical responses, and favorable safety profile of third-party EBVST banks in patients with EBV+ PTLD have led to larger trials, partnerships with industry, and attempts to integrate third-party EBVSTs earlier in treatment. For example, the Pediatric Blood and Marrow Transplant Consortium (PBMTC) has a Phase 1/2 study using third-party multivirus-specific T cells to treat EBV, CMV, and adenovirus DNAemia in pediatric patients after allogeneic HSCT or in patients with primary immunodeficiency before HSCT (NCT03475212).

Ongoing research is focused primarily on (1) protecting third-party cells from rejection by the host [54], which should in turn enhance their persistence and potentially prolong clinical responses; (2) incorporating third-party EBVSTs earlier in therapy (NCT02900976); and (3) using this therapeutic option outside the transplant setting in patients with EBV+ lymphoproliferative disease or lymphoma unrelated to prior transplant (NCT02287311).

Future Directions

While this chapter has focused on strategies to enhance the EBV specificity of the native T-cell receptor, genetic modifications can produce T cells with enhanced capabilities. In some cases, gene editing has also been used to render EBV-specific T cells resistant to the immunosuppressive tumor microenvironment (TME) or immunosuppressive medications.

Genetic modification of EBVSTs to provide resistance to destruction by commonly used immunosuppressants such as tacrolimus (FK506) and steroids is a promising preclinical strategy that has been explored by several groups [55, 56]. DeAngelis et al. silenced the FK506-binding protein (FKBP12), generating FK506-resistant EBVSTs that displayed anti-PTLD activity and FK506 resistance in vitro and in a murine xenograft model [56]. Since it is difficult to treat PTLD that occurs concurrently with GVHD, we await results from future clinical studies evaluating these and other strategies that impart immune-suppression resistance to adoptively transferred EBVSTs.

Conclusions

While PTLD has a low frequency in HSCT recipients, the incidence may increase as transplant centers treat increasingly complex patients with a wider range of transplant approaches including T-cell-depleted alternative donor and umbilical cord blood donor grafts. The diagnosis, management, and surveillance of EBV and PTLD in the post-HSCT setting continue to evolve. Rituximab has dramatically improved the outcome of PTLD after HSCT but depletes the healthy B-cell compartment and antibody production, further increasing the infectious risk for these highly immunocompromised individuals [57]. Adoptive T-cell therapy with donor-derived EBVSTs is effective, restoring EBV-specific T-cell immunity while sparing the healthy B-cell compartment. Both of these strategies can be used to treat PTLD, but there is increasing interest in implementing these strategies as preemptive measures in patients with EBV DNAemia who are at high risk for developing PLTD to avoid the toxicity of PTLD.

Despite considerable advances, the need remains to optimize the prevention and preemptive treatment of EBV DNAemia and PTLD post-HSCT and to broaden the applicability of novel treatments such as T-cell therapies beyond "boutique" centers.

Take-Home Messages
1. Preemptive rituximab is effective in reducing EBV DNAemia, but it remains to be determined what degree of EBV DNAemia warrants treatment with rituximab.
2. Both donor-derived and third-party EBV-specific T cells offer an attractive alternative to preemptive rituximab by safely reducing or eliminating EBV DNAemia without targeting healthy B cells.

3. Salvage therapy options for the treatment of relapsed/refractory PTLD can be associated with significant morbidity and mortality, and thus, there is a need for effective preventative and preemptive treatment strategies.

References

1. Comoli P, Basso S, Zecca M, Pagliara D, Baldanti F, Bernardo ME, et al. Preemptive therapy of EBV-related lymphoproliferative disease after pediatric haploidentical stem cell transplantation. Am J Transplant Off J Am Soc Transplant Am Soc Transplant Surg. 2007;7(6):1648–55.
2. Uhlin M, Wikell H, Sundin M, Blennow O, Maeurer M, Ringden O, et al. Risk factors for Epstein-Barr virus-related post-transplant lymphoproliferative disease after allogeneic hematopoietic stem cell transplantation. Haematologica. 2014;99(2):346–52.
3. Bollard CM, Tripic T, Cruz CR, Dotti G, Gottschalk S, Torrano V, et al. Tumor-specific T-cells engineered to overcome tumor immune evasion induce clinical responses in patients with relapsed Hodgkin lymphoma. J Clin Oncol. 2018;36(11):1128–39.
4. Dierickx D, Habermann TM. Post-transplantation lymphoproliferative disorders in adults. N Engl J Med. 2018;378(6):549–62.
5. Styczynski J, Gil L, Tridello G, Ljungman P, Donnelly JP, van der Velden W, et al. Response to rituximab-based therapy and risk factor analysis in Epstein Barr Virus-related lymphoproliferative disorder after hematopoietic stem cell transplant in children and adults: a study from the Infectious Diseases Working Party of the European Group for Blood and Marrow Transplantation. Clin Infect Dis. 2013;57(6):794–802.
6. Curtis RE, Travis LB, Rowlings PA, Socié G, Kingma DW, Banks PM, et al. Risk of lymphoproliferative disorders after bone marrow transplantation: a multi-institutional study. Blood. 1999;94(7):2208–16.
7. Bollard CM, Cohen JI. How I treat T-cell chronic active Epstein-Barr virus disease. Blood. 2018;131(26):2899–905.
8. Heslop HE. How I treat EBV lymphoproliferation. Blood. 2009;114(19):4002–8.
9. Landgren O, Gilbert ES, Rizzo JD, Socié G, Banks PM, Sobocinski KA, et al. Risk factors for lymphoproliferative disorders after allogeneic hematopoietic cell transplantation. Blood. 2009;113(20):4992–5001.
10. Campo E, Swerdlow SH, Harris NL, Pileri S, Stein H, Jaffe ES. The 2008 WHO classification of lymphoid neoplasms and beyond: evolving concepts and practical applications. Blood. 2011;117(19):5019–32.
11. Ruf S, Moser O, Wössmann W, Kreyenberg H, Wagner HJ. Examining the origin of posttransplant lymphoproliferative disorder in a patient after a second allogeneic hematopoietic stem cell transplantation for relapsed BCR-ABL positive acute lymphoblastic leukemia. J Pediatr Hematol Oncol. 2011;33(1):50–4.
12. Smith JM, Corey L, Healey PJ, Davis CL, McDonald RA. Adolescents are more likely to develop posttransplant lymphoproliferative disorder after primary Epstein-Barr virus infection than younger renal transplant recipients. Transplantation. 2007;83(11):1423–8.
13. Brunstein CG, Weisdorf DJ, DeFor T, Barker JN, Tolar J, van Burik JA, et al. Marked increased risk of Epstein-Barr virus-related complications with the addition of antithymocyte globulin to a nonmyeloablative conditioning prior to unrelated umbilical cord blood transplantation. Blood. 2006;108(8):2874–80.
14. Cohen JM, Cooper N, Chakrabarti S, Thomson K, Samarasinghe S, Cubitt D, et al. EBV-related disease following haematopoietic stem cell transplantation with reduced intensity conditioning. Leuk Lymphoma. 2007;48(2):256–69.
15. Gottschalk S, Rooney CM, Heslop HE. Post-transplant lymphoproliferative disorders. Annu Rev Med. 2005;56:29–44.

16. Feng WH, Hong G, Delecluse HJ, Kenney SC. Lytic induction therapy for Epstein-Barr virus-positive B-cell lymphomas. J Virol. 2004;78(4):1893–902.
17. Rickinson A, Kieff E. Epstein-Barr virus. Field virology. Philadelphia: Lippincott Williams & Wilkins; 2001. p. 2511–73.
18. Al Hamed R, Bazarbachi AH, Mohty M. Epstein-Barr virus-related post-transplant lymphoproliferative disease (EBV-PTLD) in the setting of allogeneic stem cell transplantation: a comprehensive review from pathogenesis to forthcoming treatment modalities. Bone Marrow Transplant. 2019;55(1):25–39.
19. Loren AW, Porter DL, Stadtmauer EA, Tsai DE. Post-transplant lymphoproliferative disorder: a review. Bone Marrow Transplant. 2003;31(3):145–55.
20. Fujimoto A, Hiramoto N, Yamasaki S, Inamoto Y, Uchida N, Maeda T, et al. Risk factors and predictive scoring system for post-transplant lymphoproliferative disorder after hematopoietic stem cell transplantation. Biol Blood Marrow Transplant. 2019;25(7):1441–9.
21. Dierickx D, Tousseyn T, Gheysens O. How I treat posttransplant lymphoproliferative disorders. Blood. 2015;126(20):2274–83.
22. Semenova T, Lupo J, Alain S, Perrin-Confort G, Grossi L, Dimier J, et al. Multicenter evaluation of whole-blood Epstein-Barr viral load standardization using the WHO international standard. J Clin Microbiol. 2016;54(7):1746–50.
23. Styczynski J, van der Velden W, Fox CP, Engelhard D, de la Camara R, Cordonnier C, et al. Management of Epstein-Barr Virus infections and post-transplant lymphoproliferative disorders in patients after allogeneic hematopoietic stem cell transplantation: Sixth European Conference on Infections in Leukemia (ECIL-6) guidelines. Haematologica. 2016;101(7):803–11.
24. Kanakry JA, Hegde AM, Durand CM, Massie AB, Greer AE, Ambinder RF, et al. The clinical significance of EBV DNA in the plasma and peripheral blood mononuclear cells of patients with or without EBV diseases. Blood. 2016;127(16):2007–17.
25. Hakim H, Gibson C, Pan J, Srivastava K, Gu Z, Bankowski MJ, et al. Comparison of various blood compartments and reporting units for the detection and quantification of Epstein-Barr virus in peripheral blood. J Clin Microbiol. 2007;45(7):2151–5.
26. Liu Q, Xuan L, Liu H, Huang F, Zhou H, Fan Z, et al. Molecular monitoring and stepwise preemptive therapy for Epstein-Barr virus viremia after allogeneic stem cell transplantation. Am J Hematol. 2013;88(7):550–5.
27. van Esser JW, Niesters HG, van der Holt B, Meijer E, Osterhaus AD, Gratama JW, et al. Prevention of Epstein-Barr virus-lymphoproliferative disease by molecular monitoring and preemptive rituximab in high-risk patients after allogeneic stem cell transplantation. Blood. 2002;99(12):4364–9.
28. van der Velden WJ, Mori T, Stevens WB, de Haan AF, Stelma FF, Blijlevens NM, et al. Reduced PTLD-related mortality in patients experiencing EBV infection following allo-SCT after the introduction of a protocol incorporating pre-emptive rituximab. Bone Marrow Transplant. 2013;48(11):1465–71.
29. Worth A, Conyers R, Cohen J, Jagani M, Chiesa R, Rao K, et al. Pre-emptive rituximab based on viraemia and T cell reconstitution: a highly effective strategy for the prevention of Epstein-Barr virus-associated lymphoproliferative disease following stem cell transplantation. Br J Haematol. 2011;155(3):377–85.
30. Carpenter B, Haque T, Dimopoulou M, Atkinson C, Roughton M, Grace S, et al. Incidence and dynamics of Epstein-Barr virus reactivation after alemtuzumab-based conditioning for allogeneic hematopoietic stem-cell transplantation. Transplantation. 2010;90(5):564–70.
31. Petropoulou AD, Porcher R, de Latour RP, Xhaard A, Weisdorf D, Ribaud P, et al. Increased infection rate after preemptive rituximab treatment for Epstein-Barr virus reactivation after allogeneic hematopoietic stem-cell transplantation. Transplantation. 2012;94(8):879–83.
32. McIver Z, Stephens N, Grim A, Barrett AJ. Rituximab administration within 6 months of T cell-depleted allogeneic SCT is associated with prolonged life-threatening cytopenias. Biol Blood Marrow Transplant. 2010;16(11):1549–56.

33. Heslop HE, Brenner MK, Rooney CM. Donor T cells to treat EBV-associated lymphoma. N Engl J Med. 1994;331(10):679–80.
34. O'Reilly RJ, Small TN, Papadopoulos E, Lucas K, Lacerda J, Koulova L. Biology and adoptive cell therapy of Epstein-Barr virus-associated lymphoproliferative disorders in recipients of marrow allografts. Immunol Rev. 1997;157:195–216.
35. Papadopoulos EB, Ladanyi M, Emanuel D, Mackinnon S, Boulad F, Carabasi MH, et al. Infusions of donor leukocytes to treat Epstein-Barr virus-associated lymphoproliferative disorders after allogeneic bone marrow transplantation. N Engl J Med. 1994;330(17):1185–91.
36. Doubrovina E, Oflaz-Sozmen B, Prockop SE, Kernan NA, Abramson S, Teruya-Feldstein J, et al. Adoptive immunotherapy with unselected or EBV-specific T cells for biopsy-proven EBV+ lymphomas after allogeneic hematopoietic cell transplantation. Blood. 2012;119(11):2644–56.
37. Rooney CM, Smith CA, Ng CY, Loftin SK, Sixbey JW, Gan Y, et al. Infusion of cytotoxic T cells for the prevention and treatment of Epstein-Barr virus-induced lymphoma in allogeneic transplant recipients. Blood. 1998;92(5):1549–55.
38. Leen AM, Myers GD, Sili U, Huls MH, Weiss H, Leung KS, et al. Monoculture-derived T lymphocytes specific for multiple viruses expand and produce clinically relevant effects in immunocompromised individuals. Nat Med. 2006;12(10):1160–6.
39. Heslop HE, Slobod KS, Pule MA, Hale GA, Rousseau A, Smith CA, et al. Long-term outcome of EBV-specific T-cell infusions to prevent or treat EBV-related lymphoproliferative disease in transplant recipients. Blood. 2010;115(5):925–35.
40. Leen AM, Christin A, Myers GD, Liu H, Cruz CR, Hanley PJ, et al. Cytotoxic T lymphocyte therapy with donor T cells prevents and treats adenovirus and Epstein-Barr virus infections after haploidentical and matched unrelated stem cell transplantation. Blood. 2009;114(19):4283–92.
41. Papadopoulou A, Gerdemann U, Katari UL, Tzannou I, Liu H, Martinez C, et al. Activity of broad-spectrum T cells as treatment for AdV, EBV, CMV, BKV, and HHV6 infections after HSCT. Sci Transl Med. 2014;6(242):242ra83.
42. Leen AM, Bollard CM, Mendizabal AM, Shpall EJ, Szabolcs P, Antin JH, et al. Multicenter study of banked third-party virus-specific T cells to treat severe viral infections after hematopoietic stem cell transplantation. Blood. 2013;121(26):5113–23.
43. Icheva V, Kayser S, Wolff D, Tuve S, Kyzirakos C, Bethge W, et al. Adoptive transfer of Epstein-Barr virus (EBV) nuclear antigen 1-specific t cells as treatment for EBV reactivation and lymphoproliferative disorders after allogeneic stem-cell transplantation. J Clin Oncol. 2013;31(1):39–48.
44. Uhlin M, Gertow J, Uzunel M, Okas M, Berglund S, Watz E, et al. Rapid salvage treatment with virus-specific T cells for therapy-resistant disease. Clin Infect Dis. 2012;55(8):1064–73.
45. McLaughlin LP, Bollard CM, Keller MD. Adoptive T cell therapy for Epstein-Barr virus complications in patients with primary immunodeficiency disorders. Front Immunol. 2018;9:556.
46. Neudorfer J, Schmidt B, Huster KM, Anderl F, Schiemann M, Holzapfel G, et al. Reversible HLA multimers (Streptamers) for the isolation of human cytotoxic T lymphocytes functionally active against tumor- and virus-derived antigens. J Immunol Methods. 2007;320(1–2):119–31.
47. Feucht J, Joachim L, Lang P, Feuchtinger T. Adoptive T-cell transfer for refractory viral infections with cytomegalovirus, Epstein-Barr virus or adenovirus after allogeneic stem cell transplantation. Klin Padiatr. 2013;225(3):164–9.
48. Hanley PJ, Melenhorst JJ, Nikiforow S, Scheinberg P, Blaney JW, Demmler-Harrison G, et al. CMV-specific T cells generated from naive T cells recognize atypical epitopes and may be protective in vivo. Sci Transl Med. 2015;7(285):285ra63.
49. Abraham AA, John TD, Keller MD, Cruz CRN, Salem B, Roesch L, et al. Safety and feasibility of virus-specific T cells derived from umbilical cord blood in cord blood transplant recipients. Blood Adv. 2019;3(14):2057–68.
50. Haque T, Wilkie GM, Jones MM, Higgins CD, Urquhart G, Wingate P, et al. Allogeneic cytotoxic T-cell therapy for EBV-positive posttransplantation lymphoproliferative disease: results of a phase 2 multicenter clinical trial. Blood. 2007;110(4):1123–31.

51. Eiz-Vesper B, Maecker-Kolhoff B, Blasczyk R. Adoptive T-cell immunotherapy from third-party donors: characterization of donors and set up of a T-cell donor registry. Front Immunol. 2012;3:410.
52. Vickers MA, Wilkie GM, Robinson N, Rivera N, Haque T, Crawford DH, et al. Establishment and operation of a Good Manufacturing Practice-compliant allogeneic Epstein-Barr virus (EBV)-specific cytotoxic cell bank for the treatment of EBV-associated lymphoproliferative disease. Br J Haematol. 2014;167(3):402–10.
53. Tzannou I, Papadopoulou A, Naik S, Leung K, Martinez CA, Ramos CA, et al. Off-the-shelf virus-specific T cells to treat BK virus, human herpesvirus 6, cytomegalovirus, Epstein-Barr virus, and adenovirus infections after allogeneic hematopoietic stem-cell transplantation. J Clin Oncol. 2017;35(31):3547–57.
54. Quach DH, Becerra-Dominguez L, Rouce RH, Rooney CM. A strategy to protect off-the-shelf cell therapy products using virus-specific T-cells engineered to eliminate alloreactive T-cells. J Transl Med. 2019;17(1):240.
55. Brewin J, Mancao C, Straathof K, Karlsson H, Samarasinghe S, Amrolia PJ, et al. Generation of EBV-specific cytotoxic T cells that are resistant to calcineurin inhibitors for the treatment of posttransplantation lymphoproliferative disease. Blood. 2009;114(23):4792–803.
56. De Angelis B, Dotti G, Quintarelli C, Huye LE, Zhang L, Zhang M, et al. Generation of Epstein-Barr virus-specific cytotoxic T lymphocytes resistant to the immunosuppressive drug tacrolimus (FK506). Blood. 2009;114(23):4784–91.
57. Gea-Banacloche JC. Rituximab-associated infections. Semin Hematol. 2010;47(2):187–98.

Part IV

Organ Specific Considerations and Patient Outcomes

Organ-Specific Issues of PTLD – Kidney

16

Sophie Caillard and Britta Höcker

Core Messages

- The incidence of PTLD in adult kidney transplant recipients is relatively low: 0.4% at 1 year, 1% at 5 years, and 2% after 10 years.
- In children, the incidence of PTLD is higher due to a higher rate of EBV naivety at transplantation.
- Risk factors of PTLD in kidney transplant recipients are principally EBV seronegativity and high levels of immunosuppression.
- Clinical presentation is heterogeneous, but PTLD could arise in kidney allograft in about 15% of cases and be of donor cell origin in this particular case.
- Treatment begins by immunosuppression tapering which is facilitated by the possibility of return to dialysis, and transplant nephrectomy is another option. Rituximab and chemotherapy are used in the second step but toxicity can be life-threatening. An experimental approach is EBV-specific T-cell therapy.
- In adults, prognosis is better when PTLD developed in graft kidney. For other localizations survival is between 40% and 60% after 5 years. Prognosis of PTLD in pediatric renal transplant recipients is better than in adults, with 5-year survival rates of 80%. Kidney retransplantation is possible after the cure of a previous PTLD, under specific conditions.

S. Caillard (✉)
Nephrology-Transplantation Department, Hôpitaux Universitaires de Strasbourg, Strasbourg, France
e-mail: sophie.caillard@chru-strasbourg.fr

B. Höcker
Department of Pediatrics I, University Children's Hospital of Heidelberg, Heidelberg, Germany
e-mail: Britta.Hoecker@med.uni-heidelberg.de

© Springer Nature Switzerland AG 2021
V. R. Dharnidharka et al. (eds.), *Post-Transplant Lymphoproliferative Disorders*,
https://doi.org/10.1007/978-3-030-65403-0_16

Post-transplant lymphoproliferative disorders (PTLDs) are a rare but serious complication after renal transplantation. The risk of developing PTLD in kidney transplant recipients is approximately 20-fold greater than the risk of lymphoma development in the general population. Several characteristics of PTLD occurring after kidney transplantation are common with other organs, but some are specific of kidney recipients in terms of incidence, clinical features, treatment, and outcome.

Epidemiology

The incidence of PTLD in kidney recipients is relatively low compared to heart, heart-lung, lung, or intestine recipients [1, 2]. The lower incidence observed in kidney transplantation might be explained by two points: (i) the need of fewer immunosuppression in kidney than lung or heart transplant recipients and (ii) the presence of less "donor passenger lymphocytes" in renal tissue than in lung or intestine organs. In adult kidney recipients, the PTLD incidence ranges from 0.3% to 0.5% at 1 year post-transplantation, around 1% after 5 years, and 2% after 10 years [2–6]. The risk of lymphoma is higher during the first post-transplant year, after which the annual incidence decreases from the second to the seventh post-transplant year and rises again later on, displaying a bimodal distribution [6, 7]. In children, the incidence is higher, and PTLD is the most common malignancy after pediatric kidney transplantation. According to a prospective, multicenter study among 106 pediatric renal transplant recipients, 2.8% of patients developed PTLD in the first year post-transplant [8]. In a recent US cohort, the incidence amounted to 2.2% at 5 years after transplantation [9]. It may even reach 5–10% in some series especially in pediatric recipients treated with more potent immunosuppression [10–13]. This higher frequency in children is explained by a high rate of EBV seronegativity leading to EBV primo-infection and secondary uncontrolled lymphoid proliferation. About 80% of PTLDs in childhood are EBV-associated. In a prospective study, about 41% of pediatric kidney allograft recipients were EBV-naïve at the time of transplantation, and 34% of patients had a so-called high-risk serostatus (EBV-D+/R-) [8]. Besides contracting EBV primary infection via the transplant organ, community-acquired infection, usually during adolescence, is seen. Transmission is also possible when non-leukoreduced blood products are used.

Risk factors for lymphoma in kidney transplant recipients are EBV seromismatch between donor and recipient and recipient's EBV naivety, cytomegalovirus coinfection, younger patient age, intensity of induction of immunosuppressive therapy (T-cell-depleting agents thymoglobulin, alemtuzumab, and OKT3), duration of maintenance therapy (including therapy of graft rejection episodes), calcineurin inhibitor and sirolimus-based immunosuppression [2, 14–19], and costimulatory blockade agent belatacept in EBV-negative recipients [20]. The local immune response against the transplanted organ plays an important role in the cellular dysregulation process that results in lymphomas, and HLA mismatches could be involved in the development of PTLD [21].

Clinical Presentation

The clinical presentation of PTLD is heterogeneous and sometimes nonspecific: it ranges from asymptomatic disease, discovered on a graft biopsy to a fulminant disorder. PTLD development in nodal and extranodal sites (lung, intestine) is common, often presenting with unspecific clinical signs such as fever, tonsillitis, pharyngitis, anorexia, diarrhea, and anemia [22, 23].

Nevertheless, clinical presentation can take particular patterns in kidney transplant recipients, particularly if lymphoma occurs in the allograft. A hilar tumor can be responsible for vascular compression or ureteric obstruction revealed by hydronephrosis and/or acute renal failure [24, 25]. Infiltration of kidney by the lymphoma can induce graft enlargement and creatinine elevation and mimic rejection. Sometimes, PTLD is fortuitously discovered on a systematic sonography. The differential diagnosis of a mass adjacent to a renal allograft includes hematoma or lymphocele. CT scan or MRI could be helpful showing a mild contrast enhancement of a solid mass (Fig. 16.1).

The pathological differential diagnosis of renal PTLD is acute cellular rejection. Features that distinguish PTLD include a monomorphic infiltrate of lymphoblasts, patchy area of necrosis cells, and nodular aggregates of immature lymphoid cells with nuclear atypia. Immunostaining can be helpful, showing B-cell proliferation, whereas the presence of T cells suggests an acute rejection.

In the French Registry, 500 PTLDs occurring after kidney transplantation in adults were recorded during 10 years [6]. Sixty-two occurred in the grafted kidney (12%). The PTLDs confined to the graft were more likely early-onset lymphomas with a median diagnosis after transplantation of 33 months vs. 102 months for lymphomas localized outside the graft. In other words, 53% of intragraft lymphomas occurred during the first post-transplant year (vs. 9% for other localizations). More than 70% of the PTLDs that developed in the allograft kidney were only localized in the graft area. Acute renal failure was very frequent. It has been shown that

Fig. 16.1 CT scan showing a lymphoma localized in the renal hilum and infiltrating the graft parenchyma

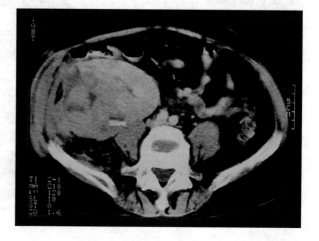

early-onset PTLDs, especially if localized near the graft kidney, are most often developed from donor passenger lymphocytes [26], conversely to the other PTLDs which are most likely of recipient origin [27]. Using fluorescence in situ hybridization and microsatellites analysis (Fig. 16.2), we showed in a French series that among 43 specimens of PTLD arising in kidney transplant recipients, 16 originated from donor cells and 27 from recipients' lymphocytes. Among the 21 graft PTLDs, a majority (67%) were of donor origin [28].

Finally, it seems that central nervous system lymphomas are more common after kidney transplantation than in general population and other organ transplant patients: 11–14% in kidney recipients vs. 3–4% in heart, heart-lung, and liver recipients in CTS report [2, 6]. In the French Registry, 14% of PTLDs were cerebral lymphomas, and the distribution of the other localizations is shown in Fig. 16.3 [6].

Fig. 16.2 Fluorescence in situ hybridization of the Y chromosome using CEP Y probes (satellite III) SpectrumGreen (Abbott, Wiesbaden, Germany) shows male tumor cells (yellow spots in red cells) in the renal allograft of female recipients (from Olagne [28])

Fig. 16.3 PTLD localizations in 500 patients of the French Kidney PTLD Registry, n=. GIT gastrointestinal tract [6]

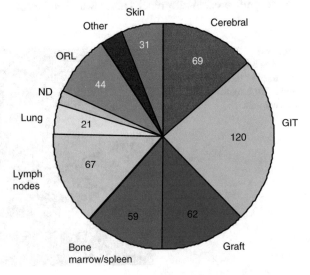

According to a report by the *North American Pediatric Renal Trials and Collaborative Studies* (NAPRTCS), in children PTLD location was distributed as follows: lymph node 59.8%, allograft 9.8%, central nervous system (CNS) 7.6%, and others 53.3% [29].

Therapeutic Aspects

Prevention

In high-risk EBV-mismatched patients, prophylaxis with anti-viral therapy, especially ganciclovir and its prodrug valganciclovir, has been proposed to reduce the risk of early-onset PTLD in kidney transplant recipients. Whereas some studies have shown a reduced incidence or a delay of EBV primary infection in patients receiving anti-viral prophylaxis [8], data on its impact on PTLD are controversial with positive results in a US case control study and a French retrospective cohort [30, 31], but negative in a recent meta-analysis combining nine studies [32].

Treatment

Management of lymphoma in kidney transplant recipients is easier than in other solid organ transplant patients because, unlike in vital organ recipients, the option of return to dialysis exists.

After lymphoma diagnosis, the first step is to reduce immunosuppression in order to reconstitute the immune system. Immunosuppression tapering is more comfortable in kidney recipients with PTLD, especially in early subsets of lymphoma (lymphoid hyperplasia or polymorphic lymphomas) [12]. For early or limited forms of PTLD, immunosuppression tapering could be progressive with careful monitoring of tumor size. Switching calcineurin inhibitors to mTOR inhibitors has been proposed because sirolimus and everolimus inhibit the in vitro proliferation of lymphoblastoid cells [33] and the growth of lymphoma in a mouse model [34]. Nevertheless, only few published cases showed regression of PTLD after switching from CNI to mTOR inhibitors as a single treatment. Furthermore, some studies from the United Network for Organ Sharing database observed unexpectedly that therapy using mTOR inhibitors was associated with a higher incidence of PTLD (RR × 2) especially in EBV-negative patients [17–19].

When reduction in immunosuppression fails, B-cell monoclonal therapy represents an attractive second-line therapeutic option because of its low toxicity. Rituximab was proposed after immunosuppression tapering, alone or in association with chemotherapy. Nevertheless, the results of a French multicenter trial assessing the efficacy of rituximab alone in PTLD were disappointing with only 44% responses in 55 SOT recipients and a 2-year actuarial survival lower than 30% [35, 36]. Hence, this strategy should be proposed in kidney transplant recipients with a good performance index and a non-aggressive form of PTLD only.

Nevertheless, the use of rituximab in combination with chemotherapy is currently the preferred treatment, especially in monomorphic PTLD, in T-cell PTLD, and in refractory patients to the first management approaches. Current therapeutic strategies are based on the injection of four doses of rituximab 1 week apart followed by a clinical reassessment. In patients achieving a remission, four additional rituximab doses are administered. In patients with disease progression, rituximab is associated with chemotherapy for 4–6 supplementary cycles, depending of the patient profile [37]. A similar approach is used in pediatric renal transplant recipients (Ped-PTLD registry, [38]).

Management of chemotherapy in kidney transplant recipients should be done with caution because of kidney dysfunction. Drug dosages must be adapted to glomerular filtration rate to avoid cumulative toxicity. In kidney transplant recipients treated by chemotherapy, toxic deaths are frequent and multifactorial: enhanced hematologic toxicity of drugs because of added myelotoxicity of immunosuppression, increased frequency and severity of infections, and accumulation of cytotoxic drugs in case of renal failure. In the French Registry, 18% of the deaths were of toxic origin. Low-dose chemotherapy has therefore been advocated in kidney transplant recipients with encouraging results [39, 40]. Advices to limit chemotherapy toxicity are the following: drastically reduce immunosuppression during chemotherapy, adapt cyclophosphamide dose to glomerular filtration rate, and systematic prophylactic use of G-CSF and clotrimazole.

In kidney transplant recipients, graft removal could be another therapeutic option. Graft nephrectomy can be proposed in case of severe graft dysfunction or when PTLD occurred in the graft. In the French Registry, graft was removed in 19 patients when lymphoma was localized in the graft (31%) leading to complete remission in all patients, at the cost of the loss of the kidney transplant [6]. On the other hand, graft loss is not the rule in patients with PTLD in whom the graft is left in place. Indeed, a recent report of the ANZDATA Registry showed that patients with PTLD did not display a decrease in graft survival after 10 years of follow-up [41].

Outcome and Prognostic Factors

In the *Collaborative Transplant Study* (CTS) report by Opelz et al., prognosis of kidney transplant patients with lymphoma was poor with a 5-year survival of 40% in the period 1995–2001 [2]. Patients' 5-year survival improved to 67% in the case of graft PTLD and decreased to 38% for patients with CNS lymphomas. In a report from the Israel Penn International Transplant Tumor Registry [42], factors negatively influencing kidney recipients' survival after PTLD were multiple sites and increasing age. Patients with graft involvement alone had better survival, especially if treated by transplant nephrectomy. In the French Registry, patients with PTLD had a 5-year survival rate of 53% and 10-year survival rate of 45%. Multivariable analyses revealed that an age >55 years, serum creatinine level >133 μmol/L, elevated lactate dehydrogenase levels, disseminated lymphoma, brain localization, invasion of serous membranes, monomorphic PTLD, and T-cell PTLD were independent prognostic indicators of poor survival [43].

In general, the prognosis of PTLD in children is better, with a 5-year survival rate of about 80–87% in pediatric kidney allograft recipients [29, 44]. However, CNS and bone marrow involvement is associated with poor survival [38]. In case of kidney graft lost, retransplantation after a PTLD is a possible option [45]. We described a series of 55 retransplantations in kidney transplant recipients with safe outcomes in terms of graft and patient survival and a very low risk of PTLD recurrence [46]. Some criteria have to be fulfilled to minimize recurrence: a 1–2 year observation period between PTLD and retransplantation depending on the widespread of the hematological disease, disappearance of monoclonal immunoglobulin, undetectable or low EBV viral load, and appearance of anti-EBNA IgG as this marker is linked to an effective cytotoxic response against EBV. After retransplantation, patients should be closely monitored, and appropriate adjustments of immunosuppression must be done in order to avoid overimmunosuppression.

Take-Home Pearls
- The incidence of PTLD in adult kidney transplant recipients is relatively low (1–1.5% at 5 years).
- The incidence of PTLD in pediatric renal transplant recipients is higher due to a higher proportion of patients with high-risk EBV serostatus.
- PTLD can be revealed by a graft dysfunction in kidney recipients.
- In adults, PTLD is often localized within or near the graft.
- Graft PTLD is more often of donor origin, developed during the first post-transplant year and localized in a single site. Its prognosis is better.
- Management of kidney transplant recipients with PTLD is easier because kidney is not a vital organ and management of immunosuppression tapering is facilitated.
- Prognosis of kidney transplant recipient is poor with a 40–60% survival after 5 years.
- Prognosis of PTLD in children is better with a 5-year survival rate of 80%.

References

1. Dharnidharka VR, Tejani AH, Ho PL, et al. Post-transplant lymphoproliferative disorder in the United States: young Caucasian males are at highest risk. Am J Transplant. 2002;2:993–8.
2. Opelz G, Dohler B. Lymphomas after solid organ transplantation: a collaborative transplant study report. Am J Transplant. 2004;4:222–30.
3. Kasiske BL, Snyder JJ, Gilbertson DT, et al. Cancer after kidney transplantation in the United States. Am J Transplant. 2004;4:905–13.
4. Caillard S, Dharnidharka V, Agodoa L, et al. Posttransplant lymphoproliferative disorders after renal transplantation in the United States in era of modern immunosuppression. Transplantation. 2005;80:1233–43.
5. Caillard S, Lelong C, Pessione F, et al. Post-transplant lymphoproliferative disorders occurring after renal transplantation in adults: report of 230 cases from the French Registry. Am J Transplant. 2006;6:2735–42.

6. Caillard S, Lamy FX, Quelen C, et al. Epidemiology of posttransplant lymphoproliferative disorders in adult kidney and kidney pancreas recipients: report of the French registry and analysis of subgroups of lymphomas. Am J Transplant. 2012;12:682–93.
7. Faull RJ, Hollett P, McDonald SP. Lymphoproliferative disease after renal transplantation in Australia and New Zealand. Transplantation. 2005;80:193–7.
8. Höcker B, Fickenscher H, Delecluse HJ, et al. Epidemiology and morbidity of Epstein-Barr virus infection in pediatric renal transplant recipients: a multicenter, prospective study. Clin Infect Dis. 2013;56:84–92.
9. Kotton CN, Huprikar S, Kumar S. Transplant infectious diseases: a review of the scientific registry of transplant patients published data. Am J Transplant. 2017;6:1–8.
10. Shapiro R, Nalesnik M, McCauley J, et al. Posttransplant lymphoproliferative disorders in adult and pediatric renal transplant patients receiving tacrolimus-based immunosuppression. Transplantation. 1999;68:1851–4.
11. Dharnidharka VR, Sullivan EK, Stablein DM, et al. Risk factors for posttransplant lymphoproliferative disorder (PTLD) in pediatric kidney transplantation: a report of the North American Pediatric Renal Transplant Cooperative Study (NAPRTCS). Transplantation. 2001;71:1065–8.
12. McDonald RA, Smith JM, Ho M, et al. Incidence of PTLD in pediatric renal transplant recipients receiving basiliximab, calcineurin inhibitor, sirolimus and steroids. Am J Transplant. 2008;8:984–9.
13. Dharnidharka VR, Ho PL, Stablein DM, Harmon WE, Tejani AH. Mycophenolate, tacrolimus and post-transplant lymphoproliferative disorder: a report of the North American Pediatric Renal Transplant Cooperative Study. Pediatr Transplant. 2002;6:396–9.
14. Absalon MJ, Khoury RA, Phillips CL. Post-transplant lymphoproliferative disorder after solid-organ transplant in children. Semin Pediatr Surg. 2017;26(4):257–66.
15. Opelz G, Naujokat C, Daniel V, et al. Disassociation between risk of graft loss and risk of non-Hodgkin lymphoma with induction agents in renal transplant recipients. Transplantation. 2003;81:1227–33.
16. Dierickx D, Habermann TM. Post-transplantation lymphoproliferative disorders in adults. N Engl J Med. 2018;378:549–62.
17. Sampaio MS, Cho YW, Shah T, Bunnapradist S, Hutchinson IV. Association of immunosuppressive maintenance regimens with posttransplant lymphoproliferative disorder in kidney transplant recipients. Transplantation. 2012;93:73–81.
18. Dharnidharka VR, Lamb KE, Gregg JA, Meier-Kriesche HU. Associations between EBV serostatus and organ transplant type in PTLD risk: an analysis of the SRTR National Registry Data in the United States. Am J Transplant. 2012;12:976–83.
19. Kirk AD, Cherikh WS, Ring M, et al. Dissociation of depletional induction and posttransplant lymphoproliferative disease in kidney recipients treated with alemtuzumab. Am J Transplant. 2007;7:2619–25.
20. Vincenti F, Larsen CP, Alberu J, et al. Three-year outcomes from BENEFIT, a randomized, active-controlled, parallel-group study in adult kidney transplant recipients. Am J Transplant. 2012;12:210–7.
21. Bakker NA, Van Imhoff GW, Verschuuren EA, et al. Early onset post-transplant lymphoproliferative disease is associated with allograft localization. Clin Transpl. 2005;19:327–34.
22. Allen UD, Preiksaitis JK. Post-transplant lymphoproliferative disorders, Epstein-Barr virus infection, and disease in solid organ transplantation: guidelines from the American Society of Transplantation Infectious Diseases Community of Practice; AST Infectious Diseases Community of Practice. Clin Transpl. 2019;23:e13652.
23. Green M. Michaels MG Epstein-Barr virus infection and posttransplant lymphoproliferative disorder. Am J Transplant. 2013;13(Suppl 3):41–54.
24. Hestin D, Claudon M, Champigneulles J, et al. Epstein-Barr-virus-associated post-transplant B-cell lymphoma presenting as allograft artery stenosis. Nephrol Dial Transplant. 1996;11:1164–7.

25. Kew CE, Lopez-Ben R, Smith JK, et al. Postransplant lymphoproliferative disorder localized near the allograft in renal transplantation. Transplantation. 2000;69:809–14.
26. Caillard S, Pencreach S, Braun L, et al. Simultaneous development of lymphoma in recipients of renal transplants from a single donor: donor origin confirmed by human leukocytes antigen staining and microsatellite analysis. Transplantation. 2005;79:79–84.
27. Petit B, Le Meur Y, Jaccard A, et al. Influence of host-recipient origin on clinical aspects of posttransplantation lymphoproliferative disorders in kidney transplantation. Transplantation. 2002;73:265–71.
28. Olagne J, Caillard S, Gaub MP, Chenard MP, Moulin B. Post-transplant lymphoproliferative disorders: determination of donor/recipient origin in a large cohort of kidney recipients. Am J Transplant. 2011;6:1260–9.
29. Dharnidharka VR, Martz KL, Stablein DM, Benfield MR. Improved survival with recent Post-Transplant Lymphoproliferative Disorder (PTLD) in children with kidney transplants. Am J Transplant. 2011;11:751–8.
30. Funch DP, Walker AM, Schneider G, et al. Ganciclovir and acyclovir reduce the risk of post-transplant lymphoproliferative disorder in renal transplant recipients. Am J Transplant. 2005;5:2894–900.
31. Ville S, Imbert Marcille BM, Coste Burel M, et al. Impact of antiviral prophylaxis in adults Epstein-Barr virus-seronegative kidney recipients on early and late post-transplantation lymphoproliferative disorder onset: a retrospective cohort study. Transplant Int. 2018;5:484–94.
32. AlDabbagh MA, Gitman MR, Kumar D, Humar A, Rotstein C, Husain S. The role of antiviral prophylaxis for the prevention of Epstein-Barr virus-associated posttransplant lymphoproliferative disease in solid organ transplant recipients: a systematic review. Am J Transplant. 2017;17:770–81.
33. Vaysberg M, Balatoni CE, Nepomuceno RR, et al. Rapamycin inhibits proliferation of Epstein-Barr virus-positive B-cell lymphomas through modulation of cell-cycle protein expression. Transplantation. 2007;83:1114–21.
34. Majewski M, Korecka M, Joergensen J, et al. Immunosuppressive TOR kinase inhibitor everolimus (RAD) suppresses growth of cells derived from posttransplant lymphoproliferative disorder at allograft-protecting doses. Transplantation. 2003;75:1710–7.
35. Choquet S, Leblond V, Herbrecht R, et al. Efficacy and safety of rituximab in B-cell post-transplantation lymphoproliferative disorders: results of a prospective multicenter phase 2 study. Blood. 2006;107:3053–7.
36. Choquet S, Oertel S, Leblond V, et al. Rituximab in the management of post-transplantation lymphoproliferative disorder after solid organ transplantation: proceed with caution. Ann Hematol. 2007;86:599–607.
37. Trappe R, Oertel S, Leblond V, et al. Sequential treatment with rituximab followed by CHOP chemotherapy in adult B-cell post-transplant lymphoproliferative disorder (PTLD): the prospective international multicentre phase 2 PTLD-1 trial. Lancet Oncol. 2012;13:196–206.
38. Maecker-Kolhoff B, Klein C. Das pädiatrische PTLD-Register (Ped-PTLD-Register). Der Nephrologe. 2009;4:339–44.
39. Fohrer C, Caillard S, Koumarianou A, et al. Long-term survival in post-transplant lymphoproliferative disorders with a dose-adjusted ACVBP regimen. Br J Haematol. 2006;134:602–12.
40. Gross TG, Hinrichs SH, Winner J, et al. Treatment of post-transplant lymphoproliferative disease (PTLD) following solid organ transplantation with low-dose chemotherapy. Ann Oncol. 1998;9:339–40.
41. Francis A, Johnson DW, Craig J, Teixeira-Pinto A, Wong G. Post-transplant lymphoproliferative disease may be an adverse risk factor for patient survival but not graft loss in kidney transplant recipients. Kidney Int. 2018;94:809–17.
42. Trofe J, Buell JF, Beebe TM, et al. Analysis of factors that influence survival in post-transplant lymphoproliferative disorder in renal transplant recipients: the Israel Penn Transplant Tumor Registry experience. Am J Transplant. 2005;5:775–80.

43. Caillard S, Porcher R, Provot F, et al. Post-transplantation lymphoproliferative disorder after kidney transplantation: report of a nationwide French registry and the development of a new prognostic score. J Clin Oncol. 2013;31:1302–9.
44. Gross TG, Orjuela MA, Perkins SL, et al. Low-dose chemotherapy and rituximab for post-transplant lymphoproliferative disease (PTLD): a Children's Oncology Group Report. Am J Transplant. 2012;12:3069–75.
45. Johnson SR, Cherikh WS, Kauffman HM, et al. Retransplantation after post-transplant lymphoproliferative disorders: an OPTN/UNOS database analysis. Am J Transplant. 2006;6:2743–9.
46. Caillard S, Cellot E, Dantal J, et al. A French cohort study of kidney retransplantation after post-transplant lymphoproliferative disorders. Clin J Am Soc Nephrol. 2017;12:1663–70.

Organ Specific Issues of PTLD – Liver

17

Françoise Smets and Carlos O. Esquivel

The incidence of post-transplant lymphoproliferative disorder (PTLD) following pediatric liver transplantation is decreasing, but it is still associated with significant morbidity and mortality. In children, PTLD mostly occurs early after transplant and is associated with Epstein-Barr virus (EBV). In adults, the incidence of PTLD is lower, frequently EBV negative, monomorphic, and of late onset. The risk factors for PTLD in children are young age, EBV seronegative status at the time of transplantation, and intense immunosuppression. The graft itself is often involved in the disease. The initial treatment consists of reduction of immunosuppression (RIS). Discontinuation of immunosuppression may be necessary in severe cases of PTLD, an approach that can be done in liver transplantation but not with other types of solid organ transplants, because the liver is more tolerogenic than other organs. Patients who are undergoing such treatment need careful surveillance for onset of acute cellular rejection. Some children stay off immunosuppression for years. Patients who experience rejection do respond well to corticosteroids, and fortunately, chronic rejection is rarely seen in this particular situation. Mortality has been reported as high as 60%, although it seems to be dropping in recent reports. Patients who do not respond to RIS or discontinuation of immunosuppression usually have monoclonal monomorphic PTLD and require a combination treatment with anti-CD20 antibodies and chemotherapy. The long-term outcomes of EBV PTLD after pediatric liver transplantation are unknown.

F. Smets (✉)
Pediatrics, Cliniques universitaires Saint-Luc – UCLouvain, Brussels, Belgium
e-mail: francoise.smets@uclouvain.be

C. O. Esquivel
Department of Surgery, Division of Abdominal Transplantation, Stanford School of Medicine, Stanford, CA, USA
e-mail: esquivel@standford.edu

© Springer Nature Switzerland AG 2021
V. R. Dharnidharka et al. (eds.), *Post-Transplant Lymphoproliferative Disorders*,
https://doi.org/10.1007/978-3-030-65403-0_17

PTLD remains a common and potentially fatal complication in liver transplant patients. The incidence is higher in children (3–20%, around maximum 10% since viral load quantification is available) than in adults (1–2%). Children who are very young at the time of transplant, with a seronegative EBV status and receiving liver graft from seropositive donor, are at higher risk to develop PTLD. Perhaps due to careful EBV surveillance with quantitative PCR, children are often diagnosed early, and consequently the PTLD is polymorphic, unlike adult patients who often present late and with EBV-negative monomorphic PTLD [1–5]. Other risk factors in children are intense immunosuppression, CMV infection, history of acute cellular rejection, and having received steroids before transplantation [1, 3]. Recently, food allergy has been reported as a potential risk factor for PTLD [6]. Hepatitis C has also been described as a risk factor in adults [3]. Hepatitis C is extremely rare in children. In a case-control study of adult transplant patients, including 60 late-onset PTLD and 166 matched controls, circulating donor-specific antibodies were inversely correlated to the risk of developing PTLD. As those antibodies could be a sign of insufficient immunosuppression, this underlies again the role of inappropriate immunosuppression in the pathogenesis of PTLD [7].

Fever, lymph nodes enlargement, and splenomegaly are common symptoms of PTLD including in recipients of liver transplantation. Multi-organ involvement is common, with frequent infiltration of the liver graft and/or the gastrointestinal tract. Anemia, neutropenia, hypoalbuminemia, and hypergammaglobulinemia are also commonly observed. If PTLD occurs in the context of EBV primary infection, tonsillitis is the most common clinical presentation, while later presentation may include laryngeal lymphoproliferation [5, 6, 8]. More than 80% of PTLD are of B-cell origin, most of them being EBV+. T-cell PTLD is described in about 15%, and among those, only 30% are EBV induced. Globally, EBV negative PTLD usually occurs late and displays aggressive clinical behavior and monomorphic histology. The prognosis is poor [1].

The first large series of PTLD in pediatric liver transplant recipients described 36 cases of PTLD [9]. All received anti-viral therapy (ganciclovir, acyclovir, or both). The immunosuppression was discontinued in 33 patients, and the remaining 3 underwent RIS. Interferon and/or chemotherapy was added in six patients. Three patients required surgery. PTLD-related survival was 86%; acute rejection was observed in 23 children with a median of 24 days. Two of these patients developed chronic rejection and one required retransplantation. Relapse of PTLD was observed in two cases. Of the 33 patients without immunosuppression, tacrolimus was restarted as monotherapy in 14 and in combination with corticosteroids in 8. Six children remained off immunosuppression. Other series are summarized in Table 17.1.

RIS is usually the first step of therapy [1, 15] (Table 17.1). Because of significant mortality, and as the liver is known to be more immunotolerant than other organs, complete immunosuppression withdrawal has been proposed in liver transplanted patients with PTLD, at least those associated with EBV [11, 15]. Most of the time corticosteroids are maintained as the only immunosuppressant. Transaminases should be carefully followed as acute rejection occurs in 60–74% of patients and

Table 17.1 PTLD in liver transplanted patients[a]

References	PTLD (n)	Population	RIS	Anti-viral γglob	Rituximab	Chemotherapy Radiotherapy	Surgery	Overall survival	Rejection/graft loss
[10]	78	Children	78	na	na	na	na	60%*	na
[11]	19	Children	19	19	2	2	–	68.4%	10/1
[12]	8	Children	6	–	2	1	–	63%	1/–
[13]	75	Children	na	na	na	na	na	93%*	na/7
[14]	18	Children	15	na	6	1	–	77.8%	9/–
[5]	45	Adults	30	na	24	27	–	71%	na/4

[a]Overall survival is survival related to PTLD when available. If not available, global survival is given and marked with an *

na not available

may evolve to chronic rejection, although rarely. Graft loss is described in 3–17% of cases [15]. Immunosuppression will be restarted in case of biopsy-proven rejection. The role of switching to immunosuppressive medications other than calcineurin inhibitors (e.g., mTor inhibitors) remains unclear. The use of antiviral medication is also a topic of debate, and surgery is seldom needed [2, 15]. Indications for rituximab or chemotherapy do not differ from other types of organ transplantation and such therapies are used after failure of RIS. Rituximab may lead to long-term hypoglobulinemia and higher rates of bacterial infections [16]. The management of PTLD in SOT recipients is reviewed in detail in Chap. 10.

Since quantitative measurement of EBV load is available, the possibility of preventing PTLD by early RIS has also been studied. Caution should be applied as we know that sensitivity of high viral load to detect PTLD is excellent, but specificity is around 50% [1]. This specificity can be improved by correlating the viral load to the EBV-specific immune response, but those tests are not yet standardized and not easily available for routine follow-up [17]. Chronic high viral load carriers exist, especially in children who may never develop EBV-related complications [1, 18]. In a study of pediatric liver transplant recipients, 43 were monitored for EBV in peripheral blood mononuclear cells. In 11 children the immunosuppression was tapered (tacrolimus trough 4–6 ng/mL and discontinuation of steroids) for high viral load [19]. Only one of them experienced acute cellular rejection. PTLD incidence was 2% among the entire series as compared to 16% in a historical control group of 30 children. Hence, RIS seems to be safe in most of pediatric liver transplant recipients; however, EBV may remain detectable even in those patients getting no immunosuppression [18]. The prevention of EBV disease and PTLD is discussed in detail in Chap. 11.

References

1. Kamdar KY, Rooney CM, Heslop HE. Posttransplant lymphoproliferative disease following liver transplantation. Curr Opin Organ Transplant. 2011;16(3):274–80.
2. Lauro A, Arpinati M, Pinna AD. Managing the challenge of PTLD in liver and bowel transplant recipients. Br J Haematol. 2015;169(2):157–72.
3. Aucejo F, Rofaiel G, Miller C. Who is at risk for post-transplant lymphoproliferative disorders (PTLD) after liver transplantation? J Hepatol. 2006;44(1):19–23.
4. Smets F, Sokal EM. Epstein-Barr virus-related lymphoproliferation in children after liver transplant: role of immunity, diagnosis, and management. Pediatr Transplant. 2002;6(4):280–7.
5. Fararjeh FA, Mahmood S, Tachtatzis P, Yallop D, Devereux S, Patten P, Agrawal K, Suddle A, O'Grady J, Heaton N, Marcus R, Kassam S. A retrospective analysis of post-transplant lymphoproliferative disorder following liver transplantation. Eur J Haematol. 2018;100(1):98–103.
6. Simakachorn L, Tanpowpong P, Lertudomphonwanit C, Anurathapan U, Pakakasama S, Hongeng S, Treepongkaruna S, Phuapradit P. Various initial presentations of Epstein-Barr virus infection-associated post-transplant lymphoproliferative disorder in pediatric liver transplantation recipients: case series and literature review. Pediatr Transplant. 2019;23(2):e13357.
7. Engels EA, Jennings LW, Everly MJ, Landgren O, Murata K, Yanik EL, Pfeiffer RM, Onaca N, Klintmalm GB. Donor-specific antibodies, immunoglobulin-free light chains, and BAFF levels in relation to risk of late-onset PTLD in liver recipients. Transplant Direct. 2018;4(6):e353.

8. Smets F, Sokal EM. Lymphoproliferation in children after liver transplantation. J Pediatr Gastroenterol Nutr. 2002;34(5):499–505.
9. Cacciarelli TV, Green M, Jaffe R, Mazariegos GV, Jain A, Fung JJ, Reyes J. Management of posttransplant lymphoproliferative disease in pediatric liver transplant recipients receiving primary tacrolimus (FK506) therapy. Transplantation. 1998;66(8):1047–52.
10. Jain A, Nalesnik M, Reyes J, Pokharna R, Mazariegos G, Green M, Eghtesad B, Marsh W, Cacciarelli T, Fontes P, Abu-Elmagd K, Sindhi R, Demetris J, Fung J. Posttransplant lymphoproliferative disorders in liver transplantation: a 20-year experience. Ann Surg. 2002;236(4):429–36; discussion 436–7.
11. Hurwitz M, Desai DM, Cox KL, Berquist WE, Esquivel CO, Millan MT. Complete immunosuppressive withdrawal as a uniform approach to post-transplant lymphoproliferative disease in pediatric liver transplantation. Pediatr Transplant. 2004;8(3):267–72.
12. Uribe M, Hunter B, Alba A, Calabrán L, Flores L, Soto P, Herzog C. Posttransplant lymphoproliferative disorder in pediatric liver transplantation. Transplant Proc. 2009;41(6):2679–81.
13. Narkewicz MR, Green M, Dunn S, Millis M, McDiarmid S, Mazariegos G, Anand R, Yin W, Studies of Pediatric Liver Transplantation Research Group. Decreasing incidence of symptomatic Epstein-Barr virus disease and posttransplant lymphoproliferative disorder in pediatric liver transplant recipients: report of the studies of pediatric liver transplantation experience. Liver Transpl. 2013;19(7):730–40.
14. Huang JG, Tan MYQ, Quak SH. Aw MM. Risk factors and clinical outcomes of pediatric liver transplant recipients with post-transplant lymphoproliferative disease in a multi-ethnic Asian cohort. Transpl Infect Dis. 2018;20(1):e12798.
15. Dufour JF, Fey MF. What is the current treatment of PTLD after liver transplantation? J Hepatol. 2006;44(1):23–6.
16. Chiou FK, Beath SV, Patel M, Gupte GL. Hypogammaglobulinemia and bacterial infections following pediatric post-transplant lymphoproliferative disorder in the rituximab era. Pediatr Transplant. 2019;17:e13519.
17. Smets F, Latinne D, Bazin H, Reding R, Otte JB, Buts JP, Sokal EM. Ratio between Epstein-Barr viral load and anti-Epstein-Barr virus specific T-cell response as a predictive marker of posttransplant lymphoproliferative disease. Transplantation. 2002;73(10):1603–10.
18. Kullberg-Lindh C, Saalman R, Olausson M, Herlenius G, Lindh M. Epstein-Barr virus DNA monitoring in serum and whole blood in pediatric liver transplant recipients who do or do not discontinue immunosuppressive therapy. Pediatr Transplant. 2017;21(5):e12875.
19. Lee TC, Savoldo B, Rooney CM, Heslop HE, Gee AP, Caldwell Y, Barshes NR, Scott JD, Bristow LJ, O'Mahony CA, Goss JA. Quantitative EBV viral loads and immunosuppression alterations can decrease PTLD incidence in pediatric liver transplant recipients. Am J Transplant. 2005;5(9):2222–8.

PTLD in Intestinal Transplant Recipients

18

Ajai Khanna and George V. Mazariegos

Introduction

Small bowel-containing allografts can be transplanted alone or in combination with other visceral organs [1]. Combinations of other organs that are commonly transplanted with small bowel include the liver and pancreas (liver, pancreas, small bowel transplantation); pancreas alone (small bowel, pancreas transplant); stomach, duodenum, and pancreas (modified multivisceral transplant); or stomach, liver, and pancreas (multivisceral transplant). Any one of the above combinations may include donor colon depending on whether the recipient has any native healthy colon remaining. A total of 4130 intestinal transplants (ITx) have been reported to the Intestinal Transplant Registry (ITR) since 1985 (Table 18.1).

Indications for Intestinal Transplantation

Common indications for ITx include short-gut syndromes, motility disorders, mucosal defects, vascular accidents, and tumors. Liver is included as part of the visceral allograft more commonly in pediatric recipients. With advances in immunosuppression and close monitoring of these patients, 1- and 5-year graft survivals have improved over time and ITx has become an established treatment for patients with nutritional failure and short-gut syndrome.

A. Khanna · G. V. Mazariegos (✉)
Division of Transplant Surgery, UPMC Children's Hospital of Pittsburgh,
Pittsburgh, PA, USA

Department of Surgery, University of Pittsburgh School of Medicine, Pittsburgh, PA, USA
e-mail: Ajai.Khanna@pitt.edu; George.mazariegos@chp.edu

© Springer Nature Switzerland AG 2021
V. R. Dharnidharka et al. (eds.), *Post-Transplant Lymphoproliferative Disorders*,
https://doi.org/10.1007/978-3-030-65403-0_18

Table 18.1 Global clinical experience: intestinal transplant

All recipients transplanted between January 1985 and December 2108	
Number of transplants	4103
Small bowel alone	1842
Small bowel + liver	1251
Multivisceral transplant	810
Modified multivisceral transplant	200
Current survivors	2060/4130 (50%)
Intestinal Transplant Registry Report 2019	

Pediatric Small bowel donors are associated
with a large lymphoid burden

Pediatric   Adult

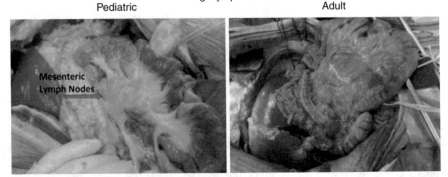

Fig. 18.1 Mesenteric lymphoid burden in pediatric and adult donors

Epidemiology and PTLD Incidence in Intestinal Transplant Patients

Immunosuppression used to promote allograft acceptance compromises immune function. This creates a milieu whereby EBV-infected B cells can result in a proliferative process that can range from non-destructive lymphoid infiltrates to a full-blown monomorphic post-transplant lymphoproliferative disorder (PTLD). The intestinal allograft, whether transplanted alone or in combination with other organs, comes with a large allogeneic lymphoid tissue burden which is unique to ITx and predisposes recipients to lymphoid malignancies like PTLD [2]. This lymphoid mass is greater in allografts from pediatric compared to adult donors and may be one of the reasons why pediatric recipients have a higher incidence of PTLD than adults (Fig. 18.1). Other reasons for the difference between pediatric and adult ITx recipients include a high frequency of recipients who are EBV naïve in this age population and the need for potent immunosuppression given their strong immune system and inherent immunogenicity of small bowel allograft. Of note, the incidence of EBV-associated PTLD in EBV-seropositive ITx recipients (at least pediatric recipients) is higher than seen in EBV-seropositive recipients of other organ types. The explanation for this observation is unknown as of this time.

The incidence of PTLD following ITx is higher compared to other solid organ transplants given the increased lymphoid allograft burden and enhanced immuno-suppression. Although 80% of PTLD lesions are EBV positive, EBV-negative PTLD lesions do occur in ITx recipients [2, 3].

The incidence of PTLD following ITx has been reported to be between 9% in the current series to 30% in older reports [4–8]. Of recipients who underwent transplant between 2005 and 2015, 9.6% of intestine recipients and 6.9% of intestine-liver recipients developed post-transplant lymphoproliferative disorder within 5 years post-transplant. Incidence was highest among recipients who were negative for Epstein-Barr virus (EBV) (11.6% of intestine recipients) [9]. While the incidence of PTLD after ITx is greater in children than adults, the SRTR report does not provide comparative data between these patient populations. Data from the UPMC Children's Hospital of Pittsburgh identifies that 59/259 (22.7%) children receiving 62 ITx between 1990 and 2019 developed PTLD. Thirty (51%) patients developed PTLD in allograft alone, 17 (20%) in allograft and native organs, and 17 (29%) in native organs (Fig. 18.2). Affected native organs included tonsils, lymph nodes, breast, bone marrow, GI tract, liver, brain, larynx, lung, and kidney.

Twenty-four of the 59 patients are alive. Of these 14 are nutritionally independent, 5 had to be started on TPN and still have the graft, and 7 underwent allograft enterectomy due to rejection when immunosuppression was reduced upon discovery of PTLD, of whom 5 are back on TPN. In another report, long-term therapeutic effects of visceral transplantation in adult and pediatric recipients were reported by the Pittsburgh group. 227 patients who survived 5 years following visceral transplantation were analyzed [10, 11]. PTLD developed at a significantly higher rate in pediatric patients compared to adults. PTLD accounted for 14/149 deaths within 5 years and 1/39 deaths between 5 and 10 years post-transplantation. Risk factors for the development of PTLD in ITx recipients include age, EBV status, splenectomy in the recipient, and immunosuppression.

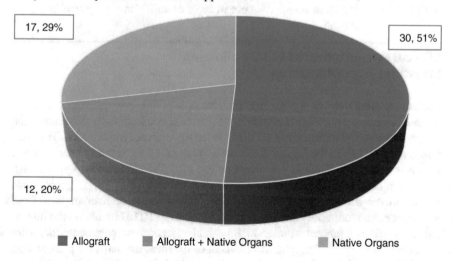

Fig. 18.2 PTLD sites following ITx at Children's Hospital of Pittsburgh 1990–2019 (*n* = 59)

The above reports describe long-term experience with PTLD in ITx recipients. However, the incidence rate of PTLD in ITx recipients has declined over time. While rates as high as 30% were noted in older reports, the incidence rate in the current series is around 9% [4–8]. The decrease in incidence of PTLD over time may be due to the clinical availability and use of EBV viral load monitoring in the blood using quantitative polymerase chain reaction (PCR) assays since the mid-1990s. The use of viral load monitoring transformed management of these patients as rising viral loads prompted clinicians to preemptively reduce immunosuppression to restore T cell defense mechanisms. An alternative explanation for the reduced incidence of PTLD in ITx recipients over time may be the evolution of immunosuppression management in this patient cohort. A report from the University of Pittsburgh reviewed 500 ITx performed between 1990 and 2008 in 453 patients (adults and children) [10]. Based on the type of immunosuppression, patients were classified as having been transplanted in Eras I–III. The combination of tacrolimus and steroids was the primary immunosuppressive regimen used in Era I followed by the addition of induction therapy, initially with cyclophosphamide but then with daclizumab, to the tacrolimus-steroid combination in Era II. A recipient preconditioning protocol with antithymocyte globulin and later alemtuzumab combined with minimal post-transplant immunosuppression was initiated during Era III. A total of 57 patients (41 pediatric and 16 adults) developed PTLD during the three eras. Cumulative PTLD-free survival was significantly greater ($P < 0.001$) in Era III compared to patients in other groups, with no instance of PTLD development beyond the fourth postoperative year. The 5-year PTLD-free survivals in Eras I–III were 64%, 81%, and 93%, respectively (Fig. 18.3). Immunosuppression, recipient age, and splenectomy were shown to be significant risk factors for the development of PTLD in this series. The reduction in PTLD incidence in Era III contributed to the overall improved patient and graft survival in this era. However, use of alemtuzumab in pediatric patients at our center was associated with a spike in the incidence of PTLD which led us to abandon its use in favor of antithymocyte globulin.

Clinical Presentation of PTLD Following Intestinal Transplantation

Pediatric patients are at a high risk of developing PTLD within the first post-transplant year. Early PTLD is commonly extranodal and frequently develops in the allograft compared to late onset PTLD that mostly affects lymph nodes. The sites affected by PTLD in the UPMC Children's Hospital of Pittsburgh experience are shown in Fig. 18.2. Clinical presentations can also include tonsillar hypertrophy, mucosal ulcers, nodular lesions on the stomal mucosa (Fig. 18.4), lymph node masses in the neck or axilla, skin nodules, lung nodules, or liver masses. CNS lesions occur uncommonly and can present as seizures. PTLD involving the intestinal allograft can present similar to intestinal rejection or gastroenteritis, with increased stoma or stool output. Involvement of the intestine may also present with protein-losing enteropathy, acute abdomen, intestinal obstruction, or intestinal perforation [7]. A rare syndrome, *fulminant PTLD*, characterized by intestinal fluid losses in association with a shock-like picture leading to multisystem organ failure,

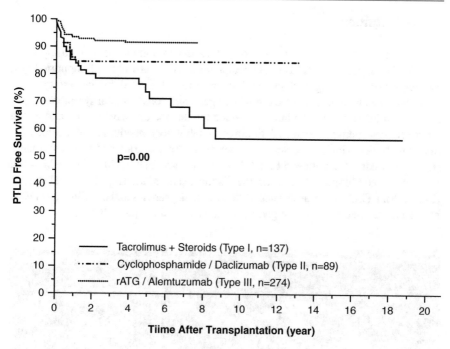

Fig. 18.3 PTLD-free survival in Eras I–III according to the type of immunosuppression (Abu-Elmagd et al. [10])

Fig. 18.4 PTLD lesion over allograft stoma

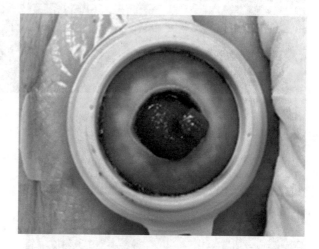

can be the presenting picture [8]. This carries a high mortality and the clinician needs to have a high index of suspicion. It is important to note that the clinical presentation of PTLD can be subtle, with the only signs and symptoms being fever, gastrointestinal symptoms, weight loss, and delayed growth. The disease can be highly lethal depending on lymphoid differentiation on histology (polymorphic vs. monomorphic) and intensity of immunosuppression. Morbidity in these patients is exacerbated by onset of rejection, protein-losing enteropathy, and translocation-related infections due to disrupted mucosal barrier of the transplanted bowel.

PTLD Diagnosis

Having a high index of suspicion is of paramount importance in diagnosing early PTLD. The diagnosis of PTLD in ITx recipients is essentially clinical, supported by a thorough history taking and physical examination followed by laboratory tests. Unaccustomed weight loss or lack of weight gain, and constitutional symptoms, especially in children, can be the only clue since the disease can have a wide and varied range of presentation. Abnormal findings or laboratory results are indications for imaging studies which are essential to detect multiple lesions and to appropriately stage the disease. CT scan and PET CT scan can show FDG-avid lesions which can be accessed and biopsied to confirm the diagnosis and establish pathological staging (Fig. 18.5). PTLD can be associated with other malignancies and the clinician should have an open mind while investigating and managing these patients [12].

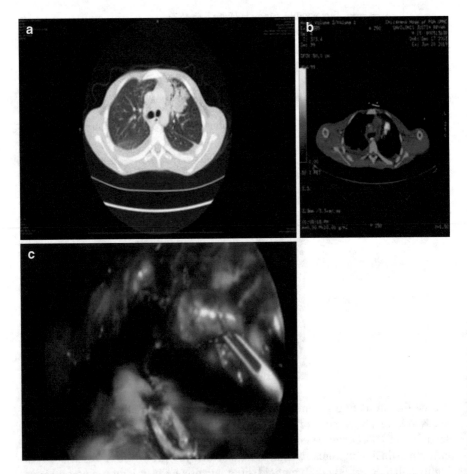

Fig. 18.5 Lung PTLD presenting as (**a**) left lung mass on CT, (**b**) FDG-avid left lung apex mass, and (**c**) thoracoscopic view of the mass in (**a**) and (**b**)

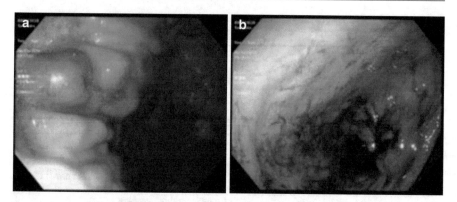

Fig. 18.6 PTLD presenting as allograft (**a**) mucosal nodules and (**b**) ulcers in the stomach in a modified multivisceral transplant recipient

In addition to these imaging studies, measurement of EBV load in the peripheral blood may also contribute to the diagnosis of EBV-associated PTLD. EBV DNAemia and rising EBV loads are PTLD unless proven otherwise in a patient with compatible symptoms. EBV loads are usually highly elevated in over 80% of patients with PTLD. However, as noted in Chaps. 6 and 8, the presence of elevated EBV loads in the peripheral blood does not necessarily confirm the presence of or lead to PTLD development. In general, while the presence of an elevated EBV load does not have a strong positive predictive value, a low or absent EBV load in the peripheral blood does have a high negative predictive value against the presence of EBV-associated PTLD.

The definitive diagnosis of PTLD requires histology. Surveillance endoscopy can discover mucosal nodules or ulcers that on biopsy prove to be PTLD (Fig. 18.6). An obvious mass or lymphadenopathy is an indication to perform excision or incision biopsy. Biopsy can be from a superficial mucosal or skin lesion or deeper sites through the use of CT-guided interventions, thoracoscopy or laparoscopy. PTLD can initially present as a bowel perforation in the transplanted allograft with the diagnosis being made at the time of surgery. This also occurs in patients with PTLD in the visceral allograft who are undergoing chemotherapy as the lesion involutes. The histologic appearance of PTLD lesions varies and can range from mild non-destructive lesions like infectious mononucleosis to a full-blown Hodgkin's lymphoma. PTLD is inherently mostly of recipient origin and 80% are related to EBV. A detailed description of PTLD pathology is discussed in Chap. 2 of this textbook.

Management

The management of PTLD in ITx recipients is challenging. While reduction of immune suppression is always considered as a first-line option, intestinal allograft recipients are unique in that they may present with concomitant PTLD and

Table 18.2 PTLD management in intestinal transplantation

Diagnosis	Treatment
EBV PCR monitoring	*Medical*
Frequent enteroscopy for allograft monitoring	Reduction in immunosuppression
	IVIG
	Ganciclovir[a]
	Rituximab
	Radiation for local disease
	Chemotherapy
	Optimize nutritional status and hydration
	Surgical
	Local resection of lesion
	Small bowel resection
	Allograft enterectomy

[a]Evidence supporting the efficacy associated with the use of ganciclovir is questionable

rejection, limiting or even eliminating the ability to reduce or stop immune suppression as initial management. Additionally, compared to other solid organ transplants (e.g., liver allografts in which one can temporarily hold immunosuppression and monitor liver enzymes to diagnose rejection), the highly immunogenic intestinal graft may rapidly progress to significant rejection after reduction of immune suppression before the host immune system has time to control the PTLD. Accordingly, rituximab (either as initial therapy or as second-line therapy if rejection develops) is frequently used in this population. While many centers may also use an antiviral agent like ganciclovir, their efficacy in the treatment of EBV disease and PTLD is unproven [13]. Patients with localized disease may benefit from local radiation or surgical resection depending upon the site of the lesion. Advanced disease is treated with a chemotherapeutic regimen, usually cyclophosphamide and prednisone in combination with rituximab (Table 18.2). Biopsy histopathology confirms the grade of the PTLD and helps in determining whether the patient needs chemotherapy in addition to or as an alternative to rituximab.

We recommend involvement of the multidisciplinary tumor board to include hematology-oncology, infectious diseases, gastroenterology, and surgery to optimize delivery of the best available therapy for each individual patient. In cases of PTLD recurrence or relapse or monomorphic PTLD and Hodgkin's lymphoma, intensive chemotherapy regimens are indicated.

Throughout treatment, particular attention needs to be paid to patient's hydration and nutritional status. Depending on the integrity of the intestine, patients may need to be fed enterally or parenterally for extended periods of time while diagnosis is ascertained, and treatment is being instituted. Systemic symptoms may be from bacterial translocation from inflamed or rejecting intestine and the team should have a low threshold to start patients on antimicrobial therapy.

Annual PET scanning surveillance can identify the extent of the metastatic disease and is of immense value in monitoring treatment response. This is especially important in helping the clinician decide and actively monitor immunosuppressive

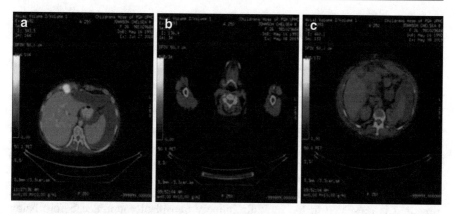

Fig. 18.7 Recurrent PTLD in a patient following modified multivisceral transplantation. (**a**) Rt lower chest wall. (**b**) Neck. (**c**) Posterior abdominal wall

Table 18.3 Allograft enterectomy: indications

| Acute abdomen/perforation necessitating laparotomy |
| Extensive PTLD |
| Vascular thrombosis |
| Exfoliative rejection recalcitrant to treatment |
| Persistent rejection with no regeneration on intestinal biopsy |
| Onset of multisystem organ failure due to translocation |
| Hemorrhage associated with rejection |

therapy given the highly immunogenic nature of the intestinal allograft. Annual PET scan following initial therapy for PTLD is also instrumental in detecting recurrent lesions (Fig. 18.7).

Allograft Enterectomy

Surgical management of advanced PTLD involving the small bowel can range from exploratory laparotomy and local resection of stricture or perforation to allograft enterectomy depending on allograft integrity and presence of local or advanced disease. Indications for allograft enterectomy are shown in Table 18.3. When small bowel transplant is included as part of the multivisceral graft, modified or full, segmental resection of the involved small bowel component of the allograft, although technically challenging, may be possible in carefully selected patients.

Allograft enterectomy will allow for cessation of immunosuppression in cases of isolated ITx but will result in TPN dependence. Indications for enterectomy also may include acute abdomen from perforation or bleeding that necessitates mandatory exploration, and intraoperative findings reveal extensive PTLD involvement of the allograft, obvious ischemia from vascular thrombosis, or severe exfoliative rejection in the presence of sepsis.

It is uncommon for the stomach or liver to reject in multivisceral or modified multivisceral transplant setting. Hence, if it is identified that the small bowel is the most affected organ, it may be possible to perform a limited resection of the affected bowel. The surgical approach in these patients has to be carefully executed to avoid injury to the porto-mesenteric system draining the liver.

Overall prognosis depends upon the extent of the disease. Mortality is high in PTLD associated with visceral transplantation since allograft injury from PTLD or from rebound rejection leads to bacterial translocation and systemic sepsis with capillary leak syndrome.

Re-transplantation following allograft enterectomy should be entertained only if the patient has demonstrated steady improvement in general condition and has been screened carefully for recurrent PTLD. The patient is maintained on TPN during this time and is presented to the multidisciplinary transplant committee before being accepted for re-transplantation. At this point in our experience, re-transplantation after PTLD cannot be recommended as 4 of the 59 patients who developed PTLD were re-transplanted but succumbed to infection, rejection, or recurrent PTLD.

EBV Surveillance and the Prevention of EBV-Associated PTLD

Viral load measurements help in deciding preemptive interventions and to monitor response of PTLD and EBV disease to therapeutic strategies. Measurement of EBV serostatus prior to transplant identifies EBV-naïve candidates who will require careful observation due to their risk for EBV and PTLD. However, as previously noted, EBV disease and PTLD do occur with some frequency in EBV-seropositive ITx recipients. The monitoring strategy used at the UPMC Children's Hospital of Pittsburgh includes obtaining viral loads every 2 weeks for the first 3 months, every month for the next 3 months, every 2 months for the next 6 months, and then every 3–4 months thereafter. Of course, more frequent monitoring is indicated for those with elevated and/ or climbing loads or those with suspicious symptoms. This protocol helps to identify recipients with DNAemia and require enteroscopy, imaging studies, and treatment [5, 13, 14]. Rising EBV loads and EBV DNAemia are typically managed by lowering immunosuppression with or without initiation of intravenous ganciclovir, although there is lack of data to support the efficacy of ganciclovir. Preemptive anti-B cell therapy with the chimeric anti CD-20 monoclonal antibody rituximab is indicated in the presence of concurrent rejection. IVIG is also used to augment passive immunity [15–18]. Additional details on the prevention of EBV-associated PTLD are discussed in Chap. 11.

Conclusion

The incidence of PTLD in recipients of ITx has decreased in the current era but continues to present unique challenges and is associated with a high mortality. A high index of suspicion and early diagnosis coupled with EBV titer monitoring, frequent surveillance endoscopy, and image-guided or surgical biopsy are integral to early diagnosis and treatment. Multidisciplinary approach involving medical oncology, gastroenterology, infectious disease, radiology, and pathology is instrumental in comprehensive management of the patient. Better immunosuppression strategies of initial induction followed by low-dose maintenance immunosuppression aimed at keeping the immune surveillance system intact can prevent the development of this morbid and lethal disease.

Take-Home Pearls

- Incidence of PTLD in recipients of intestinal transplants (ITx) continues to present unique challenges and is associated with increased mortality and graft loss.
- EBV disease and PTLD can occur in EBV-seropositive ITx recipients.
- ITx patients can have concomitant PTLD and allograft rejection.
- A high index of suspicion and early diagnosis coupled with EBV titer monitoring, frequent surveillance endoscopy, and image-guided or surgical biopsy are integral to early diagnosis and treatment.
- Multidisciplinary approach involving medical oncology, gastroenterology, infectious disease, radiology, and pathology is instrumental in comprehensive management of the patient.

References

1. Abu-Elmagd K, Bond G, Reyes J, Fung J. Intestinal transplantation: a coming of age. Adv Surg. 2002;36:65–101. Review. PubMed PMID: 12465547.
2. Fujieda M, Hattori M. Cancer-infection interface in children after transplantation: post-transplant lymphoproliferative disorder and Epstein-Barr virus infection. Curr Opin Organ Transplant. 2013;18:549–54.
3. Stanley K, Friehling E, Ranganathan S, Mazariegos G, McAllister-Lucas LM, Sindhi R. Post-transplant lymphoproliferative disorder in pediatric intestinal transplant recipients: a literature review. Pediatr Transplant. 2018;22(5):e13211. https://doi.org/10.1111/petr.13211.
4. Hawksworth J, Zimmerman A, Kroemer A, Radkani P, Guerra J, Khan K, Yazigi N, Kaufman S, Subramanian S, Sagedy H, Fishbein T. Post-transplant proliferative disorder following intestine transplantation: contemporary single center experience transplantation. Transplantation. 2019;103(7S2):S79.
5. Nalesnik M, Jaffe R, Reyes J, et al. Posttransplant lymphoproliferative disorders in small bowel allograft recipients. Transplant Proc. 2000;32:1213.
6. Hurwitz M, Desai DM, Cox KL, Berquist WE, Esquivel CO, Millan MT. Complete immunosuppressive withdrawal as a uniform approach to post-transplant lymphoproliferative disease in pediatric liver transplantation. Pediatr Transplant. 2004;8:267–72.
7. Sullivan BJ, Kim GJ, Sara G. Treatment dilemma for survivors of rituximab-induced bowel perforation in the setting of post-transplant lymphoproliferative disorder. BMJ Case Rep. 2018;11(1):e226666. https://doi.org/10.1136/bcr-2018-226666.
8. Green M, Michaels MG, Webber SA, Rowe D, Reyes J. The management of Epstein-Barr virus associated post-transplant lymphoproliferative disorders in pediatric solid-organ transplant recipients. Pediatr Transplant. 1999;3:271–81.
9. Smith JM, Weaver T, Skeans MA, Horslen SP, Noreen SM, Snyder JJ, Israni AK, Kasiske BL. OPTN/SRTR 2017 annual data report: intestine. Am J Transplant. 2019;19(Suppl 2):284–322.

10. Abu-Elmagd KM, Costa G, Bond GJ, Soltys K, Sindhi R, Wu T, Koritsky DA, Schuster B, Martin L, Cruz RJ, Murase N, Zeevi A, Irish W, Ayyash MO, Matarese L, Humar A, Mazariegos G. Five hundred intestinal and multivisceral transplantations at a single center: major advances with new challenges. Ann Surg. 2009;250(4):567–81. https://doi.org/10.1097/SLA.0b013e3181b67725.
11. Abu-Elmagd KM, Kosmach-Park B, Costa G, Zenati M, Martin L, Koritsky DA, Emerling M, Murase N, Bond GJ, Soltys K, Sogawa H, Lunz J, Al Samman M, Shaefer N, Sindhi R, Mazariegos GV. Long-term survival, nutritional autonomy, and quality of life after intestinal and multivisceral transplantation. Ann Surg. 2012;256(3):494–508. https://doi.org/10.1097/SLA.0b013e318265f310.
12. Aida N, Ito T, Maruyama M, Saigo K, Akutsu N, Aoyama H, Kitamura H, Kenmochi TA. Case of epstein-barr virus-associated leiomyosarcoma concurrently with posttransplant lymphoproliferative disorders after renal transplantation. Clin Med Insights Case Rep. 2019;12:1179547619867330. https://doi.org/10.1177/1179547619867330. eCollection 2019. PubMed PMID: 31391783; PubMed CentralPMCID: PMC6669837.
13. Green M, Michaels MG. Epstein-Barr virus infection and posttransplant lymphoproliferative disorder. Am J Transplant. 2013;13(Suppl 3):41–54; quiz 54.
14. Abu-Elmagd KM, Mazariegos G, Costa G, et al. Lymphoproliferative disorders and de novo malignancies in intestinal and multivisceral recipients: improved outcomes with new outlooks. Transplantation. 2009;88:926–34.
15. Berney T, Delis S, Kato T, et al. Successful treatment of posttransplant lymphoproliferative disease with prolonged rituximab treatment in intestinal transplant recipients. Transplantation. 2002;74:1000–6.
16. Messahel B, Taj MM, Hobson R, et al. Single agent efficacy of rituximab in childhood immunosuppression related lymphoproliferative disease: a United Kingdom Children's Cancer Study Group (UKCCSG) retrospective review. Leuk Lymphoma. 2006;47:2584–9.
17. McGhee W, Mazariegos GV, Sindhi R, Abu-Elmagd K, Reyes J. Rituximab in the treatment of pediatric small bowel transplant patients with posttransplant lymphoproliferative disorder unresponsive to standard treatment. Transplant Proc. 2002;34:955–6.
18. Choquet S, Leblond V, Herbrecht R, et al. Efficacy and safety of rituximab in B-cell post-transplantation lymphoproliferative disorders: results of a prospective multicenter phase 2 study. Blood. 2006;107:3053–7.

PTLD After Heart Transplantation

19

Anne I. Dipchand and Michael McDonald

Introduction

This chapter will address organ-specific issues regarding PTLD in adult and pediatric heart transplant recipients. Overall, PTLD following heart transplantation is more common than following kidney or liver, but not as common as after lung, intestinal, or multivisceral transplantation [1–3]. PTLD is a more frequent concern in children compared to adults [4]. There are potential influencing factors including age, immunosuppression, and EBV infection history which will be explored herein. Graft involvement is extremely rare but survival is impacted by a diagnosis of PTLD in a child or adult heart transplant recipient.

Incidence/Prevalence

There are multiple international single-center reports citing PTLD in 1–10% of adult heart transplant recipients [5–10]. Malignancy itself is much more common in adult patients with PTLD making up the minority (5–10%) of the reported malignancies [6, 7, 9]. These reports, however, include relatively small numbers of heart transplant recipients.

A. I. Dipchand (✉)
Labatt Family Heart Centre, Hospital for Sick Children, Department of Paediatrics,
University of Toronto, Toronto, ON, Canada
e-mail: anne.dipchand@sickkids.ca

M. McDonald
Department of Medicine, Advanced Heart Failure and Transplant Program, Peter Muck
Cardiac Centre/UHN Transplant, Division of Cardiology, Toronto, ON, Canada
e-mail: michael.mcdonald@uhn.ca

© Springer Nature Switzerland AG 2021
V. R. Dharnidharka et al. (eds.), *Post-Transplant Lymphoproliferative Disorders*,
https://doi.org/10.1007/978-3-030-65403-0_19

The earliest adult registry report of PTLD ($n = 274$) came from the Israel Penn International Transplant Tumor Registry (IPITTR) in 2004 in response to the limited single-center data reported to that point in the literature ($n = 84$ patients) on incidence (0.7–6.8%), and the marked variability in reported patient survival (0–68%) [11]. Though incidence/prevalence data is not available, valuable observations from this cohort are noted below. Sampiano explored the US Organ Procurement Transplantation Network/United Network for Organ Sharing (UNOS) database up to Sept 2010 for all organs and reported any post-transplant malignancy in 11% (1073/16,511) of adult heart transplant recipients; PTLD made up 16% ($n = 172$) [1]. Subsequently, Higgins reported the incidence and types of malignancy from 35 US centers in the Cardiac Transplant Research Database (CTRD) between 1993 and 2008 compared to the general population. Primary post-transplant malignancy occurred in 8% of patients, of which PTLD made up 17% [12]. Though there was an overall decline in malignancies over the eras with prevalence not different compared to the general population, this did not apply to PTLD. The largest non-North American cohort ($n = 3393$; 1984–2003) comes from the 16 centers contributing to the Spanish Post-Heart-Transplant Tumour Registry (SPHTTR) in which 490 (14%) patients developed malignancy of which 13% ($n = 62$) were PTLD [13]. The most contemporary cohort (2006–2015) comes from the UNOS database with 120 (1%) PTLD cases in 14,487 adult heart transplant recipients [14].

PTLD is by far the most common malignancy occurring in the pediatric heart transplant population, making up well over 95% of the malignancies reported to both the registry of the International Society for Heart and Lung Transplantation (ISHLT) and to the Pediatric Heart Transplant Study (PHTS) [15, 16]. Time-unadjusted frequency estimates from single-center reports range from 5% to 16% [2, 3, 17–19]. Webber reported the earliest multi-institutional registry data from the PHTS (1993–2002) with a 5% incidence (56/1184 primary transplants) and a freedom from PTLD of 98%, 94%, and 92% at 1, 3, and 5 years respectively [20]. Data from the UNOS registry (1987–2013) revealed a 7% (360/5169) incidence of PTLD [14].

In an attempt to model prevalence over time and the natural history, Manlhiot used a competing risk hazard model in a single-center cohort and reported PTLD affecting 9% of patients surviving 3 years after transplant, 15% of those surviving 5 years, and 28% of those surviving 10 years after transplant (time-adjusted prevalence). Data from the PHTS (1993–2009) was also used to try to model natural history in a much larger cohort of 3170 pediatric transplant recipients, 147 of whom developed PTLD (4.64%) [16]. Freedom from PTLD was 98.5%, 94%, and 90% at 1, 5, and 10 years, respectively. However, 2 distinct phases of risk were identified using parametric multiphase hazard analysis; the first in the first 2 years post-transplant that peaked at 5.6 months and then declined into a second phase (2–18 years post-transplant) in which the hazard gradually increased over time, depicting a gradual decline in freedom from PTLD over time (Fig. 19.1).

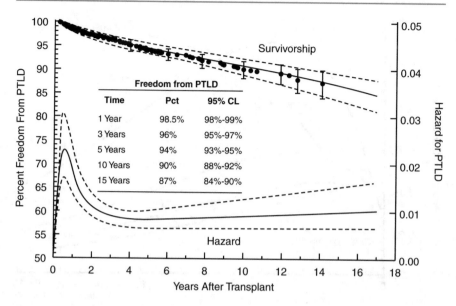

Fig. 19.1 A Kaplan–Meier estimate of freedom from PTLD and the hazard for PTLD as a function of time post-pediatric heart transplantation. A steady decline in freedom from PTLD was observed over time. The peak hazard for PTLD occurred at 5.6 months post-transplantation. Dotted lines depict the 95% confidence limits. (Data from the Pediatric Heart Transplant Study. Used with permission R. Chinnock)

Risk Factors for PTLD

Determination and interpretation of risk factors for PTLD in both adult and pediatric heart transplant recipients is challenging and the literature is varied and conflicting as summarized below [14, 21].

Age

In adult recipients, there were no age-related differences for a diagnosis of PTLD in the cohort from the Spanish registry [13]. Although older age is reported in adult studies as a risk factor for all malignancy, most do not look specifically at PTLD which occurs in a younger cohort of patients [7, 9]. The most robust age-related analysis comes from CTRD in which PTLD was increased in the younger age group (18–35 years), in addition to having the largest observed difference of a 27-fold increased incidence compared with the general US population of the same age range and demographics [12].

In pediatric recipients, the hypotheses around the role of age and the development of PTLD are challenged by the potential impact of changes in the developing immune system over time, in addition to EBV serostatus, the ability to assess EBV

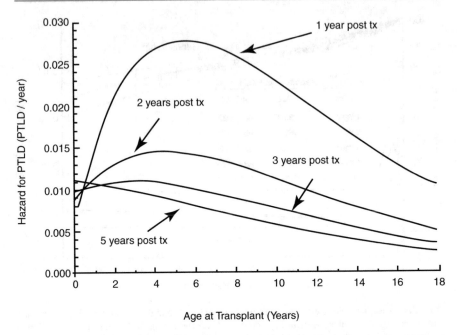

Fig. 19.2 The hazard for PTLD as a function of age at the time of transplantation in childhood. Hazard functions are predicted for children at 1 year, 2 years, 3 years, and 5 years post-transplant. (Data from the Pediatric Heart Transplant Study. Used with permission R. Chinnock)

serologic status in the youngest recipients using serological testing (due to placental transfer), and timing of acquisition of primary EBV disease. All of these factors are impacted upon and inseparable from age, making it hard to determine the role of age alone. There are multivariable risk factor analyses that have not shown age to be a risk factor for the development of PTLD [19]. The focused PHTS analysis looking specifically at age at transplant showed a complex relationship, with young children aged 1 to <10 years being at higher risk than infants (RR 2.4) or adolescents (RR 1.7), for at least the first 5 years post-transplant (Fig. 19.2) [16]. This was hypothesized to be related to passively transferred immunity in the infants and an increasingly competent immune system in the older age group.

Gender

There is no data demonstrating a difference in PTLD by gender in adult or pediatric heart recipients.

Timing

Timing of PTLD is often referred to in the literature as early versus late; by convention this is generally referring to <1 year post-transplant compared to later post-transplant. Adult data is limited with small numbers, but Khedmat reported that

PTLD occurred early in 37% of cases, using pooled data from the existing literature on 180 adult heart transplant recipients, though there were many limitations to the study [22]. In a small but more robust analysis, the majority of adult heart transplant recipients presented late (>80%) at a mean of 3.2 years post-transplant [8].

The timing of PTLD in pediatric reports is varied with small single-center reports citing occurrence at an average of 2.8–3.3 years post-transplant [2, 3, 8]. In the larger PHTS analysis, the mean age was 23.9 months (3–91.1 months) though the peak instantaneous risk was highest at 6 months post-transplant and then slowly decreased but never reached 0 [20]. Finally, in the expanded PHTS dataset and more sophisticated analysis, time post-transplant had a complex relationship with both age (Figs. 19.1 and 19.2) and EBV status (see below) [16].

EBV Status

EBV status has long been hypothesized to play a role in the development of PTLD post-transplant as detailed elsewhere in this book. The actual evidence in the literature regarding heart transplant recipients is varied but supportive of increased risk in donor-positive, recipient-negative combinations [23]. In the large UNOS cohort of adult recipients, EBV serostatus was not associated with the development of PTLD in multivariable analysis despite differences on univariate analysis [21]. Opelz reported EBV-negative serostatus associated with increased risk (HR 3.6) of non-Hodgkin lymphoma in a cohort of 2042 adult heart recipients [24].

In pediatric recipients, an EBV-positive donor is a strong risk factor for PTLD development in the negative recipient [2] with a complex interaction with age; nearly 25% of EBV-negative recipients between the ages of 4 and 7 years with EBV-positive donors developed PTLD in the PHTS analysis (Fig. 19.3) [16].

Katz reported an association between EBV seronegativity and EBV seroconversion with the development of PTLD in a small cohort of pediatric heart transplant recipients [18]. Higher EBV load or a chronic carrier state has been reported to be associated with a higher risk of PTLD after pediatric heart transplantation, in some cases irrespective of recipient serostatus at the time of transplant [2, 17, 19, 25].

Immunosuppression

Induction therapy has historically been a presumptive risk factor for PTLD, but reports are conflicting. Early reports in the adult literature reported a high incidence with OKT3 use (11%) [26]. Subsequently, reports showed no association, though dose may have played a factor [5, 13]. The association with anti-thymocyte globulin also varies in the literature with reportedly no association [6] versus an increased risk in the first year [22] in adults and reportedly an association with a higher dose [2] and longer duration [19] in pediatrics versus no association [27].

Despite multiple attempts to find an association between the type of immunosuppression and PTLD, no clear relationship has been identified with either type of calcineurin inhibitor or mTOR inhibitor in heart transplant recipients. There is

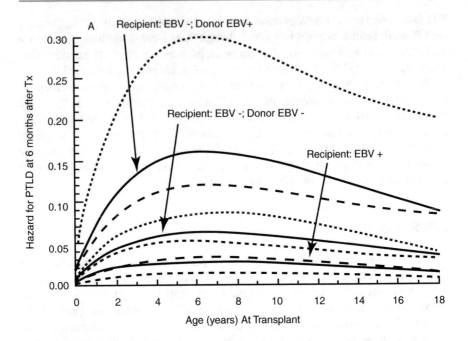

Fig. 19.3 Influence of EBV serology of donor and recipient on the predicted hazard for PTLD and freedom from PTLD at 5 years post-pediatric heart transplantation. (A) The predicted hazard for PTLD at 6 months post-transplantation for different EBV serologies in donor/recipient pairs as a function of age at time of transplant. (Data from the Pediatric Heart Transplant Study. Used with permission R. Chinnock)

limited data in 454 adult heart transplant recipients (1999–2015), suggesting less malignancy with everolimus (1.8%) compared with MMF (9.9%) but a similar 2-year survival [10]. There, however, remains a paucity of data in the literature.

Site of Involvement

The site of involvement of PTLD can vary widely and there are no unique features specific to heart transplant recipients. Reports in adults are limited but extranodal involvement has been reported in up to 82%, most commonly gastrointestinal [8]. The distribution from IPITTR included lymph nodes (34%), lung (32%), GI (24%), liver (23%), and CNS (13%) with 2 or more sites involved at presentation in 51% [11]. For children, in the PHTS cohort, single versus multiple sites at presentation were equally reported and sites included gastrointestinal (39%), lung (25%), cervical adenopathy (18%), and CNS 3.6% [20].

Allograft involvement of PTLD following heart transplantation is very rare and reports are scarce. Involvement has been reported of the mitral valve, intracavitary (LV), infiltrating the myocardium and/or epicardium and involving the coronary arteries and arterioles in a vasculitic nature [28].

Rejection

One of the mainstays of PTLD treatment is a reduction in immunosuppression with its obligate risk of rejection. There is limited literature looking specifically at rejection post-PTLD diagnosis other than as a cause of death (see below). It has been reported in 24% of adult recipients [8]. In the PHTS cohort, 61% of children treated with reduced immunosuppression had rejection; this was higher (71%) when the immunosuppression was discontinued, compared to just lowered (53%) [20].

Outcomes

A diagnosis of PTLD confers a decreased survival in both adult and pediatric heart transplant recipients though reported estimates vary based on many of the risk factors noted above, in addition to the actual type of PTLD (discussed elsewhere in this book). Overall reported mortality in adults ranges from 30% to 80% [5, 13]. In adults, reported 1- and 5-year survival for early versus late PTLD was 65% and 46% versus 53% and 41% [22]. The 5-year survival from the CTRD cohort was 32%, and survival from the IPITTR was 45%, 33%, 30%, and 13% at 1, 3, 5, and 10 years, respectively [11]. In the most contemporary cohort (2006–2015) of 14,487 adult heart transplant recipients of whom 120 developed PTLD, PTLD almost tripled the hazard of death [14].

Decreased survival has also been reported in children with about two times the hazard in the largest cohort from UNOS [21]. Recurrence of PTLD is a significant problem with a freedom from death or recurrence reported of 72%, 58%, and 50% at 1, 3, and 5 years [19]. In the PHTS cohort, probability of survival was 75%, 68%, and 67% at 1, 3, and 5 years with an event-free survival (death, rejection, or PTLD recurrence) of 76%, 73%, 61%, and 56% at 6 months and 1, 3, and 5 years, respectively [20].

Reported causes of death are PTLD, rejection, and infection. Rejection/graft loss has been reported to be as frequent a cause of death as PTLD itself in children [20]. Reported causes of death in adults was PTLD (51%), rejection (21%), sepsis (5%), and other infection (5%) in IPITTR [11].

Conclusions

PTLD in heart transplant recipients remains poorly understood but is associated with double the mortality in adults and children. PTLD makes up the minority of malignancies in adults post-heart transplant, and, other than younger age, there is a clear paucity of data in the literature regarding risk factors for development and/or outcomes. In children, PTLD is a more frequent problem with a gradual increase in the likelihood of getting PTLD over time post-transplant. EBV status and the age of the child at the time of transplant are important risk factors. There remain significant gaps in the literature regarding PTLD post-heart transplantation.

References

1. Sampaio MS, Cho YW, Qazi Y, Bunnapradist S, Hutchinson IV, Shah T. Posttransplant malignancies in solid organ adult recipients: an analysis of the U.S. National Transplant Database. Transplantation. 2012;94(10):990–8.
2. Schubert S, Renner C, Hammer M, Abdul-Khaliq H, Lehmkuhl HB, Berger F, Hetzer R, Reinke P. Relationship of immunosuppression to Epstein-Barr viral load and lymphoproliferative disease in pediatric heart transplant patients. J Heart Lung Transplant. 2008;27(1):100–5.
3. Tai CC, Curtis JL, Szmuszkovicz JR, Horn MV, Ford HR, Woo MS, Wang KS. Abdominal involvement in pediatric heart and lung transplant recipients with posttransplant lymphoproliferative disease increases the risk of mortality. J Pediatr Surg. 2008;43(12):2174–7.
4. Gao SZ, Chaparro SV, Perlroth M, Montoya JG, Miller JL, DiMiceli S, Hastie T, Oyer PE, Schroeder J. Post-transplantation lymphoproliferative disease in heart and heart-lung transplant recipients: 30-year experience at Stanford University. J Heart Lung Transplant. 2003;22(5):505–14.
5. Peraira JR, Segovia J, Fuertes B, Fernández JA, Escudier JM, Salas C, Pulpón LA. Current induction immunosuppression and post-heart transplant lymphoproliferative disorders. Transplant Proc. 2003;35(5):2009–10.
6. El-Hamamsy I, Stevens LM, Carrier M, Pelletier G, White M, Tremblay F, Perrault LP. Incidence and prognosis of cancer following heart transplantation using RATG induction therapy. Transpl Int. 2008;18(11):1280–5.
7. Doesch AO, Müller S, Konstandin M, Celik S, Kristen A, Frankenstein L, Ehlermann P, Sack FU, Katus HA, Dengler TJ. Malignancies after heart transplantation: incidence, risk factors, and effects of calcineurin inhibitor withdrawal. Transplant Proc. 2010;42(9):3694–9.
8. Kumarasingh G, Lavee O, Parker A, Nivison-Smith I, Milliken S, et al. Post-transplant lymphoproliferative disease in heart and lung transplantation: defining risk and prognostic factors. J Pediatr Surg. 2015;34(11):1406–14.
9. Van Keer J, Droogné W, Van Cleemput J, Vörös G, Rega F, Meyns B, Janssens S, Vanhaecke J. Cancer after heart transplantation: a 25-year single-center perspective. Transplant Proc. 2016;48(6):2172–7.
10. Wang YJ, Chi NH, Chou NK, Huang SC, Wang CH, Wu IH, Yu HY, Chen YS, Tsao CI, Shun CT, Tsai JT, Wang S-S. Malignancy after heart transplantation under everolimus versus mycophenolate mofetil immunosuppression. Transplant Proc. 2016;48(3):969–73.
11. Aull MJ, Buell JF, Trofe J, First MR, Alloway RR, Hanaway MJ, Wagoner L, Gross TG, Beebe T, Woodle ES. Experience with 274 cardiac transplant recipients with posttransplant lymphoproliferative disorder: a report from the Israel Penn International Transplant Tumor Registry. Transplantation. 2004;78(11):1676–82.
12. Higgins RS, Brown RN, Chang PP, Starling RC, Ewald GA, Tallaj JA, Kirklin JK, George JF. A multi-institutional study of malignancies after heart transplantation and a comparison with the general United States population. J Heart Lung Transplant. 2014;33(5):478–85.
13. Crespo-Leiro MG, Alonso-Pulpón L, Vázquez de Prada JA, Almenar L, Arizón JM, Brossa V, Delgado JF, Fernandez-Yañez J, Manito N, Rábago G, Lage E, Roig E, Diaz-Molina B, Pascual D, Muñiz J. Malignancy after heart transplantation: incidence, prognosis and risk factors. Am J Transplant. 2008;8(5):1031–9.
14. Hayes D Jr, Tumin D, Foraker RE, Tobias JD. Posttransplant lymphoproliferative disease and survival in adult heart transplant recipients. J Cardiol. 2017;69(1):144–8.
15. Rossano J, Cherikh WS, Chambers DC, Goldfarb S, Hayes D, et al. The International Thoracic Organ Transplant Registry of the International Society for Heart and Lung Transplantation: twenty-first pediatric heart transplantation report—2018; focus theme: multiorgan transplantation. J Heart Lung Transplant. 2018;37(10):1184–95.
16. Chinnock R, Webber SA, Dipchand AI, Brown RN, George JF. A 16-year multi-institutional study of the role of age and EBV status on PTLD incidence among pediatric heart transplant recipients. Am J Transplant. 2012;12(11):3061–8.

17. Das B, Morrow R, Huang R, Fixler D. Persistent Epstein-Barr viral load in Epstein-Barr viral naïve pediatric heart transplant recipients: risk of late-onset post-transplant lymphoproliferative disease. World J Transplant. 2016;6(4):729–35.
18. Katz BZ, Pahl E, Crawford SE, Kostyk MC, Rodgers S, Seshadri R, Proytcheva M, Pophal S. Case-control study of risk factors for the development of post-transplant lymphoproliferative disease in a pediatric heart transplant cohort. Pediatr Transplant. 2007;11(1):58–65.
19. Manlhiot C, Pollock-Barziv SM, Holmes C, Weitzman S, Allen U, Clarizia NA, Ngan BY, McCrindle BW, Dipchand AI. Post-transplant lymphoproliferative disorder in pediatric heart transplant recipients. J Heart Lung Transplant. 2010;29(6):648–57.
20. Webber SA, Naftel DC, Fricker FJ, Olesnevich P, Blume ED, Addonizio L, et al. Lymphoproliferative disorders after paediatric heart transplantation: a multi-institutional study. Lancet. 2006;367(9506):233–9.
21. Hayes D Jr, Breuer CK, Horwitz EM, Yates AR, Tobias JD, Shinoka T. Influence of posttransplant lymphoproliferative disorder on survival in children after heart transplantation. Pediatr Cardiol. 2015;36(8):1748–53.
22. Khedmat H, Taheri S. Heart allograft involvement by posttransplant lymphoproliferative disorders: report from the PTLD. Int Surv Exp Clin Transplant. 2011;9(4):258–64.
23. Dharnidharka VR. Comprehensive review of post-organ transplant hematologic cancers. Am J Transplant. 2018;18(3):537–49.
24. Opelz G, Daniel V, Naujokat C, Döhler B. Epidemiology of pretransplant EBV and CMV serostatus in relation to posttransplant non-Hodgkin lymphoma. Transplantation. 2009;88(8):962–7.
25. Bingler MA, Feingold B, Miller SA, Quivers E, Michaels MG, et al. Chronic high Epstein-Barr viral load state and risk for late-onset posttransplant lymphoproliferative disease/lymphoma in children. Am J Transplant. 2008;8(2):442–5.
26. Swinnen LJ, Costanzo-Nordin MR, Fisher SG, O'Sullivan EJ, Johnson MR, Heroux AL, Dizikes GJ, Pifarre R, Fisher RI. Increased incidence of lymphoproliferative disorder after immunosuppression with the monoclonal antibody OKT3 in cardiac-transplant recipients. N Engl J Med. 1990;323(25):1723–8.
27. Castleberry C, Pruitt E, Ameduri R, Schowengerdt K, Edens E, Hagin N, Kirklin JK, Naftel D, Urschel S. Risk stratification to determine the impact of induction therapy on survival, rejection and adverse events after pediatric heart transplant: a multi-institutional study. J Heart Lung Transplant. 2018;37(4):458–66.
28. Murray DL, Pereira NL, Miller DV. An unusual presentation of post-transplant lymphoproliferative disorder mimicking vasculitis in heart transplantation. J Heart Lung Transplant. 2008;27(11):1257–61.

PTLD after Lung Transplantation

20

Allan R. Glanville and Gary Visner

Abbreviations

ACR	Acute cellular rejection
AMR	Antibody-mediated rejection
BAL	Bronchoalveolar lavage
BSSLTx	Bilateral sequential single lung transplant
CF	Cystic fibrosis
CHD	Congenital heart disease
CLAD	Chronic lung allograft dysfunction
EBV	Epstein-Barr virus
HLTx	Heart-lung transplantation
HTx	Heart transplantation
ISHLT	International Society for Heart and Lung Transplantation
LTx	Lung transplantation
PTLD	Post-transplant lymphoproliferative disorder
RAS	Restrictive allograft syndrome
SLTx	Single lung transplant

A. R. Glanville (✉)
The Lung Transplant Unit, St. Vincent's Hospital, Sydney, NSW, Australia
e-mail: allan.glanville@svha.org.au

G. Visner
Department of Pediatrics, Boston Children's Hospital, Harvard Medical School, Boston, MA, USA
e-mail: gary.visner@childrens.harvard.edu

© Springer Nature Switzerland AG 2021
V. R. Dharnidharka et al. (eds.), *Post-Transplant Lymphoproliferative Disorders*,
https://doi.org/10.1007/978-3-030-65403-0_20

Introduction

The incidence and importance of post-transplant lymphoproliferative disorder (PTLD) after heart-lung transplantation (HLTx) have been recognized for over 30 years, but with the evolution of lung transplantation (LTx) to encompass initially single lung transplantation (SLTx) and latterly bilateral sequential single lung transplantation (BSSLTx), recent literature has focused largely on these two modalities [1, 2]. Both appear to have a slightly lower incidence than HLTx which may be due to the larger volume of lymphatic tissue transplanted within the HLTx bloc, but the overall rate of PTLD in recipients of LTx remains higher than other forms of solid organ transplantation at 6–9.5% [3–6]. Alternative explanations for the apparent higher rate after HLTx include the possibility that recipients of HLTx have a lower rate of Epstein-Barr virus (EBV) seropositivity at the time of transplantation due to a lower rate of pediatric acquisition in light of the previous tendency to sequester children with congenital heart disease (CHD), in particular away from some of the common sites of community exposure such as kindergartens and preschool where EBV is often acquired, leading to a higher rate of primary EBV infection with an attendant risk of PTLD approaching 50% [7]. With better diagnostic rates for CHD, combined with early surgical and enhanced medical therapies, the demand for HLTx has fallen so that few centers worldwide perform more than 3–4 cases per annum [8]. Although difficult to prove, another risk factor which may have changed over time is the level of immune suppression employed and local factors such as avoiding transplanting EBV-naïve recipients or, where possible, transplanting them with a matched EBV-negative graft, allowing the risk that EBV might be acquired later from other sources. Early supporting evidence to support the principles discussed above was well described by Aris et al. in 1996, who set out to quantify the risk of PLTD based on pre-LTx EBV serostatus in a small single center series of LTx patients, in 80 of whom pre- and post-lung transplant EBV serostatus was determined [5]. Six of 94 (6.4%) LTx patients who survived >1 month developed PTLD. All cases of PTLD involved thoracic structures at presentation and occurred in the first post-operative year. EBV-naïve (EBV−) recipients were much more likely to develop PTLD than those who were seropositive (EBV+) (5/15 [33%] vs. 1/60 [<2%], $p < 0.001$). Consistent with the prevailing adult (donor) EBV+ (EBV D+) rate of 85%, two of the EBV-naïve patients remained EBV naïve after LTx, presumably reflecting the fact that they received a matched EBV− graft (EBV D−/R−). Therefore, the rate of PTLD was 42% in those with primary EBV infection. As compared with EBV− patients that remained tumor-free, those who developed PTLD had similar levels of immunosuppressants and doses of antiviral therapy. Aris et al. concluded PLTD occurred predominantly in EBV-naïve patients, who therefore should be monitored more closely after LTx and, possibly, managed with lower immunosuppression. Importantly they opined that as PTLD could be successfully treated in most cases, EBV-naïve patients should not be excluded from LTx because their risk of death from PTLD was <15%. This position was supported by Wigle et al. in 2001 who concluded that although EBV seronegativity carried a 6.8-fold increase in the relative risk of developing PTLD, long-term survival could be achieved, and thus, EBV seronegativity, by itself, should not be considered a contra-indication to LTx [9]. A recent retrospective cohort study of adults listed in the Scientific Registry of Transplant Recipients between May 5, 2005, and August 31, 2016, concluded that despite increased rates of PTLD and associated mortality in the EBV D+/R− population, EBV-seronegative patients did not have worse mortality when transplanted with lungs from EBV-seropositive donors compared with lungs from EBV-seronegative donors [10]. The incidence of PTLD was 6.2% (79 of 1281) versus 1.4% (145 of 10,352) in EBV D+/R− versus all other recipients (adjusted odds ratio 4.0; 95% confidence interval, 2.8–5.9, $p < 0.001$). Among EBV D+/R− recipients, age less than 40 years and white race were associated with PTLD.

Paranjothi et al., in 2001, provided the largest and most comprehensive assessment of PTLD post-LTx to date, in a retrospective single center study [11]. PTLD was identified in 30/494 (6.1%) adult LTx recipients, 14 of which cases were diagnosed during the first year after LTx and 16 subsequently. The incidence density was significantly higher in the first year than in later years (3.3 cases/100 patient-years vs. 1.3 cases/100 patient-years; $p < 0.008$), which may in part reflect the overall survival and the relatively short median follow-up of 2.8 years. Presentation in the thorax and involvement of the allograft were significantly more common in the early cases (thorax, 12/14, 86%; allograft, 9/14, 64%) than in the late cases (thorax, 2/16, 12%; allograft, 2/16, 12%). There was no difference in survival after the diagnosis of PTLD between the early and late cases, but survival time after diagnosis was significantly longer in cases with, than those without, allograft involvement (median 2.6 years vs. 0.2 years, respectively; log rank $p = 0.007$). They concluded disease in the thorax and involvement of the allograft were common in the first year after LTx, but other sites, especially the gastrointestinal tract, predominated later. PTLD confined to the allograft appeared to have a somewhat better prognosis than disease involving other sites. A small report of primary central nervous system PTLD described a particularly poor prognosis which perhaps is to be expected [12]. In 2015, Kumarasinghe et al. published a large single center retrospective series detailing outcomes in 70 cases of PTLD (41 heart [HTx], 22 LTx, 6 HLTx, and 1 HTx-kidney transplant) 1984–2013 [4]. The incidence of PTLD was 7.59% in heart-lung, 5.37% in HTx, and 3.1% in LTx recipients. Extranodal disease (82%) with diffuse large B-cell lymphoma (72%) was the most common presentation. Bone marrow involvement (13%) and central nervous system disease (3%) were uncommon. Poor prognostic markers were bone marrow involvement (HR 6.75, $p < 0.001$) and serum albumin <30 g/liter (HR 3.18, $p = 0.006$). Improved survival was seen with a complete response within 3 months of treatment (HR 0.08, $p < 0.001$). Five-year overall survival was 29%.

Risk Factors for PTLD Acquisition

Whether the burden of immune suppression is a critical factor in determining the risk of PTLD is uncertain as the reported evidence is variable. However, most studies are small, single center retrospective studies that are poorly controlled. Montone et al. in 1996 reported that cyclosporine and azathioprine dosages and cyclosporine levels were similar between patients with and without PTLD, but PTLD was more prevalent in patients with high cumulative doses of antilymphocyte globulin [13]. Conversely in the same year Mihalov et al. reported no apparent effect of the withdrawal of prophylactic OKT3 from the immunosuppression regimen of HTx transplant recipients on the incidence of all tumors, PTLD, or skin/lip tumors [6]. Perhaps one should not extrapolate from heart to lung. Gao et al. reported their experience with both HTx and LTx and concluded recipient age and rejection frequency, as well as high-dose cyclosporine immunosuppression, were significantly ($p < 0.02$) associated with PTLD development [14]. In 2002, Malouf et al. reported a reduction in the apparent rate of PTLD in EBV-naïve recipients [15]. None of 15 EBV-naïve recipients who received continuous antiviral prophylactic therapy developed PTLD during a mean follow-up of 806 ± 534 (39–1084) days compared with 1/3 who did not receive antiviral prophylactic therapy. A sophisticated strategy of pre-emptive EBV viral load monitoring was reported by Bakker et al. in 2007 [16]. Serial monitoring used a threshold of 10,000 EBV copies/ml to determine the trigger point for reducing immune suppression. They concluded pre-emptive reduction of immunosuppression after lung transplantation guided by EBV-DNA load appeared to be a safe approach for the prevention of PTLD in lung transplant recipients late after transplantation. The same confidence cannot be assumed in the pediatric population where the rate of PTLD after pediatric LTx remains higher than in adults. The NIH-sponsored Clinical Trials in Organ Transplantation in Children (CTOTC-03) prospectively obtained serial quantitative measurements of EBV PCR in both whole blood and BAL fluid after pediatric LTx [17]. Of 61 patients, 34 (56%) had an EBV + PCR (at least once in WB or BAL). EBV donor (D)+ patients more often had a positive PCR (D+/recipient (R)−: 13/18; D+/R+: 14/23) compared to EBV D− patients (6/17). Several D−/R− (5/12) patients developed EBV, but none developed PTLD. All four PTLD patients were D+/R− with EBV + PCR. Having an EBV-seropositive donor was associated with increased risk of EBV + PCR in whole blood, but EBV load in BAL was not predictive of developing PTLD.

Leyssens et al. provided interesting data from a case control series of 31 LTx recipients with PTLD [18]. PTLD prevalence was 3.9%, time to PTLD was 323 (166–1132) days, and 54.8% had early-onset PTLD versus 45.2% late-onset PTLD. At LTx, more EBV− patients were present in PTLD (42%) compared to controls (5%) ($P < 0.0001$). EBV viral load was higher in PTLD versus controls ($p < 0.0001$). EBV status at LTx ($p = 0.0073$) and EBV viral load at PTLD ($p = 0.0002$) were the most important risk determinates for later PTLD. Patients with PTLD demonstrated shorter time to onset of chronic lung allograft dysfunction (CLAD) ($p = 0.0006$) and poorer 5-year survival post-LTx (66.6% vs. 91.5%), resulting in worse CLAD-free survival (HR 2.127, 95% CI 1.006–4.500; $p = 0.0483$) and overall survival (HR 3.297 95% CI 1.473–7.382; $p = 0.0037$) compared to controls. Late-onset PTLD had worse survival compared to early-onset PTLD ($p = 0.021$). They concluded primary EBV infection is a risk for PTLD and that PTLD is associated with worse long-term outcome post-LTx.

These conclusions were supported by a recent meta-analysis by Cheng et al. analyzing 14 studies published in 2005–2015 which included 164 LTx recipients [19]. The main finding was that SLTx was associated with a 7.67-fold risk of death after PTLD compared with BSSLTx (pOR 7.67 95% CI 1.98–29.70; $p = 0.003$). Risk of death for early-onset (<1 year post-LT) vs. late-onset (>1 year post-LT) PTLD was not different (pOR 0.62, 95% CI 0.20–1.86, $p = 0.39$). Survival in polymorphic vs. monomorphic PTLD and extranodal vs. nodal disease was similar.

Clinical and Histopathological Features

LTx recipients have a predilection for developing PTLD in the allograft, perhaps related to the transplantation of donor lymphoid tissue. The development of PTLD in donor-derived cells has been elegantly demonstrated by Mentzer et al. in 1996 in an EBV− LTx recipient who developed an immunoblastic lymphoma 4 months after LTx from an EBV+ donor [20]. The neoplastic cells expressed B lymphocyte markers (CD19+, CD20+, sIgM+, kappa+) as well as the EBV antigen EBNA-2. A cell line with similar cytologic features spontaneously grew from in vitro cultures of the patient's peripheral blood mononuclear cells. The cell line and the lymphoma were EBV+, expressed a similar spectrum of B-cell surface proteins, and had the donor's HLA haplotype. Analysis of immunoglobulin gene rearrangements and viral terminal repeat sequences revealed that the cell line and the tumor represented distinct B-cell clones. More sophisticated tools are now available to confirm donor origin, but this early case provides conclusive evidence of donor origin. However, a subsequent study by Peterson et al. in 2006 showed PTLD may be either of donor or of host origin using molecular techniques [21]. Four PTLD cases were identified from autopsy files, and each underwent restriction fragment length polymorphism analysis using polymerase chain reaction-based genotyping for CYP2D6. Epstein-Barr virus (latent membrane protein 1) immunostaining and polymerase chain reaction analysis were performed on PTLD-involved tissues. Three cases were shown to be of host origin and one of donor origin.

It appears early PTLD predominantly affects the allograft but late disease is often extra-pulmonary or disseminated [22]. Hence, a high index of suspicion should be entertained in the otherwise healthy LTx recipient who develops lymphadenopathy or a bowel obstruction. Late disease can also involve the allograft and a case of an obstructive endobronchial lesion in a young patient, which developed 6 years after BSSLTx for cystic fibrosis (CF) has been reported [23]. Wudhikan in 2010 described the largest series to date, with 32 cases (5%) of PTLD in 639 LTx patients [24]. The median interval after LTx to diagnosis was 40 (3–242) months. Eight patients (25%) were diagnosed within 1 year of transplantation and had PTLD predominantly within the thorax and allograft. Twenty-four patients (75%) were diagnosed more than 1 year after transplantation and their tumors mainly affected the gastrointestinal tract. Monomorphic PTLD, diffuse large B-cell lymphoma, was diagnosed in 91%. Median overall survival was 10 (0–108) months. Subsequently Kremer et al. reported 34/705 LTx recipients developed PTLD which involved the allograft in

49% and the gastrointestinal tract lumen in 23% [25]. Histologically, 39% of tumors were monomorphic and 48% polymorphic. Of 17 patients diagnosed within 11 months of transplantation, PTLD involved the allograft in 12 (71%) and the GI tract in 1 ($p = 0.01$). "Early" PTLD was 85% polymorphic ($p = 0.006$). Conversely, of the 18 patients diagnosed more than 11 months after transplant, the lung was involved in 5 (28%) and the gastrointestinal tract in 7 (39%; $p = 0.01$). "Late" PTLD was 71% monomorphic ($p = 0.006$). Median overall survival after diagnosis was 18.6 months.

Recognizing the importance of making a firm distinction between PTLD and acute cellular rejection (ACR) by transbronchial biopsy (TBBx), the standard means of monitoring the status of the lung allograft, Rosendale et al., in 1995, analyzed TBBx from 11 cases of ACR and 1 case of PTLD and open lung biopsies from 4 cases of PTLD in the allograft [3]. Areas of particular interest were the main tumor mass of the PTLD and the pulmonary parenchyma adjacent to the mass where perivascular mononuclear infiltrates predominated and mimicked ACR. The main tumor mass in the PTLD cases revealed consolidation of lung parenchyma by a monomorphous lymphocytic infiltrate, which was composed of large lymphoid cells that marked as B lymphocytes. The ACR cases and peripheral areas of the PTLD lesions were composed of polymorphous, perivascular lymphocytic infiltrates with similar numbers of B and T cells. All cases of PTLD, both the main mass and the peripheral infiltrates, had lymphocytes that stained positively with antibody to Epstein-Barr virus latent membrane protein, while none of the ACR cases was positive. Occasionally both ACR and PTLD may occur concurrently. In 2010, Calabrese et al. described a convincing case of a young CF patient who developed multiple pulmonary nodules 2 months post-BSSLTx shown on needle biopsy to be PTLD, while surveillance TBBx was typical for ACR [26]. Each sample had different lymphocyte characteristics: the perivascular lymphoid cells in TBBx were mainly T lymphocytes (CD3 positive), while a larger number of lymphocytes in the needle biopsy were B cells (CD20 positive).

Radiological Features

Collins et al., in 1996, retrospectively reviewed the computed tomographic (CT) and histologic findings of lymphoproliferative disease (LPD) associated with the EBV [27]. The findings are relevant to our discussion given the stereotypic radiological features of LPD even though the patient population involved 5 patients with acquired immunodeficiency syndrome and 4 with other conditions as well as 15 post-HTx, LTx, or HLTx. Final diagnoses included malignant lymphoma ($n = 15$), polyclonal LPD ($n = 8$), and hyperplasia of bronchus-associated lymphoid tissue ($n = 1$). CT findings included multiple nodules ($n = 21$), lymphadenopathy ($n = 9$), areas of ground-glass opacification ($n = 8$), septal thickening ($n = 7$), consolidation ($n = 5$), pleural effusion ($n = 4$), and solitary endobronchial lesion ($n = 2$). The nodules were 2–4 cm in diameter, involved mainly the middle and lower lung zones, and frequently had a predominantly peribronchovascular ($n = 15$) or subpleural

($n = 14$) distribution. They concluded EBV-associated LPD may range from benign lymphoid hyperplasia to high-grade lymphoma, and the most common CT manifestation comprised multiple nodules, frequently in a predominantly peribronchovascular or subpleural distribution. Of course, in the immunocompromised patient, the pulmonary nodule remains a diagnostic and therapeutic challenge [28]. The differential diagnosis is broad, and infectious causes such as aspergillosis and bacterial/fungal lung abscess should be considered as opined by Lee et al. who reviewed 234 LTx in 1990–2000 and found that solitary pulmonary nodules were most commonly due to bronchogenic carcinoma and PTLD, while multiple pulmonary nodules were often due to invasive pulmonary aspergillosis, cytomegalovirus pneumonitis, bronchiolitis obliterans, and metastatic carcinoma [29].

Therapeutic Options and Outcomes

Therapeutic options for PTLD have been discussed previously in this book, so only a brief lung-focused discussion will be presented here. One major difference, as mentioned above, is that PTLD in LTX recipients often occurs in the allograft, which may limit some therapeutic endeavors, including systemic chemotherapy and radiotherapy. A traditional strategy has been to reduce or completely stop all immune suppression on the diagnosis of PTLD, but this risks the development of significant ACR and antibody-mediated rejection with subsequent CLAD which may demonstrate a restrictive allograft syndrome (RAS) phenotype, making retransplantation a potentially hazardous undertaking. Monoclonal antibody therapy with rituximab, an anti-CD20 monoclonal antibody based on the premise that PTLD would have a significant population of CD-20-positive B cells, was initially trialed by Cook et al. in 1999 who reported 2/3 patients with diffuse large B-cell PTLD after LTx developed complete remissions [30]. Seven years later Knoop et al. provided further support for the successful use of rituximab in a 4/6 patients, concluding that a reduction in immunosuppression combined with first-line treatment with rituximab may induce long-term complete remission in LTx recipients with PTLD. In 1999 Schoch et al. described a promising case report using extracorporeal photochemotherapy (ECP) in a LTx recipient with a history of ACR and EBV-associated PTLD [31]. ECP in combination with a moderate reduction of immunosuppressive therapy resulted in complete remission which persisted at 1-year follow-up, without further ACR.

As mentioned elsewhere in this book, it is important to distinguish between the lytic and latent stages of EBV. As noted by Mentzer et al. in 2001, immunologic and antiviral therapies are moderately effective for treating EBV-associated infections in the lytic phase, but less useful in the more common latent phase [32]. The lack of virus-specific enzyme thymidine kinase (TK) expression in EBV+ tumor cells, due to viral latency, makes antiviral therapy alone ineffective as an anti-neoplastic therapy. Based on a promising case report from their unit in 1998, Mentzer et al. developed a strategy for the treatment of EBV-associated PTLD using pharmacologic induction of the latent viral TK gene and enzyme in the tumor cells, using arginine butyrate which selectively activates the EBV TK gene in latently EBV-infected human lymphoid cells and tumor cells [32, 33]. In a phase I/II trial employing an intra-patient dose escalation of arginine butyrate combined with ganciclovir in 6 patients with PTLD, all of which were resistant to conventional radiation and/or chemotherapy, this combination produced complete clinical responses in 4/6 patients. In an exciting pre-clinical study just published by Sang et al., combination therapy with rapamycin and a PI3K inhibitor, or an Akt inhibitor, was found to hold promise of being an efficacious treatment for EBV-associated PTLD while simultaneously promoting allograft survival [34].

Conclusions

The transplanted lung has a rich population of lymphoid tissues which conveys an increased risk of EBV acquisition with LTx and thereby an increased risk of PTLD especially in the EBV-naïve recipient. Allograft disease predominates early after LTx with gastrointestinal and disseminated disease as late manifestations of PTLD. There is no convincing prophylactic therapy but a high index of suspicion, and where available serial EBV viral load dynamics monitoring holds the promise of early diagnosis which may be associated with an enhanced chance of successful therapy. Despite the known risks, the broad LTx community has not supported avoidance of transplanting the EBV-naïve population, and this strategic policy is beginning to show increased benefit with the development of a number of therapies under trial.

Financial Conflict of Interest Disclosure The authors report no potential financial conflict of interest and attest that no funding has been received from any source for this work.

References

1. Yousem SA, Randhawa P, Locker J, et al. Posttransplant lymphoproliferative disorders in heart-lung transplant recipients. Hum Pathol. 1989;20:361–9.
2. Colby TV, Yousem SA. Pulmonary lymphoid neoplasms. Semin Diagn Pathol. 1985;2:183–96.
3. Rosendale B, Yousem SA. Discrimination of Epstein-Barr virus-related posttransplant lymphoproliferations from acute rejection in lung allograft recipients. Arch Pathol Lab Med. 1995;119:418–23.
4. Kumarasinghe G, Lavee O, Parker A, et al. Post-transplant lymphoproliferative disease in heart and lung transplantation: defining risk and prognostic factors. J Heart Lung Transplant. 2015;34:1406–14.
5. Aris RM, Maia DM, Neuringer IP, et al. Post-transplantation lymphoproliferative disorder in the Epstein-Barr virus-naive lung transplant recipient. Am J Respir Crit Care Med. 1996;154:1712–7.
6. Mihalov ML, Gattuso P, Abraham K, Holmes EW, Reddy V. Incidence of post-transplant malignancy among 674 solid-organ-transplant recipients at a single center. Clin Transpl. 1996;10:248–55.
7. Kurland G, Orenstein DM. Complications of pediatric lung and heart-lung transplantation. Curr Opin Pediatr. 1994;6:262–71.

8. Chambers DC, Cherikh WS, Goldfarb SB, et al. The International Thoracic Organ Transplant Registry of the International Society for Heart and Lung Transplantation: thirty-fifth adult lung and heart-lung transplant report-2018; focus theme: multiorgan transplantation. J Heart Lung Transplant. 2018;37:1169–83.

9. Wigle DA, Chaparro C, Humar A, Hutcheon MA, Chan CK, Keshavjee S. Epstein-Barr virus serology and posttransplant lymphoproliferative disease in lung transplantation. Transplantation. 2001;72:1783–6.

10. Courtwright AM, Burkett P, Divo M, et al. Posttransplant lymphoproliferative disorders in Epstein-Barr virus donor positive/recipient negative lung transplant recipients. Ann Thorac Surg. 2018;105:441–7.

11. Paranjothi S, Yusen RD, Kraus MD, Lynch JP, Patterson GA, Trulock EP. Lymphoproliferative disease after lung transplantation: comparison of presentation and outcome of early and late cases. J Heart Lung Transplant. 2001;20:1054–63.

12. Gifford G, Fay K, Jabbour A, Ma DD. Primary central nervous system posttransplantation lymphoproliferative disorder after heart and lung transplantation. Intern Med J. 2015;45:583–6.

13. Montone KT, Litzky LA, Wurster A, et al. Analysis of Epstein-Barr virus-associated posttransplantation lymphoproliferative disorder after lung transplantation. Surgery. 1996;119:544–51.

14. Gao SZ, Chaparro SV, Perlroth M, et al. Post-transplantation lymphoproliferative disease in heart and heart-lung transplant recipients: 30-year experience at Stanford University. J Heart Lung Transplant. 2003;22:505–14.

15. Malouf MA, Chhajed PN, Hopkins P, Plit M, Turner J, Glanville AR. Anti-viral prophylaxis reduces the incidence of lymphoproliferative disease in lung transplant recipients. J Heart Lung Transplant. 2002;21:547–54.

16. Bakker NA, Verschuuren EA, Erasmus ME, et al. Epstein-Barr virus-DNA load monitoring late after lung transplantation: a surrogate marker of the degree of immunosuppression and a safe guide to reduce immunosuppression. Transplantation. 2007;83:433–8.

17. Parrish A, Fenchel M, Storch GA, et al. Epstein-Barr viral loads do not predict post-transplant lymphoproliferative disorder in pediatric lung transplant recipients: a multicenter prospective cohort study. Pediatr Transplant. 2017;21:e13011.

18. Leyssens A, Dierickx D, Verbeken EK, et al. Post-transplant lymphoproliferative disease in lung transplantation: a nested case-control study. Clin Transpl. 2017;31:e12983.

19. Cheng J, Moore CA, Iasella CJ, et al. Systematic review and meta-analysis of post-transplant lymphoproliferative disorder in lung transplant recipients. Clin Transpl. 2018;32:e13235.

20. Mentzer SJ, Longtine J, Fingeroth J, et al. Immunoblastic lymphoma of donor origin in the allograft after lung transplantation. Transplantation. 1996;61:1720–5.

21. Peterson MR, Emery SC, Yung GL, Masliah E, Yi ES. Epstein-Barr virus-associated posttransplantation lymphoproliferative disorder following lung transplantation is more commonly of host origin. Arch Pathol Lab Med. 2006;130:176–80.

22. Angel LF, Cai TH, Sako EY, Levine SM. Posttransplant lymphoproliferative disorders in lung transplant recipients: clinical experience at a single center. Ann Transplant. 2000;5:26–30.

23. De Giacomo T, Venuta F, Anile M, Diso D, Rolla M, Coloni GF. Non-Hodgkin's lymphoma, presenting as an isolated endobronchial mass after bilateral lung transplantation: a case report. Transplant Proc. 2007;39:3541–4.

24. Wudhikarn K, Holman CJ, Linan M, et al. Post-transplant lymphoproliferative disorders in lung transplant recipients: 20-yr experience at the University of Minnesota. Clin Transpl. 2010;25(5):705–13.

25. Kremer BE, Reshef R, Misleh JG, et al. Post-transplant lymphoproliferative disorder after lung transplantation: a review of 35 cases. J Heart Lung Transplant. 2012;31:296–304.

26. Calabrese F, Loy M, Lunardi F, Marino D, Aversa SM, Rea F. Acute cellular rejection and Epstein-Barr virus-related post-transplant lymphoproliferative disorder in a pediatric lung transplant with low viral load. Transpl Infect Dis. 2010;12:342–6.

27. Collins J, Muller NL, Leung AN, et al. Epstein-Barr-virus-associated lymphoproliferative disease of the lung: CT and histologic findings. Radiology. 1998;208:749–59.

28. End A, Helbich T, Wisser W, Dekan G, Klepetko W. The pulmonary nodule after lung transplantation. Cause and outcome. Chest. 1995;107:1317–22.
29. Lee P, Minai OA, Mehta AC, DeCamp MM, Murthy S. Pulmonary nodules in lung transplant recipients: etiology and outcome. Chest. 2004;125:165–72.
30. Cook RC, Connors JM, Gascoyne RD, Fradet G, Levy RD. Treatment of post-transplant lymphoproliferative disease with rituximab monoclonal antibody after lung transplantation. Lancet. 1999;354:1698–9.
31. Schoch OD, Boehler A, Speich R, Nestle FO. Extracorporeal photochemotherapy for Epstein-Barr virus-associated lymphoma after lung transplantation. Transplantation. 1999;68:1056–8.
32. Mentzer SJ, Perrine SP, Faller DV. Epstein--Barr virus post-transplant lymphoproliferative disease and virus-specific therapy: pharmacological re-activation of viral target genes with arginine butyrate. Transpl Infect Dis. 2001;3:177–85.
33. Mentzer SJ, Fingeroth J, Reilly JJ, Perrine SP, Faller DV. Arginine butyrate-induced susceptibility to ganciclovir in an Epstein-Barr-virus-associated lymphoma. Blood Cells Mol Dis. 1998;24:114–23.
34. Sang AX, McPherson MC, Ivison GT, et al. Dual blockade of the PI3K/Akt/mTOR pathway inhibits posttransplant Epstein-Barr virus B cell lymphomas and promotes allograft survival. Am J Transplant. 2019;19:1305–14.

Part V

The Future

Research Priorities and Future Directions

21

Vikas R. Dharnidharka, Michael Green, Steven A. Webber, and Ralf Ulrich Trappe

Introduction

The preceding chapters of this book emphasize how much has been learned about PTLD in the past few decades. Yet so much still remains to be learned. Listed below are some of the unanswered questions regarding PTLD. Each of these areas is ripe for future research and the gain of new knowledge.

V. R. Dharnidharka (✉)
Division of Pediatric Nephrology, Hypertension and Pheresis,
Washington University School of Medicine, St. Louis, MO, USA
e-mail: vikasd@wustl.edu

M. Green
Departments of Pediatrics, University of Pittsburgh School of Medicine,
UPMC Children's Hospital of Pittsburgh, Pittsburgh, PA, USA

Departments of Surgery, University of Pittsburgh School of Medicine,
UPMC Children's Hospital of Pittsburgh, Pittsburgh, PA, USA

Division of Infectious Diseases, UPMC Children's Hospital of Pittsburgh,
Pittsburgh, PA, USA
e-mail: Michael.green@chp.edu

S. A. Webber
Department of Pediatrics, Vanderbilt University School of Medicine,
Monroe Carell Jr. Children's Hospital at Vanderbilt, Nashville, TN, USA
e-mail: steve.a.webber@vumc.org

R. U. Trappe
Department of Hematology and Oncology, Christian-Albrechts-University Kiel,
Kiel, Germany

Division of Hematology and Oncology, Department of Medicine,
DIAKO Ev. Diakonie-Krankenhaus Bremen, Bremen, Germany
e-mail: rtrappe@gwdg.de

© Springer Nature Switzerland AG 2021
V. R. Dharnidharka et al. (eds.), *Post-Transplant Lymphoproliferative Disorders*,
https://doi.org/10.1007/978-3-030-65403-0_21

Etiology/Pathogenesis of PTLD

1. *What is the point at which proliferation of EBV-infected B cells becomes uncontrolled and what measurable markers identify that this has occurred?*

We know that EBV inserts into the B-cell genome and drives cellular proliferation. Under normal circumstances, this proliferation is controlled primarily by cytotoxic CD8+ T cells, which are impaired by extrinsic immunosuppressive agents. Yet less than 10% of transplant recipients develop PTLD. Is this just an issue of degree of cumulative immunosuppression or is it also related to the organs themselves? If so, why are intestinal and lung transplants associated with the highest rates of PTLD? Is it the presence of lymphoid tissue, antigenic drive by the organ and/or associated pathogens, or something else? Is cumulative immunosuppression over time most important, or exceeding some threshold of total immunosuppression at any one point in time? How do the different immunosuppressive agents combine to suppress the immune system? Is the combination synergistic in a linear fashion, exponential fashion, or otherwise? Is the use of certain immunosuppressive agents (e.g., belatacept) more likely to lead to PTLD, and are any such agents (e.g., mTOR inhibitors) actually protective? To address these important questions, prospective observational studies could be implemented to follow patients, their immune suppression, immune function, and status of EBV infection over time in an effort to clarify the events and factors defining who progresses to PTLD and who does not.

Do the factors that determine progression to PTLD differ in organ and stem cell transplant recipients?

2. *Why is primary EBV infection so much more likely to lead to PTLD and why don't all recipients develop PTLD?*

Multiple studies have shown that the EBV-seronegative recipient is much more likely to develop PTLD. What are the unique features of primary infection under an immunosuppressed state that make it different from a reactivation of primary infection that developed in an immunocompetent host? Does the delayed recovering immune response against EBV in stem cell recipients present a similar or quantitatively different setting and risk compared to the seronegative recipient's efforts to control primary EBV infection after organ transplant? Are there measurable features of the EBV-seronegative organ recipient or the patients receiving stem cells from an EBV-seropositive donor which predict progression to PTLD after primary infection after organ transplant? Are these features present prior to or after infection? (e.g., EBV-specific CTL response). The proposed observational studies mentioned above could potentially attempt to answer these questions as well *if* funding is available to answer the questions.

3. *What are the etiologic agent(s) or factors involved in the genesis of EBV-negative PTLD?*

While we have strong evidence for the role of EBV in the pathogenesis of PTLDs, we have minimal knowledge about the triggers for EBV-negative PTLDs. Are these entities also induced by some microbial infection? Why do they manifest considerably later than EBV-positive PTLDs and why does their incidence not peak? If this is not attributable to a microbe, then what else could drive uncontrolled immune-cell proliferation? Why are EBV-negative PTLDs so rare after stem cell transplant, and do they differ from EBV-negative PTLDs after organ transplantation? Our current answer that EBV-negative PTLDs are typical lymphomas that just happen to occur in a transplant recipient seems unsatisfactory, as their response to treatment – including their response to immunosuppression reduction for SOT – is very different from NHL in the immune-competent population.

4. *What are the differences in pathophysiology for late PTLD or non-B-cell PTLD compared to typical early EBV-driven B-cell PTLD? Why do they behave so differently?*

Why are some PTLDs of T-cell or NK-cell origin? Compared to B-cell PTLD, these other types such as T-cell PTLD tend to occur later, are less likely to be EBV-associated, and have a poor response to therapy and higher mortality. What makes the presentation, response, and outcomes so different?

Surveillance and Monitoring

1. *How intense should the PTLD monitoring be? What is both scientifically valid and cost-effective?*

The role and optimal methods for viral infection surveillance, whether for EBV, CMV, or BK virus, are being intensively discussed by transplant professionals at this time, but the optimal timing is still not known. Serial measurements of viral load by PCR can be quite expensive and few studies have addressed cost-effectiveness. For CMV and BK virus, DNAemia is due to viral replication, and there is a clear progression of DNAemia to virus-induced organ involvement that can be prevented in many cases. However, for EBV, DNAemia may reflect B-cell proliferation with or without viral replication. The determinants of progression to EBV disease/PTLD are less clear and many cases of chronic high load carrier do not progress to clinical disease. So what does a single high viral load mean? What do repeated high viral loads mean? Why is it different for different transplanted organs, such as heart versus liver, and between adults and children?

2. *Is viral load monitoring indicated in patients who are EBV seropositive prior to transplantation?*

Finally, should optimal surveillance combine viral load monitoring with some assessment of the patients' immunological status (e.g., cytotoxic T-cell frequency and function)? If this were done, what would be their combined performance as tests to predict progression to disease as well as what role would measurement have as a marker of treatment response? The evidence is incomplete at this point and more research is needed in order to define optimal and cost-effective surveillance programs. While many of the above questions could be raised for recipients of stem cells from EBV-seropositive donors, additional ones would include whether measurement of load and/or markers of host-immune response differ for recipients of identical, haploidentical, or umbilical cord transplants.

Treatment of PTLD

1. *What are the optimal treatment strategies for PTLD, and how should these be individualized for factors such as patient age, EBV status, histopathology, time of onset post-transplant, and prior rejection history and disease stage?*

Currently, the accepted initial approach for SOT recipients with PTLD is to reduce immunosuppression in nearly all cases. However, it is unclear when this should be the only initial therapy or when other treatments are indicated at presentation. Only a few cases of PTLD, such as Burkitt's type or CNS location, have a clear consensus to move immediately to therapies beyond immunosuppression reduction.

2. *There also remains disagreement as to what is an adequate trial of reduction in immunosuppression. Which agents, what order, for how long, and how much? When should immunosuppression be completely withheld? How should the allograft be best protected from acute and chronic rejection?*

Rituximab has certainly gained ground as a first-line therapy in CD-20-positive tumors, but it remains unclear under what circumstances reduced immunosuppression alone might be used as first-line therapy without rituximab. Rituximab may be used as monotherapy in many situations, but some patients need more intensive treatment including chemotherapy, and factors to identify these patients already have been established in SOT in adults. For SOT, the role of cellular (adoptive) immunotherapy and whether it can replace rituximab or chemotherapy in this setting are currently under study in several prospective clinical trials. Antiviral agents, such as ganciclovir, are frequently used at diagnosis, but there is only limited evidence for lytic EBV transcripts in PTLD cases. Also, when should chemotherapy be introduced and which agents are optimal in different clinical settings? When should second-line therapies be introduced, and what should they be? With increasing incidences of central nervous system disease in recent years, there is also a clear need for prospective clinical trials specifically in primary CNS-PTLD to define treatment in this still devastating disease. Rituximab, antiviral therapy, and chemotherapy clearly are effective in this setting and also radiotherapy is an option, but it is still unclear how to balance efficacy and toxicity to optimize patient outcome.

For stem cell transplant recipients, strong evidence exists for the efficacy of the use of EBV-specific T-cell therapy, from the donor or third party, in the treatment of EBV-associated PTLD. For recipients in whom adoptive immune therapy is not available, rituximab has been shown to be effective though in some cases rituximab combined with traditional chemotherapy is necessary to control EBV-associated PTLD. Determining upfront who will require more aggressive therapy and defining the optimal regimen for a given stem cell recipient present important opportunities for research in this area.

Summary

While we have clearly learned much about EBV and its role in the pathogenesis of PTLDs, a large number of critically important and clinically relevant questions remain unanswered. With limited number of patients, the priorities for clinical trials might be how best to prevent PTLD development. Advanced molecular pathology studies such as detailed host and microbial gene sequencing might advance the field. Similarly, detailed molecular sequencing of tumor cells might be the strategy for studying causes of non-EBV PTLDs. We hope that bringing together this state-of-the-art collection of chapters, reflecting much of what has been learned, will help to inform those who search for answers to these and other questions in the years to come.

Index

© Springer Nature Switzerland AG 2021
V. R. Dharnidharka et al. (eds.), *Post-Transplant Lymphoproliferative Disorders*,
https://doi.org/10.1007/978-3-030-65403-0

Printed in the United States
by Baker & Taylor Publisher Services